Dear Colleague:

This is the ninth volume in the popular Cummings Foundation for Behavioral Health series beginning in 1991 that addresses healthcare utilization and costs. The Nicholas & Dorothy Cummings Foundation, in association with Context Press, is pleased to continue the tradition of distributing complimentary copies to the directors of American Psychological Association approved doctoral programs, to selected leaders in psychology, and to key persons in the field of behavioral healthcare.

Once again the Cummings Foundation for Behavioral Health has selected a timely topic that we hope you will find useful in your work. The debate over universal healthcare will occupy and dominate political and professional discussion from Washington to the treatment office, and changes are inevitable as our current system is broken. Every provider would do well to heed these harbingers and position practice to meet the future exigencies.

We request that after you have finished reading this volume, you donate it to a library of the institution with which you are affiliated. Additional copies for qualified individuals and libraries only, may be obtained by sending $5.00 to cover postage and handling to the address below. Regretfully, repeat, multiple and bulk requests cannot be accommodated.

Sincerely,

Janet L. Cummings, Psy.D., President
The Nicholas & Dorothy Cummings Foundation, Inc.
4781 Caughlin Parkway, Reno, NV 89509
E-mail: CummFound@aol.com
www.thecummingsfoundation.com

Library and Institutional copies may be ordered from CONTEXT PRESS for a charge of $29.95 plus shipping and handling.

Universal Healthcare:
Readings for Mental Health Professionals

Universal Healthcare:
Readings for Mental Health Professionals

Editors:
Nicholas A. Cummings, Ph.D., Sc.D.
William T. O'Donohue, Ph.D.
Michael A. Cucciare, M.A.

With a Special Update of the Dörken Report
of the National Academies of Practice

Cummings Foundation for Behavioral Health:
Healthcare Utilization and Cost Series,
Volume 9
2005

CONTEXT PRESS
Reno, Nevada

✳ 61115488

Universal Healthcare: Readings for Mental Health Professionals

Hardback   pp. 263

Library of Congress Cataloging-in-Publication Data

Universal healthcare : readings for mental health professionals / editors, Nicholas A. Cummings, William T. O'Donohue, Michael A. Cucciare.
   p. cm. – (Healthcare utilization and cost series ; v. 9)
   ISBN 1-878978-55-1 (hardcover)
   1. Mental health services–United States. 2. Mental health services–Economic aspects–United States. 3. Mental health policy–United States 4. Health services accessibility–United States. 5. Health care reform–United States. I. Cummings, Nicholas A. II. O'Donohue, William T. III. Cucciare, Michael A., 1976- IV. Series.
   RA790.6.U65 2005
   362.1'0425'0973–dc22

                                                      2005019979

© 2005 CONTEXT PRESS
933 Gear Street, Reno, NV   89503-2729

Printed in the United States of America

The Healthcare Utilization and Cost Series
of the Cummings Foundation for Behavioral Health

Volume 1 (1991):
> *Medical Cost Offset: A Reprinting of the Seminal Research Conducted at Kaiser Permanente, 1963-1981*
> Nicholas A. Cummings, Ph.D. and William T. Follette, M.D.

Volume 2 (1993):
> *Medicaid, Managed Behavioral Health and Implications for Public Policy: A Report of the HCFA-Hawaii Medicaid Project and Other Readings.*
> Nicholas A. Cummings, Ph.D., Herbert Dorken, Ph.D., Michael S. Pallak, Ph.D. and Curtis Henke, Ph.D.

Volume 3 (1994):
> *The Financing and Organization of Universal Healthcare: A Proposal to the National Academies of Practice.*
> Herbert Dorken, Ph.D.

Volume 4 (1995):
> *The Impact of the Biodyne Model on Medical Cost Offset: A Sampling of Research Projects.*
> Nicholas A. Cummings, Ph.D., Sc.D., Editor.

Volume 5 (2002):
> *The Impact of Medical Cost Offset on Practice and Research: Making It Work for You.* A Report of the Second Reno Conference, May 2002.
> Nicholas A. Cummings, Ph.D., Sc.D., William T. O'Donohue, Ph.D., and Kyle E. Ferguson, M.S., Editors.

Volume 6 (2003):
> *Behavioral Health as Primary Care: Beyond Efficacy to Effectiveness.*
> A Report of the Third Reno Conference, May 2003.
> Nicholas A. Cummings, Ph.D., Sc.D., William T. O'Donohue, Ph.D., and Kyle E. Ferguson, M.S., Editors.

Volume 7 (2004):
> *Early Detection and Treatment of Substance Abuse within Integrated Primary Care.*
> A Report of the Fifth Reno Conference, May 2004.
> Nicholas a. Cummings, Ph.D., Sc.D., William T. O'Donohue, Ph.D., Melanie Duckworth, Ph.D., and Kyle E. Ferguson, M.S.

Volume 8 (2005):
  Psychological Approaches to Chronic Disease Management.
  A Report of the Fifth Reno Conference, May 2004.
  Nicholas A. Cummings, Ph.D., Sc.D., William T. O'Donohue, Ph.D., and
  Elizabeth Naylor, Editors.

The Reno Conferences

Co-sponsored by the University of Nevada, Reno and
The Nicholas & Dorothy Cummings Foundation, Inc.

The Topics of the Conferences has been some aspect
of the integration of Behavioral health in primary care,

The First Reno Conference on Organized Behavioral Healthcare Delivery was convened at the University of Nevada, Reno in January 1999.

The Second Reno Conference on Medical Cost Offset was convened at the University of Nevada, Reno in January 2001.

The Third Reno Conference on Medical Cost Offset and Behavioral Health in Primary care was convened at the University of Nevada, Reno in May 2002.

The Fourth Reno Conference on Substance Abuse Treatment in Primary Care was convened at the University of Nevada, Reno in May 2003.

The Fifth Reno Conference on Disease Management in Integrated Primary Care was convened at the University of Nevada, Reno in May 2004.

Preface

The United States is currently facing a healthcare crisis. Over the last four decades, the United Sates has increased its spending on healthcare from 5% to 14% of its total Gross Domestic Product (GDP). This translated into dollars means that $1 out of every $7 dollars in the U.S. is spent for healthcare.

One important factor contributing to the U.S. healthcare crisis is high utilization of healthcare resources or when small subgroups of individuals use disproportionate amounts of healthcare services. Several researchers have described psychosocial pathways that can lead to high utilization. Some of these pathways include: (a) consumers' lack of information about how to most effectively use the healthcare system and thus how to most effectively manage their psychological and physical health; (b) the presence of stress and its impact on the onset and management of chronic disease conditions; and (c) undiagnosed behavioral health problems such as depression and substance abuse (Friedman, Sobel, Myers, Caudill, & Benson, 1995).

Consistent with these pathways, in 2002, President George W. Bush identified three obstacles preventing Americans from accessing the mental healthcare they need. These are: (1) the stigma surrounding mental illnesses; (2) unfair treatment limitations and financial requirements placed on mental health benefits; and (3) the fragmented mental health service delivery system. In response to these obstacles, the President charged the New Freedom Commission to make recommendations on resolving these problems by creating improved mental health policy and service delivery. From June 2002 to April 2003, the 22 Commissioners met monthly to analyze the public and private mental health systems, visit innovative model programs across the country and hear testimony from the systems' many stakeholders, including dozens of consumers of mental healthcare, families, advocates, public and private providers, and administrators and mental health researchers. The Commission received feedback, comments and suggestions from nearly 2,500 people from all 50 states via personal testimony, letters, emails and a comment section on their website. In addition to public comment, the Commission consulted with nationally recognized professionals with expertise in diverse areas of mental health policy. The Commission established 15 subcommittees to examine specific aspects of mental health services and offer recommendations for improvement.

In their final report, the New Freedom Commission recommended six goals to remedy the inadequacies of mental health service delivery. The six goals are that (1) Americans understand that mental health is essential to overall health; (2) mental health care is consumer and family driven; (3) disparities in mental health services are eliminated; (4) early mental health screening, assessment, and referral to services are common practice; (5) excellent mental healthcare is delivered and research is accelerated; and (6) technology is used to access mental health care and information (New Freedom Commission, 2003).

There is little debate that the current healthcare system is inadequately addressing the mental health needs of Americans. Critics of the present healthcare system have suggested that the various problems identified by the President's New Freedom Commission can be most effectively remedied through system and policy changes such as *integrated care* and *universal healthcare*. The former is a system of care in which behavioral health is integrated into primary care medicine, while the latter describes a system (and policy) of healthcare in which everyone is entitled to receive care.

There was a time in which healthcare was solely the responsibility of individuals and families. However, over the last century we have seen a transition of healthcare financing from that of individuals to third party payors and the Federal government—the Federal government currently pays approximately 50% of our nation's healthcare costs. An important legislative factor contributing to this change was the passing of state workmen's compensation laws (the first of those laws passed in 1911) that required employers to pay for healthcare needed for employees who were hurt while working. The passing of workmen's compensation laws also contributed to the need for group health insurance. After the Second World War group healthcare coverage became a major factor of the collective bargaining process. A major wage-price freeze during WW II forced employers to offer non wage benefits such as healthcare insurance to keep and attract employees (Henderson, 2005). Furthering the popularity of employer provided group healthcare insurance, in 1954, the Internal Revenue Service ruled that employer contributions to employee healthcare insurance were exempt from taxation, which is still in affect today. This tax law provides a subsidy to healthcare insurance which lowers the cost of insurance, thus having the effect of increasing its demand among consumers (Phelps, 1997). Moreover, during the 1950's and 1960's employers began to add improvements such as dental care, prescription drugs, and vision care to employee healthcare insurance plans (Henderson, 2005).

Similarly, two decades earlier, the government officially undertook more of a "caretaker" role with the signing of the Social Security Act by President Franklin D. Roosevelt in 1935, which guaranteed retirement income, healthcare for older adults, and disability coverage for eligible individuals and their dependents. This, of course, was (and still is) an issue of debate among many individuals in the U.S. Among the opposition's arguments against Social Security is that the Federal government has no moral ground to justify forcing an individual to set aside a portion of their earned income for retirement (Williams, 2005).

Although the U.S. has never adopted a comprehensive universal healthcare plan, it did make a significant move in that direction in 1965 with the passing of the Medicare and Medicaid Act. Medicare is a government program that was developed to guarantee healthcare services to elderly Americans' regardless of their economic circumstances. In 2001, Medicare provided coverage to approximately 41 million Americans. Medicare provides its healthcare benefits to 46 million enrollees—and this upward trend is accelerating at a worrisome rate. These services come through two programs: Part A and Part B. Part A is medical hospital insurance and Part B is supplemental medical insurance that covers medical costs associated with physicians and surgeons but does not cover eye and hearing exams, foot care, immunizations, or physical exams. Medicaid was developed in 1965 as part of the same legislative package as Medicare and is financed through both state and federal funding. Persons eligible for Medicaid services typically have a low income and fall into one of the following five categories: pregnant women; children and teenagers; and persons who are aged, blind and/or disabled.

Approximately thirty years later, then First Lady Hillary Clinton proposed a nationwide healthcare plan that many consider a failed attempt at developing a system of universal healthcare. Specifically, Clinton's plan would have required every business in the U.S. to provide healthcare coverage to its employees, despite the cost. Tanner (1996) argued that such a mandate would have been financially devastating to businesses and would have resulted in the loss of thousands of jobs. Clinton's plan would have also required that American's give up their current healthcare insurance even if they were pleased with the plan; and alternatively accept a federally designed healthcare benefit package that had the potential to be more expensive. Furthermore, the specific healthcare services covered under the proposed benefit package would be determined not by the healthcare needs or preferences of individuals, but by the lobbying power of special interests (Tanner, 1996). Another unfortunate characteristic of Clinton's plan was that all individuals covered would have paid the same premium regardless of health status and/or lifestyle, which would have resulted in huge premiums being paid by young and healthy individuals.

Many nations have implemented universal healthcare systems. The first nation to implement a comprehensive universal healthcare plan was Great Britain in 1948, followed by Japan in 1958, Canada in 1966, France in 1967, and Italy and Germany in 1978. One advantage of universal healthcare is that it (theoretically) allows for equal access to healthcare by all individuals, while a disadvantage is that with little supply side constraints the demand for services increases. Another important disadvantage is that it eliminates competition which some argue is key for innovation and consumer satisfaction.

The present volume attempts to discuss and address the goals outlined by President George W. Bush's New Freedom Commission that were set forth to remedy the inadequacies of mental health service delivery in the U.S. Important systems and policy issues such as integrated care and universal healthcare are discussed within the context of reshaping the American healthcare system to meet its citizens healthcare needs.

This book owes a special thanks to many people. First and foremost our special thanks are due to the chapter authors who furnished this volume with their excellent work. We are exceedingly grateful to Emily Neilan for her outstanding effort in preparing this manuscript and keeping us on schedule. Lastly (but certainly not least), we would like to thank our families and friends for their patience and support during this project.

References

Friedman, R., Sobel, D., Myers, P., Caudill, M., & Benson, H. (1995). Behavioral medicine, clinical health psychology, and cost offset. *Health Psychology, 14,* 509-518.

Henderson, J. W. (2005). *Health economics and policy* (3rd ed). Mason, OH: South-Western (Thompson Corporation).

New Freedom Commission on Mental Health. (2003). *Achieving the promise: Transforming mental health care in America. Final Report.* Rockville, MD: DHHS Pub. No. SMA-03-3832. Available at www.mentalhealthcommission.gov/reports/final report/fullreport-02.htm

Phelps, C. E. (1997). *Health economics* (2nd ed.). Reading, MA: Addison Wesley Longman, Inc.

Tanner, M. (1996, September). Back to Clintoncare. *Cato Institute.* Retrieved May 25, 2005, at http://www.cato.org/dailys/9-06-96.html

Williams, W. (2005, March). A principled argument against social security. *Hispanic Pundit.* Retrieved May 25, 2005, at http://hispanicpundit.com/archives/2005/03/10/a-principled-argument-against-social-security/

Contributing Authors

Scott J. Adams, Psy.D. is Senior Research Associate for the WICHE Mental Health Program. His specialties include psychotherapy and personality assessment. Dr. Adams has helped states re-design systems of care for children and families, integrate primary care and mental health, and teach behavioral observation and recovery principles. He is a lead researcher in a HRSA-funded mental health research center. Dr. Adams is co-author of the upcoming book *Mental Health and Rural America: 1994-2004.*

Mimi M. Bradley. Psy.D. is a Postdoctoral Fellow at the Western Interstate Commission on Higher Education (WICHE) through the Administration and Public Psychology program at the University of Colorado Health Sciences Center, Department of Psychiatry. She earned her degree from California School of Professional Psychology, San Francisco Bay Area campus. She completed her pre-doctoral internship at the University of Colorado Health Sciences Center in Denver, Colorado. She co-authored the upcoming book *Mental Health and Rural America: 1994-2004.*

Carlos Brandenburg, Ph.D. has held the position of Administrator for the Nevada State Division for Mental Health and Developmental Services (Department of Human Services) since 1995. He has also served as Director of Forensic Services for Lake's Crossing Center for the Mentally Disordered Offender in Reno, Nevada from 1979-1995. In this position he developed internal policies and procedures for the agency, and supervised 54 staff members in the implementation and management of a comprehensive forensic mental health service program for the State of Nevada.

Blake Chaffee, Ph.D. is currently Vice President of Behavioral Health for TriWest Healthcare Alliance. Dr. Chaffee is a clinical psychologist who left clinical practice to implement the first TRICARE managed care program in southern California for Aetna. He has since worked on six TRICARE procurements as a consultant or managed care executive. Dr. Chaffee received his bachelor's degree from Wesleyan University, his Doctorate from the American University in Washington, D.C. and completed his internship at the National Naval Medical Center in Bethesda, Maryland.

Judi Chamberlin is a psychiatric survivor and an activist since 1971 in the survivor/consumer/ex-patient movement. She is the author of *On Our Own: Patient-Controlled Alternatives to the Mental Health System* and has written numerous articles about the movement, self-help, and patients' rights. She helped to found the Ruby Rogers Advocacy and Drop-In Center, affiliated with the Center for Psychiatric

Rehabilitation, and co-founder of the National Empowerment Center. Judi is also a board member of the National Association for Rights Protection and Advocacy; the American Association of People with Disabilities; the Center for Public Representation; and Mental Disability Rights International.

Michael A. Cucciare, M.A. received his master's degree and is currently a doctoral candidate in clinical psychology at the University of Nevada, Reno. He has co-authored the book *Integrated Behavioral Healthcare: A Guide to Effective Intervention* (Prometheus Books) and is co-author of over 10 journal articles and book chapters in the areas of integrated behavioral healthcare delivery, health psychology, and clinical gerontology.

Nicholas A. Cummings, Ph.D., Sc.D. is Distinguished Professor, University of Nevada, Reno and President, Cummings Foundation for Behavioral Health, Inc. He chairs the boards of CareIntegra and The Nicholas & Dorothy Cummings Foundation. He is the founder of over two dozen organizations, including the California school of Professional Psychology (four campuses), American Biodyne, National Council of Schools and programs in Professional Psychology (NCSPP), and the National Academies of Practice (NAP). He is a former president of the American Psychological Association and the recipient of the Gold Medal for a Lifetime of Achievement in Practice. He is the author of over 450 journal articles and book chapters, and has authored, edited or co-edited 34 books.

Herbert Dörken, Ph.D. received his Ph.D. at McGill University. He is a Life Fellow of the American Public Health Association, and of the divisions of public service, clinical psychology, health psychology and independent practice of the American Psychological Association, An ABPP diplomat in clinical psychology, he has been licensed in Minnesota, California and Hawaii. He pioneered in research on senile decline, on the development and direction of a state wide community mental health program, and 8/62 was appointed by the Governor of California to be Deputy Director of the Department of Mental Hygiene. He went on to become a Research Psychologist and Professor at the University of California, San Francisco School of Medicine. Later with Nicholas Cummings in a HCFA funded research they showed that psychology organized and delivered services, demonstrated reduced total healthcare costs in both Medicaid and employed populations. He has drafted and successfully lobbied to enactment 43 legislative bills. He was among the first to write and lecture on the industrialization of healthcare, cost as the driving force in healthcare reform and the impact of law and regulation on practice. His predominant interest is the organization and development of effective healthcare services and the potential of universal healthcare, covered in 2 books, 35 book chapters and over 150 articles. He has been actively involved in healthcare since his in-residence clinical and research internship from 6/46 and remains active 59 years later.

Melanie Duckworth, Ph.D. is an associate professor in the Clinical Psychology Training Program at the University of Nevada, Reno. She received her doctorate in clinical psychology from the University of Georgia in 1992. She completed an internship in clinical psychology and a one-year postdoctoral fellowship in behavioral medicine at the Brown University School of Medicine. Dr. Duckworth's current research examines posttraumatic stress reactions, coping styles and strategies, and psychological disability in the context of interpersonal violence, motor vehicle accidents, and chronic medical conditions.

Daniel B. Fisher, M.D., Ph.D. earned a Ph.D. in Cancer Research at the University of Wisconsin and an MD from George Washington University. He then completed a residency in psychiatry at Harvard Medical School and has practiced as a board certified psychiatrist in community mental health for 25 years. He presently works as a psychiatrist at Riverside Community Mental Health Center in Wakefield, MA. He has been Executive Director of the National Empowerment Center, Lawrence, MA, for 13 years. He has carried out research and published numerous articles and chapters in books in the area of recovery from mental illness. He was a member of the New Freedom Commission on Mental Health.

Anil Godbole, M.D. is chairman of Psychiatry at Advocate Illinois Masonic and Bethany Hospitals. He is a distinguished Life Fellow of the American Psychiatric Association and Clinical Associate Professor of Psychiatry at University of Illinois at Chicago. He was a member of President's 'New Freedom Commission on Mental Health' and he chaired the subcommittee on evidence-based practices. He has held leadership positions in National Association of Psychiatric Health Systems and American Hospital Association. He has published a dozen articles and is a frequent national speaker on subjects of behavioral health delivery systems and evidence based practices.

Sheila Leslie, M.A. is the state Assemblywoman for District #27 in central Reno. She serves as the Assistant Majority Whip for the state Assembly and the Chair of the Health and Human Services Committee. Sheila has a Masters Degree in Spanish Literature from the University of Nevada, Reno and is the author of many articles and studies on human services issues such as teen pregnancy, mental health, and youth gangs.

Dennis A. Mohatt, M.A. received his undergraduate training at the University of Oregon, and earned his master's degree in community-clinical psychology at the University in Pennsylvania. Dennis is currently the Director of the Mental Health Program for the Western Interstate Commission for Higher Education (WICHE). He has also served on the Nebraska Department of Health and Human Services (Deputy Director); National Rural Health Advisory Committee, to the United States Secretary of Health and Human Services; and the Rural Issues Subcommittee of the

President's New Freedom Commission on Mental Health. Dennis has been a member of the Board of Directors for the National Association for Rural Mental Health since 1987, and served as the association's President from 1992-1995.

William T. O'Donohue, Ph.D. is the Nicholas Cummings Professor of Organized Behavioral Healthcare Delivery in the Department of Psychology at the University of Nevada, Reno. He is also president and CEO of Care Integra, a company selling integrated care services, and executive director of the Cummings Foundation for Behavioral Health. He holds adjunct appointments in the Departments of Philosophy and Psychiatry at the University of Hawaii, Manoa. He received his doctorate in clinical psychology from the State University of New York at Stony Brook and a master's degree in philosophy from Indiana University. He has authored, edited or co-edited over forty books and has written numerous book chapters and journal articles.

John A. Talbott, M.D., Professor of Psychiatry and Director of the Professionalism Project, University of Maryland School of Medicine is Editor-Emeritus of Psychiatric Services, past president of the American Association of Chairmen of Departments of Psychiatry, past president of the American Psychiatric Association (1984-85) and former vice president of the American Board of Psychiatry and Neurology. He's published twenty books and two hundred articles about mental health services, public policy and the chronic mentally ill.

Table of Contents

Chapter 1

Behavioral Health Economics and Policy: An Overview

William O'Donohue and Michael A. Cucciare
University of Nevada, Reno

Introduction

It is important for mental health professionals to understand the macroeconomics of behavioral healthcare to better understand the issues involved in the ongoing debate on how to best address problems facing the current U.S. healthcare system. This understanding can lead not only to intellectual satisfaction but also to understanding how to position oneself to take advantage of opportunities and to avoid catastrophes. This chapter attempts to do this by first providing the reader with the general overview of the economics of the current U.S. healthcare system including how the current system is financed, how the budget for both physical and mental health is allocated, and how the U.S. compares to other industrialized nations on health spending. Second, a brief history and overview of healthcare insurance is presented. This section presents and discusses some of the major policy and economic events that have affected how current healthcare services are delivered and financed, presents an overview of healthcare insurance, and some of the fundamental problems and concepts inherit in the way healthcare is currently insured. Third, several key policy issues such as universal healthcare and tort reform are discussed that are at the heart of the current debate on how to best fix the current healthcare crisis.

Healthcare Economics:
How Does the Current U.S. Healthcare System Work?

Healthcare Dollars Spent as a Percentage of Gross Domestic Product

Currently the United States spends an estimated 14% of its gross domestic product (GDP) on healthcare (Wurman, 2004). This means that roughly $1 out of every $7 dollars currently spent in the United States is spent for healthcare. Healthcare spending as a portion of the U.S Gross Domestic Product (GDP) has increased alarmingly over the last four decades. The following are healthcare dollars spent in the U.S. over the last four decades given as a percentage of GDP (see Centers for Medicare and Medicaid Services (CMS), 2004a).

- 5% in 1960
- 7% in 1970
- 9% in 1980
- 12% in 1990
- 13% in 2000

This trend in healthcare spending is expected to continue. Specifically, by the year 2010, it is expected that 17% of our Nation's GDP or $1 out of every $6 dollars will be spent on healthcare (CMS, 2004a). What is of particular concern is not the absolute percent of GDP (although this is a concern) but the increase in the rate in which healthcare costs are rising. This is one of the key dimensions of the current healthcare crisis.

The U.S. also spends more on healthcare as a percentage of GDP than any other country. Germany, Canada, and France are ranked second, third, and fourth, while the United Kingdom (UK) and Japan are tied at fifth. In the year 2001, Germany spent 10.7% of their GDP on healthcare, Canada spent 9.7%, France spent 9.5%, and the UK and Japan spent 7.6% (Japan's figure is for 2000) (Henderson, 2005).

It is important to note that the U.S. is not the only industrialized nation that has watched its healthcare financing (as a percentage of GDP) grow over the last three decades. Between the years of 1970 and 1999, U. S. healthcare spending expressed as a percentage of GDP grew by 6% (however U.S. spending on healthcare nearly doubled in dollar amount). During the same period of time, Switzerland's healthcare spending grew by 5%; Japan by 3%; the United Kingdom by 3%; and Canada by 2% (CMS, 2004a). It is clear that the financing of healthcare, especially trying to keep up with the rate at which healthcare costs are increasing, is becoming an important issue for many nations.

Per Capita Spending on Healthcare in the U.S and Other Countries

Per capita spending on healthcare in the U.S. is also rapidly increasing. In 1986, per capita spending on healthcare was approximately $2,000; this increased to approximately $5,000 in the year 2001, and is expected to increase further to approximately $7,000 per person by the year 2006 (CMS, 2004a, Henderson, 2005). The U.S. spends more on healthcare in terms of per capita spending than many other countries such as Germany, Canada, France, and the UK (CMS, 2004a, Henderson, 2005). In particular, in 2001, Germany spent $2,808, Canada spent $2,792, France spent $2,561, and the UK spent $1,992 on per capita healthcare expenditures (Henderson, 2005).

Per capita healthcare spending in the U.S. increased 11.5 times between the years of 1970 and 1999. Other nations such as Japan, United Kingdom, Switzerland, and Canada have also observed increases in per capita spending during this time period. For example, Japan's per capita healthcare spending increased 13.5 times;

the United Kingdom's increased 10.6 times; Switzerland's increased 9.7 times; and Canada's increased 8.4 times between the years of 1970 and 1999 (CMS, 2004a).

Healthcare Spending in the U.S. by Age Group and as a Percentage of Annual Income

Some age and income groups have a greater impact upon healthcare costs than others. U.S. citizens over the age of 65 and with annual incomes of less than $20,000 spend a much higher percentage of their income on healthcare than any other age group. For example, the Centers for Medicare and Medicaid Services (2004a) report that individuals over the age of 65 spend 13% of their annual income on healthcare. Similarly, persons with annual incomes of less than $20,000 spend approximately 15% of their annual income on healthcare. These percentages are put into greater perspective when compared to the 5% of income afforded to healthcare by persons between the ages of 55 and 64, and 6% for individuals with annual incomes between $20,000 and $49,999 (CMS, 2004a).

How is the U.S. Healthcare System Financed?

The total healthcare budget in the U.S. in the year 2000 was 1.3 trillion dollars (Wurman, 2004). Wurman reports that the healthcare budget in 2000 was financed through multiple sources including private health insurance (34%), federal government (32%), consumer out-of-pocket (15%), state and local government (13%), and other sources (6%). The percentage of healthcare financing from private health insurance has skyrocketed in recent decades, while out-of pocket spending has decreased. In 1960, 21% of healthcare was covered by employer provided health insurance, while 55% was paid for through out-of-pocket spending (Schilling, 2004). In contrast, Schilling (2004) reports that in 2001 employer provided health insurance paid for 35% of healthcare expenditures and out-of-pocket spending decreased to 17%. Clearly, private health insurance is funding the largest percentage of current healthcare spending which is a trend that has been increasing since 1960. In recent years, in order to control healthcare costs employers have been purchasing policies with higher deductibles, more exclusions and higher co-payments (Henderson, 2005). Thus out of pocket expenditures appear to be on the rise in the last few years.

How is the $1.4 Trillion Dollar Healthcare Budget Allocated?

In 2001, the U.S. healthcare budget was allocated in the following manner (percentages may not sum due to rounding) (Henderson, 2005):

- 31% hospital care
- 22% physicians' services
- 11% other professional services
- 11% pharmacy and supplies
- 7% administration
- 7% nursing home

- 7% research and construction
- 3% public health
- 3% other medical products
- 2% home health

The last two decades reveal that healthcare expenditures for hospital services have declined from 47% of the total healthcare budget in 1980 to roughly 31% in 2001. In contrast, healthcare expenditures for prescription medications and home healthcare services have increased from 6% and 1% in 1980 to 11% and 2% in 2000, respectively (CMS, 2004a).

A major share (or 7.8%) of the U.S. healthcare budget is spent on treating mental illness and substance abuse (MH/SA). Mark et al. (2000) reported that the U.S. spent $85.3 billion dollars on MH/SA in the year 1997. The majority of the mental health budget went toward paying for mental health treatment ($73.4 billion dollars) with the remaining $11.9 billion dollars paying for the treatment of substance abuse.

The largest percentage of MH/SA dollars in 1997 went toward paying for hospitals and independent practicioners, $26.5 billion dollars and $22.3 billion dollars respectively. Breaking these figures down further reveals that of the $26.5 billion spent on hospitals, approximately $24 billion dollars paid for specialty hospitals treating mental illness and substance abuse, and $2 billion dollars paid for nonspecialty care in general hospitals. Of the $22.3 billion dollars that paid for independent practicioners, approximately $7 billion dollars paid for services provided by psychiatrists, $5 billion dollars paid for nonpsychiatric physicians, and $10 billion dollars paid for other professionals such as psychologists, social workers, counselors, and nurse practicioners. The remaining MH/SA budget dollars paid for multiservice mental health organizations ($12 billion dollars); prescription medications ($9 billion dollars); nursing homes ($4.7 billion dollars); specialty substance abuse treatment centers (e.g., methadone clinics) ($4 billion dollars); residential treatment centers for children ($3 billion dollars); home health ($428 million dollars); and insurance administration ($3.5 billion dollars) (dollar amounts may not sum due to rounding) (Mark et al., 2000).

Spending trends for MH/SA between 1987 and 1997 reveal a shift away from hospital care spending and increased spending on prescription medications. For example, spending on hospital care dropped from 42.5% in 1987 to 31% of total MH/SA spending in 1997. In contrast, spending for prescription medications rose from 7.5% of total MH/SA spending to 12.3% in 1997. It is interesting to note that the number of prescriptions written by physicians rose from 44.5 million in 1987 to 73.2 million in 1997 (Mark et al., 2000). Although figures are not available for more recent years, all indications point to a continuation of this trend.

It is important to note that in contrast to expenditures for physical medicine, the percentage of the U.S. total healthcare budget paying for MH/SA services has dropped from 8.8% in the year 1988 to 7.8% in 1997 (CBS News, 2000).

Furthermore, U.S. MH/SA financing trends indicate that the government is paying for increasing amount of MH/SA treatment services. Mark et al. (2000) reported that Medicare, Medicaid, and other state and local health programs spent $47.9 billion dollars (or 56% total spending) and private sources such as out-of pocket, private insurance, and other private sources spent $37.5 billion dollars (or 43%) on MH/SA in the year 1997.

It is also useful to look at more specific allocations in the overall Health and Human Services budget. Stossel (2004) has argued that specific allocations are influenced by political pressures and do not rationally follow actual risks to health and life. He states:

In the '80s, when the National Institutes of Health were slow to spend money on AIDS research, activists in Washington, D.C., heckled President Reagan, stopped traffic marched on Congress, and accused politicians of discriminating against gays. It worked. AIDS now gets more research money per patient than any other diseases. The success of the AIDS lobby became a model for the breast cancer lobby. Women marched on the Capitol, accusing politicians who resisted increasing funding of being "anti-woman". Who wants to be "anti-woman"? Funding for breast cancer research joined AIDS near the top of the list of per-patient expenditures. But breast cancer and AIDS are not the leading killers. Among diseases, breast cancer is ninth. AIDS 18th, Yet in 2001, AIDS research got $4,439 per patient from NIH, breast cancer $290, and Parkinson's $175. Diabetes, which killed more people than AIDS and breast cancer combined, got $41. Heart disease, the number one killer, got just $58 per patient. (p. 91-92)

Public and Private Financing of Healthcare

The percentage of public sector (i.e., Medicare and Medicaid) dollars used to fund the U.S. healthcare system have increased, while out-of-pocket dollars (i.e., private) have decreased. 40% of total healthcare dollars in 1970 came from out-of-pocket spending; 27% in 1980; 23% in 1990; and 17% in the year 2000. In contrast, the percentage of Medicare and Medicaid spending on healthcare has increased from 20% of healthcare dollars in 1970 paid for by these public services to 28% in 1980; 29% in 1990; and 36% in the year 2000 (CMS, 2004a). The budget for Medicare for the year 2001 shows that 39% of Medicare spending went toward paying for inpatient hospital services; 18% managed care; 17% physician services; 8% outpatient healthcare services; 7% labs, medical supplies, and related services; and the remaining 10% paid for services such as home health and hospice (CMS, 2004b). The budget for Medicaid for the year 1999 shows that 29% of Medicaid spending went toward paying for institutional long-term care; 19% inpatient and outpatient hospital services; 17% home health and other community based healthcare services; 14% capitated payments and primary care case management services; 11% prescription drugs; 5% clinics, lab and X-rays; and the remaining 5% paid for physician and other practitioner services (CMS, 2004b).

Decreases in out-of-pocket spending on healthcare are illustrated when examining sources of payment for prescription medications. CMS (2004a) reports that during the year 1965, 93% of prescription drug financing was made by out-of-pocket payments, while the rest was covered by public and private health insurance. In contrast, in 1985, 63% (a decrease of 30%) of the financing for prescription drugs was made by out-of-pocket spending while 14% and 24% was covered by private and public health insurance respectively. Decreases in out-of-pocket spending continued in the year 2000 with 32% of the financing for prescription drugs paid for with out-of-pocket spending, while the rest was covered by private and public health insurance (22% and 46% respectively) (CMS, 2004a).

One factor contributing to the increased public financing of the U.S. healthcare system is the increasing number of Medicare and Medicaid enrollees. For example, in the year 1970, 20.4 million individuals were eligible for Medicare services (all of these individuals were elderly). In the year 2000, the number jumped to 40 million, with 34.1 million elderly and 5.4 million disabled individuals enrolled in Medicare. The number of Medicare enrollees is projected to continue to increase through the next three decades with 76.8 (68.2 million elderly and 8.6 million disabled) million by the year 2030 (CMS, 2004b).

Public Spending: Medicare and Medicaid. The U.S. Congress passed comprehensive healthcare coverage for the indigent and elderly in 1965. This coverage is known as Medicare and Medicaid (see www.cms.gov). Both Medicare and Medicaid were established by the Social Security Act. Medicare was a responsibility of the Social Security Administration (SSA) and federal financing to state Medicaid programs was managed by the Social and Rehabilitation Service (SRS). Both the SSA and SRS were agencies in the Department of Health, Education, and Welfare (HEW). In 1977, the HEW created the Health Care Financing Administration (HCFA) to organize Medicare and Medicaid. The HCFA was later renamed the Centers for Medicare & Medicaid Services (CMS) in 2001 (see http://www.cms.hhs.gov/about/history).

Medicare is a government program that was developed to guarantee healthcare services to elderly Americans' regardless of their economic circumstances. Currently, Medicare provides coverage to approximately 40 million Americans. To be eligible for Medicare services, an individual must meet one of the two following criteria: be at least 65 years of age or be under the age of 65 with a certain disability such as end stage renal disease. Briefly, Medicare provides its enrollees healthcare benefits through two programs: Part A and Part B. Part A is medical hospital insurance and Part B is supplemental medical insurance. Persons over the age of 65 and that are eligible to receive Social Security or Railroad Retirement benefits automatically receive Medicare Part A benefits. Elderly persons that are not eligible for Social Security may enroll in Medicare Part A for a monthly premium. Part A covers inpatient hospital services for a maximum of 90 days for each benefit period. A benefit period starts on the first day benefits are received (e.g., date of hospital admission) and ends 60 days after being released (1st Insured, 1999). Part B (also known as supplementary medical insurance or Medigap plans) is a voluntary plan whereby an individual who elects to pay a monthly premium, deductible, and 20 percent of all medical expenses is eligible (the remaining 80 percent is paid by Part B). Part B covers medical costs associated with physicians and surgeons; however, it does not cover eye, hearing and physical exams, foot care, or immunizations. Medicare beneficiaries receive four categories of benefits – inpatient hospital care, medically necessary inpatient care in a skilled nursing facility after an acute inpatient hospital stay, home healthcare, and hospice care (see Henderson, 2005 and the Centers for Medicare and Medicaid Services (CMS) website www.cms.gov for a more thorough discussion of Medicare's features).

Since 1966, the number of Medicare beneficiaries has grown from 19 million to approximately 41 million Americans in 2001, which is approximately 14% of the U.S. population (Henderson, 2005). The 41 million Medicare beneficiaries in 2001 included approximately 35 million individuals over the age of 65, 6 million disabled persons, and 320,000 individuals with end stage kidney disease (Henderson, 2005). In addition to the increasing number of enrollees, annual expenditures for Medicare have grown substantially since it first year of operation. In its first year, Medicare's expenditures totaled $1.6 billion; however, by the year 2005 costs grew to $309 billion and are projected to increase to a staggering $495 billion dollars by the year 2012 (Henderson, 2005).

Public programs (such as Medicare and Medicaid) accounted for 45% of total healthcare spending in the U.S. in 2001 (CMS, 2004b). Spending on the part of public programs such as Medicare has shifted substantially away from paying for inpatient to paying for outpatient services. During the year 1980 (total spending was $37 billion dollars), 67% of total Medicare spending went toward paying for inpatient hospital services with this percentage decreasing to 39% of total spending in 2001 (total spending was $236 billion dollars). Alternatively, Medicare has increased its spending on outpatient programs such as hospice, health centers and rehabilitation facilities, and home health services (CMS, 2004b).

Medicaid was developed in 1965 as part of the same legislative package as Medicare. Medicaid is financed through both state and federal funding. Persons eligible for Medicaid services typically have a low income and fall into one of the following five categories: pregnant women; children and teenagers; and persons who are aged, blind and/or disabled. How does Medicaid work? Briefly, each state receives different levels of Medicaid funding depending on the per capita income of individuals living in a given state relative to the nation's average per capita income (note: average U.S. per capita income in 2003 was $31,459, average three year U.S. household income for 2001-2003 was $43,527, U.S. Census Bureau, 2004).

States are generally allowed to develop their own Medicaid programs as long as they follow federal guidelines such as being accessible to low-income individuals (see Henderson, 2005 and the Centers for Medicare and Medicaid Services (CMS) website www.cms.gov for a more thorough discussion of Medicaid's features).

Medicaid had 10 million low-income enrollees in 1967, which increased to 46 million in the year 2001 (CMS, 2004b). Medicaid's spending has increased from $1.7 billion in 1966 to $180 billion in 1999, with spending expected to increase to whopping $500 billion by the year 2012 (Henderson, 2005).

Total Medicaid spending in the year 1999 illustrates a similar emphasis on financing outpatient healthcare services with 17% percent (or $26 billion) of dollars going toward home health and other community-based services. The largest percentage or 29% of total Medicaid spending in 1999 paid for institutionalized long-term care (CMS, 2004b).

In addition to Medicare and Medicaid, the Department of Defense (DoD) spends billions of dollars each year on providing healthcare to active duty, retired members, and their dependents. It is estimated that in 2005, the DoD will spend $37 billion dollars on healthcare with costs expected to exceed $50 billion by the year 2010 (Gilmore, 2005).

Private Spending: Out-of-Pocket and Private Health Insurance. Since the 1960s, out-of-pocket spending for healthcare has decreased from 55% of the total national healthcare budget to 17% in the year 2001 (Shilling, 2004). As a result, private health insurance, along with public programs such as Medicare and Medicaid, are increasingly paying for a larger percentage of total national healthcare costs. It is estimated that in the year 2005, as much as 35% of U.S. healthcare costs (compared to 28% in 1980) will be paid for by private health insurance (CMS, 2004c; Schilling, 2004). It is important to note that although generally out-of-pocket per capita spending on healthcare is decreasing in the U.S., out-of-pocket spending on inpatient hospital and outpatient services, and home health are on the rise (CMS, 2004a).

One of the unfortunate consequences of increased healthcare spending by private insurance is that employees are now spending more of their income on health insurance premiums. Employees of small businesses (e.g., businesses with between 3 - 24 employees) appear to be the greatest hit by these increases. In the year 1988, the average monthly employee contribution to their healthcare premium was $8 for single and $52 for a family insurance plan; while in the year 2001, the average monthly contribution tripled to $30 and $150, respectively (CMS, 2004c). Increases in premiums have also been observed for all types of healthcare plans including Health Maintenance Organizations (HMOs) and Preferred Provider Organizations (PPOs). The average annual premium costs for all healthcare plan types in the year 2001 were $2,650 for single and $7,053 for a family plan (CMS, 2004c).

Healthcare Insurance Coverage in Relation to Organization Size

Recent data from the CMS (2004c) show that small businesses are less likely to offer healthcare benefits to their employees when compared to larger businesses. Data from 2001 show that 58% of small businesses (i.e., less than ten employees) provided healthcare benefits to their employees, while in the same year, 99% of large businesses (i.e., 200 plus employees) provided healthcare insurance coverage to their employees (CMS, 2004c). In addition to being more likely to provide healthcare insurance, large or "jumbo" size companies are more likely to provide their employees with a choice of healthcare plans. For example, the CMS reports that in the year 2001 roughly 60% of jumbo size businesses (5,000 or more employees) provided their employees with three or more healthcare plans, with only 2% of small businesses (3-199 employees) offering the equivalent. Larger businesses are also more likely to provide healthcare insurance to their retirees. However, over the last 14 years, the number of large businesses providing retiree healthcare benefits has declined from 66% in 1988 to 34% in 2002 (CMS, 2004c).

The Uninsured

It comes as no surprise that individuals without healthcare insurance coverage spend more out-of-pocket on their health than those with healthcare coverage. In the year 1998, the uninsured paid approximately 48% of their healthcare costs out-of-pocket as opposed to 20% by those with healthcare insurance coverage (CMS, 2004d). The CMS (2004d) reports that in the year 2000, 18% of individuals in the U.S. did not have healthcare coverage, which is an increase of 4% since the year 1987. Individuals with income levels below the federal poverty level are the most likely to not have healthcare coverage, i.e., 33% of these individuals did not have coverage in 2001. This is compared to the 11% of uninsured individuals with incomes exceeding 200% of the federal poverty level (CMS, 2004d).

Ethnic background is associated with a lack of healthcare coverage. The CMS (2004d) reports that in the year 2000, 34% of Hispanics; 29% of Native Americans; 20% of African-Americans; 19% of Asians; and 11% of Caucasians in the U.S. did not have healthcare insurance coverage. The greatest increases in noninsured populations by ethnicity since the year 1987 occurred in Native Americans, Asians (both with a 6% increase), and Hispanics (5% increase) (CMS, 2004d).

Also, certain age groups are more likely to be uninsured. Between the years of 1987 and 2000, the percentage of individuals without healthcare coverage by age group has not changed significantly. Individuals between the ages of 18-34 are the most likely to not have healthcare insurance (representing 41% of uninsured U.S. individuals in the year 2002, Henderson, 2005), which some have argued attenuates the problem of the uninsured as individuals in this age range tend to be a healthy demographic. In addition, the overwhelming majority of individuals without coverage are between the age of 18 and 54, making up approximately 69% of all uninsured individuals in the year 2000. The other 31% is accounted for by those individuals under the age of 18 (22%) and between the ages of 55 and 64 (9%) (CMS, 2004d). The impact of not having health insurance can be great and take many forms. The Centers for Medicare and Medicaid Services (2004d) report that in the year 2000, 39% of the uninsured under the age of 65 had to postpone medical care due to cost; 36% had no consistent source of healthcare; 30% were unable to fill prescriptions due to cost; 20% did not get healthcare care for a serious medical problem; 27% reported that medical bills impacted their life significantly; and 39% reported being contacted by a collection agency regarding their healthcare bills.

Finally, individuals living in western and southern states are more likely to be uninsured than persons living in the mid-western and eastern United States (CMS, 2004d).

A Brief History and Introduction to Healthcare Insurance

The last three decades have witnessed several major changes in the way healthcare services are delivered and financed. Specifically, the transition from private to public sector and out-of-pocket to third-party spending, and deregulation and the growth of managed care have substantially impacted the current way healthcare services are delivered and funded (Henderson, 2005). Each of these developments is discussed below.

Transition from Private to Public Financing

Henderson (2005) argues that the most important factor impacting the current status of healthcare service delivery is the transition from private-sector (e.g., out-of-pocket and private health insurance) to public-sector (e.g., federal, state, and local) financing. For example, in 1960, the private-sector financed 75% of healthcare costs; in contrast, the government was responsible for only 25% of every medical dollar. With the introduction of Medicare and Medicaid in the mid-1960s came increases in government financing of healthcare. By the end of the 1960s, the federal share of the healthcare budget almost reached 40%, although currently the total (including federal and state spending) share of government healthcare spending has reached approximately 50% (Henderson, 2005; Levit, Smith, Cowan, Sensing, & Catlin, 2004).

Transition from Out-of-Pocket to Third Party Spending

Over the last forty years, there has been a substantial decrease in the amount of out-of-pocket with a large increase in third party spending on healthcare. Approximately 50% of total healthcare spending came from out-of-pocket in the 1960s, which has decreased to 14% in the year 2002 (Levit et al., 2004). It is important to note that not all private-sector funding has decreased since 1960. For example, private health insurance spending has increased from 22% in the 1960s to 35% in 2002 (Levit et al., 2004). With greater spending on the part of federal programs and private insurance providers, healthcare costs at the point of purchase are virtually nonexistent for the insured individual (Henderson, 2005).

Rising healthcare costs are, to some extent, due to a lack of disincentives to spend on the part of insured individuals and healthcare providers. Insured individuals have little financial incentive to control their healthcare spending. Schilling (2004) argues that American's are notable for demanding what can be phrased "recreational medicine" or for example, in response to a minor ache or pain, an individual might take a half day off from work and demand/receive a battery of medical tests – all for little or no cost to the patient. In addition, Americans often demand the newest and subsequently most expensive medications, a practice that has increased greatly since the Food and Drug Administration, starting in 1997, allowed pharmaceutical companies to advertise directly to consumers (Schilling, 2004). This trend is illustrated in the recent demand for the painkiller Vioxx, which Schilling points out is only appropriate for a small group of individuals experiencing bleeding ulcers, yet demanded by a wide variety of individuals experiencing pain. Insured individuals have little incentives to limit their demand for healthcare services as long as insurers are willing to pay their bills. Henderson (2005) argues that even if the expected benefit of a healthcare procedure is small, it is unlikely that the insured will limit the demand of such services as long as their share of the expense is little or none.

Consequences of third party payment systems can be observed in the varying costs of insured and uninsured healthcare procedures. For example, the cost of hospital services have increased sixteen times between the 1970s and the year 2001, while the cost of purchasing eye glasses (not usually covered by health insurance) has increased only ten times (Henderson, 2004).

High Utilization and Concentration of Healthcare Expenditures. Another factor contributing to rising healthcare costs (and insurance premiums) is "high utilization" (Cummings, Cummings, & Johnson, 1997; O'Donohue & Cucciare, 2005). High utilization is a phrase used to describe the finding that large amounts of healthcare expenditures are concentrated in a relatively small group of individuals (Anderson & Knickman, 1984; Ash, Zhao, Ellis, & Kramer, 2001; Liptzin, Regier, & Goldberg, 1980). For example, Berk and Monheit (2001) found that the most expensive 1% of health care consumers accounted for 27% of total health care costs in 1996, the most expensive 5% accounted for 55%, and the top 10% accounted for 69%. Similarly, Ash et al. (2001) reported that healthcare costs for the year 1998 was highly skewed with the top .8% costing more than $25,000 per individual while the median healthcare cost per individual was $240.

Who are the High Utilizers? Various psychological and medical conditions have been linked to high utilization of healthcare services (Liptzin et al., 1980). In one study, researchers examined annual treatment costs during the year of 1995 for 284,060 Medicaid patients diagnosed with chronic psychological and medical problems (Garis & Farmer, 2002). The researchers found that the most expensive psychological problems to treat were (dollar amounts represent mean annual costs) some form of psychosis ($6,964) and depression ($5,505). The most expensive medical conditions to treat were cardiovascular disease ($2,320), congestive heart failure ($2,318), diabetes ($2,114), acid peptic disease ($1,811), asthma ($1,634), and hypertension ($1,351). Finally, researchers found that greater treatment costs for psychological problems is mostly due to costs for (a) nonphysician healthcare (e.g., mental health) provided in patients' homes and (b) inpatient hospital costs.

Garis and Farmer (2002) also examined mean annual healthcare costs for individuals with co-occurring psychological and medical problems. The most expensive comorbid conditions to treat were psychosis and depression ($18,316), psychosis and anxiety ($10,425), psychosis and diabetes ($9,947), diabetes and acid peptic illness ($9,927), asthma and depression ($5,448), and acid peptic illness and anxiety ($5,099).

Deregulation and the Growth of Managed Care

Deregulation or the removal of hospital rate regulation followed by the growth of managed care has resulted in a decline of hospital services usage (Jordan, 2004) and an increase in the existence and use of outpatient facilities and medical practices (Henderson, 2005). Accordingly, since deregulation, there has been an increase in freestanding outpatient medical facilities such as ambulatory surgery centers (or surgicenters) and clinics (Lynk & Longley, 2002). Also, more physicians are advertising directly to individual consumers and providing medical practices such as evening and weekend hours, and house-calls (Henderson, 2005).

Managed care insurance plans are becoming increasingly more popular among employer-based group insurance plans. Henderson (2005) reported that in the year 1999 nine out of ten employees covered by employer-based group insurance were covered by a managed care plan (i.e., HMO or PPO). The rise and popularity of managed care organizations (MCOs) occurred in response to the growing need to control escalating healthcare costs, increase the effectiveness and efficiency in which healthcare services are delivered, and reduce incentives for providers to deliver unnecessary medical services (Cummings et al., 1997; Hayes, Barlow, & Nelson-Gray, 1999). Many types of MCOs are in existence including Health Maintenance Organizations (HMOs), Preferred Provider Organizations (PPOs), Individual Practice Associations (IPAs), and Employee Assistance Programs (EAPs). Briefly, in HMOs individuals or groups of individuals contract with an HMO to provide all healthcare services over the course of a year for a prepaid set monthly fee. In a PPO, the focus is on managing the delivery of services by a "panel" of providers who have been approved to provide healthcare services to individuals and who have discounted rates in exchange for a large volume of service. An IPA consists of a group of independent practitioners who contract directly with companies or other groups to provide healthcare services. It is argued by some that small IPAs are not exactly MCOs in that the practitioner contracts directly with an organization to provide healthcare services thereby eliminating the need for third party management, however, as IPAs grow in size they require more complex management that is involved in traditional MCOs. Furthermore, in smaller IPAs, the practitioners absorb any risk associated with healthcare utilization. And finally, EAPs were designed by large companies for the purpose of early identification and treatment of high prevalence behavioral health problems such as substance use and depression. EAPs contract with a group of providers in which employees with behavioral health problems are referred (see Cummings et al., 1997; Hayes et al., 1999 for more discussion on types of managed care organizations). Unfortunately, as noted by Schilling (2004), managed care companies such as HMOs have become less popular over recent years due to consumer complaints and doctors' groups, while more expensive PPOs have become more favorable.

Introduction to Healthcare Insurance

Healthcare insurance coverage in the U.S. first became available in 1798. Insurance was made available by the U.S. Marine Hospital and insured eligible seaman against accidents and disability. It was not until 1847 that a company offered sickness insurance to its employees. The first insurer to offer insurance coverage beyond accidents and disability was The Massachusetts Health Insurance Company of Boston (Henderson, 2005).

Group healthcare insurance was first offered in 1910 by Montgomery Ward and Company to its employees. The policy provided enrollees with a financial benefit in the event of illness or disability. However, it was not until after the Second World War that group healthcare coverage became a major factor of the collective bargaining process. A major wage-price freeze during WW II forced employers to offer non wage benefits such as healthcare insurance to keep and attract employees (Henderson, 2005). Furthering the popularity of employer provided group healthcare insurance, in 1954, the Internal Revenue Service ruled that employer contributions to employee healthcare insurance were exempt from taxation, which is still in affect today. This tax law provides a subsidy to healthcare insurance which lowers the cost of insurance, thus having the effect of increasing its demand among consumers (Phelps, 1997). Moreover, during the 1950's and 1960's employers began to add improvements such as dental care, prescription drugs, and vision care to employee healthcare insurance plans (Henderson, 2005).

Types of Healthcare Insurance: Indemnity and Social Insurance

Much of the growing debate over healthcare policy reform involves two conflicting types of healthcare insurance – indemnity and social insurance (Henderson, 2005). *Indemnity* insurance plans reimburse healthcare users for financial loss due to certain events and medical expenses. Indemnity insurance can cover loss due to fire, theft, casualty, life, and healthcare costs (Henderson, 1995; Insurance Finder, 2005). In indemnity plans, payments or premiums are paid by the insured to the insurer. Premiums are financial payments made to an insurance company to purchase and maintain a policy. Individuals who demonstrate a greater risk for loss typically pay higher premiums (see Sowell, 2004 for a discussion on the relationship between risk and insurance). A second type of insurance or *social* insurance is the basis of all federal and state healthcare assistance programs including Medicare and Medicaid. This type of insurance ignores expected financial loss to set premium rates and instead allocates costs based on the financial capabilities of eligible individuals (Henderson, 2005).

Henderson (2005) points out that both indemnity and social insurance strategies are employed in the United States today. Individuals (or their employers) covered by private healthcare insurance pay premiums set by the indemnity strategy. Many healthcare insurance policies are written as group policies and premiums are the same for everyone belonging to the group. Premiums within groups, however, will most often vary as a consequence of family size. Also, premium rates across groups may vary as consequence of expected utilization of healthcare services, often determined by examining past claims data. Individuals with past patterns of high utilization (and thus have higher healthcare costs) will more likely pay higher premiums than individuals with less expected future utilization. Those that favor indemnity insurance argue it is more equitable than the social approach because the cost of insurance is based on lifestyle decisions of the individual. For example, an individual who chooses to exercise, eat healthy, and avoid tobacco use is less likely to need/utilize expensive healthcare services and therefore, should pay a lower insurance premium than someone who is unwilling to make these lifestyle choices.

Healthcare insurance programs such as Medicare and Medicaid are illustrative of social insurance. Federal programs provide healthcare insurance to many of our nation's elderly, indigent, and disabled, and to many individuals with chronic illnesses such as renal failure. Those that argue for the social insurance strategy take the point of view that healthcare insurance is an individual right and a social responsibility (Henderson, 2005).

Healthcare insurance plans generally fall into two categories – medical expense insurance and disability income insurance. The former provides financial reimbursement for healthcare expenditures, while the latter provides financial payments when a person is unable to work. Most healthcare insurance policies, regardless of type, provide the eligible individual with insurance in a few or all of the following areas (see Henderson, 2005):

- Hospitalization – covers room and board and all hospital services such as lab fees, nursing care, use of operating and recovery rooms, outpatient services, medications, and medical supplies involved in a "normal" hospital stay.
- Physician and surgical – covers surgical procedures and inpatient hospital visits within an allowable dollar amount.
- Regular medical benefits – covers general physician services and other surgical procedures.
- Major medical – covers large medical expenses with few limitations on specific items covered. This type of insurance is commonly offered as a supplement to hospital, physician and surgical insurance coverage and employs deductibles, coinsurance, and a maximum limit on out-of-pocket spending.
- Dental – covers many common dental procedures such as fillings, extractions, and dentures. Dental insurance covers preventative procedures such as X – rays and routine cleanings and often comes with a co-payment.
- Disability – covers the eligible individual in the event they are longer able to work in their usual occupation due to an illness, accident, or injury. Disability insurance commonly covers a set dollar amount based on the needs of the

policy holder. Also, these policies often have a waiting period and allow for a maximum number of years in which the individual may receive benefits.

- Long-term care – covers the eligible individual in the event that long – term care (e.g., skilled nursing) is needed due to chronic medical and psychological illness and disability.

Historically, healthcare coverage for physical and behavioral health has not been equal. Healthcare insurance plans have traditionally placed greater limits on spending for behavioral health services than for services related to physical medicine. For example, many plans place greater limits on the number of inpatient hospital days and outpatient visits an individual might require for behavioral health purposes. Plans also commonly have greater co-payments related to behavioral services (Hennessey & Barry, 2005). Co-payments are meant to force consumers to have a stake in purchasing decisions.

As a result of these discrepancies in coverage, many individuals have advocated for the passing of mental health parity laws or laws requiring healthcare insurance plans to provide equal coverage for both physical and behavioral health (Frank, Goldman, & McGuire, 2001); thus, as many as 34 state parity laws and one federal law has been passed mandating partial parity. Partial parity as stated in the 1996 Federal Partial Parity law bans the practice of using annual or lifetime dollar limits to control the use of behavioral health services unless equal dollar limits are placed on other services such as physical medicine (Hennessey & Barry, 2005). At the time this chapter was written, federal laws requiring full parity for behavioral health services had not been passed.

Healthcare Insurance: Fundamental Problems and Concepts

One of the most challenging problems occurring in the transaction between insurance purchaser and provider is unequal access to relevant information. Phelps (1997) calls this the problem of *asymmetric knowledge*. The phrase "symmetric knowledge" in the context of healthcare refers to the extent to which both sides of an economic negotiation (e.g., insurance provider and insurance purchaser) have equal amounts of relevant information. Asymmetries of knowledge occur when bargaining in an economic exchange (as in the case with someone interested in purchasing health insurance) takes place and one side (usually the insurance provider) has less relevant information than the other (Phelps, 1997). For example, imagine an individual interested in purchasing dental insurance does so while knowing that he or she has several expensively treated dental problems. This person may be attempting to obtain dental insurance to have these procedures covered and thus avoid having to pay for these services out-of-pocket. In this case, one side of the negotiation, namely the health insurance purchaser, has considerably more relevant information about their likelihood of using expensive dental procedures than the insurance provider.

Henderson (2005) argues that several problems can arise from asymmetric knowledge including imperfect consumer knowledge, lack of discretionary utilization, and adverse selection. Each of these problems is discussed below.

Imperfect Consumer Knowledge

This problems stems from the difficulties consumers have in collecting and interpreting healthcare information. The quality of information that consumers have regarding healthcare services is often poor, with much of their information coming from other consumers. Also, the nature of healthcare information is often technical, requiring years of training to understand in such a manner as to make appropriate diagnostic and treatment decisions. This leads most healthcare consumers to have little or no understanding regarding the technical aspects of healthcare services (e.g., what blood tests can determine and how they are interpreted). When consumers have access to only imperfect knowledge regarding aspect of healthcare they are likely to have problems making informed decisions about which services, providers, etc., are most appropriate. Henderson (2005) argues that this can lead to the problem of dual role or when a physician become both the consumer's adviser and provider of healthcare services. Henderson further argues that dual role in this context can lead to abuse of the healthcare system on the part of the provider (e.g., providing unnecessary services or services that have little relative benefit to the consumer).

Lack of Discretionary Utilization

The second problem with asymmetric knowledge occurs when one party to a contract (e.g., insurance provider) cannot monitor the behavior of the second party (e.g., insurance consumer). Specifically, once an agreement between two parties such as the insurance provider and consumer has been reached, the latter party may engage in opportunistic behavior when not monitored. In this context opportunistic behavior may take the form of engaging in unnecessary utilization with little regard for cost. For example, a person visiting a physician for a battery of tests will behave differently when they have healthcare insurance. The patient with insurance might ask questions such as what are the benefits of the tests?, are there complications?, and what is the length of the time required for tests? The provider with knowledge that the patient is insured will most likely provide the tests with confidence that the insurance will cover the cost. In contrast, patients without insurance are more likely to ask questions regarding the cost of the tests, costs of alternative tests, whether the recommended tests are absolutely necessary, and the consequences of failing or postponing the tests. In contrast, the provider that knows a patient in uninsured will most likely take the patient's financial situation into account when determining what tests to conduct.

Adverse Selection

This problem occurs when insurance purchasers have more information about their healthcare utilization (and therefore costs) than the insurance provider. This can result in insurance providers having a disproportionate number of high utilizers.

This issue leads to a number of economic problems such as increased (a) premiums for all individual covered within the group and (b) incentives for low-risk individuals in the group (and low utilizers of healthcare services) to cancel their coverage in search of less expensive insurance.

What Might be Wrong with the Current U.S. Healthcare System?

The present healthcare system has been criticized on a number of grounds including its efficiency, its effectiveness, and its fairness. Critics have suggested what are in general major reforms that they argue will improve healthcare in the U.S. What follows is a brief summary of the major criticisms and suggestions for reforms.

Universal Healthcare

Some argue that healthcare is a right and individuals who are deprived of needed healthcare are being deprived of a basic right. While it is beyond the scope of this chapter to critically summarize these arguments, some basic questions can be asked of this position:

1. How are claims that a certain right exists to be justified? What kind of right is this (a right by virtue of being human, a right by virtue of being an American citizen, i.e., a constitutional right, etc). Do all people have this right? If so, what are our obligations for citizens of other countries?
2. Can these rights be overridden or abrogated in any way? For example, if an individual smokes for their entire life and knows of the increased risk of emphysema and cancer, can they claim the right to have treatment paid for when they get these diseases?
3. How is universal healthcare to be paid for? Are savings from reforms below really sufficient? If economics represents how to choose and allocate scarce resources, what do we have to give up in order to pay for universal healthcare?
4. How worried should we be that universal healthcare can increase expenditures because consumers are spending other people's money and thus are no longer constrained by the normal inhibitions associated with spending one's own money?
5. How worried should we be that the universal healthcare plans attempted in other countries have serious problems, e.g., long waits, excluded conditions, lack of innovation, slow to adopt expensive new technologies?

Tort Reform

Healthcare professionals and organizations are sued for the damages they allegedly have inflicted due to their malpractice. It is certainly the case that a large number of medical errors are made, with some estimates indicating approximately

60,000 unnecessary deaths occurring each year due to these errors (American Medical Association, 1989). Medical malpractice also results in prolonged suffering due to inappropriate treatment or new morbidity caused by incorrect treatment. It also results in economic damages due to inability to function or impairment in functioning.

The present system rests on patients hiring attorneys and filing lawsuits to gain redress for any alleged damages. Some have argued that this system is problematic for the following reasons:

1. Only a small portion of patients who are victims of medical errors file a claim. One study found 1.5% of those injured by medical negligence filed a claim (Physician Insurers Association of American, 2003).
2. Malpractice suits can results in physicians practicing defensive medicine and prescribing unnecessary tests. One estimate shows that the federal government alone pays about $29-$48 billion dollars a year due to defensive medicine (Institute of Medicine, 2001).
3. Healthcare professionals pay large sums for malpractice insurance, eventually passing on these costs to consumers and insurance providers. In 2003, physicians alone spent $6.3 billion dollars on malpractice premiums (Physician Insurers Association of America, 2003). In many states, these rates are increasing many multiples of inflation.
4. The threat of malpractice has been regarded as the number one impediment to meaningful quality improvement methods in healthcare. Healthcare professionals are reluctant to disclose problems due to the threat of suits. Quality improvement methods have been regarded as a better more significant way to reduce errors than the present litigation based system.
5. It has forced physicians and clinics to close because they could not afford premiums. In Nevada, for example, a state which has had no limits on non-economic damages, increases in premiums (to about $200,000/yr) has forced many obstetricians to leave the state. This limits choice for patients and can result in underserved areas.

There have been a variety of suggestions for reforms including:

6. The elimination of venue shopping in which attorneys attempt to move cases into more plaintiff friendly areas.
7. Placing limits on the practice of "joint and several liabilities" often called the "deep pockets rule" by which an entity such as a hospital can be found to be one percent at fault but can be required to pay all of the judgment because they have the most assets.

8. Placing a cap on non-economic damages (often the cap is $250,000). Thus, economic damages (decreases in earning potential as well as increases in expenditures) can be fully compensated, but the "pain and suffering" damages are limited. This can make insurers costs more predictable by allowing them to avoid mega-judgments of many millions of dollars.

9. Decreasing coverage for behaviors such as sexual contact with patients so that healthcare providers have more of a disincentive for these kinds of misbehaviors.

10. The use of quality improvement techniques and technology to decrease medical errors. Specifically, the Bush Administration has focused on: Developing the Consumer Assessment of Health Plans Survey (CAHPS) that provides information on consumers' descriptive ratings of health plans as well as evaluative ratings of care.

    a.   Providing quality information about nursing homes on the internet to enable families to make comparisons and informed judgments.

    b.   Examining how information technology, such as decision support systems embedded in clinicians' personal digital assistants (PDAs), can improve safe patient care.

    c.   Promoting the introduction and use of bar coding for dispensing prescription drugs to reduce errors.

    d.   Developing voluntary standards necessary to make the creation of an electronic healthcare record possible; this would make a patient's medical records available across different care sites, and to the patient.

    e.   Examining model disease management programs that can improve the quality of care for people with asthma and diabetes.

    f.   Developing computer software that hospitals can use to identify quality problems, assisting in quality improvement activities.

    g.   Developing a program called "Put Prevention into Practice" in order to assure that evidence-based recommendations for clinical prevention are actually translated into improved delivery of services.

Administrative Costs

Healthcare administrative costs generally represent the transaction costs incurred in exchanging the information and resources necessary to provide healthcare services. In 1999, health administration costs totaled at least $294.3 billion in the United States, or $1,059 per capita, as compared with $307 per capita in Canada. After exclusions, administration accounted for 31% of healthcare expenditures in the United States and 16.7% percent of healthcare expenditures in

Canada (Woolhandler, Campbell, & Himmelstein, 2003). At a micro-level a study by the American Medical Association estimates that a physician spends an average of six minutes on each claim while the physician's staff spends an average of one hour. Those physicians who contract with outside billing services pay about $8 per claim (American Medical Association Center for Health Policy Research, 1989). These costs can escalate dramatically as unintended consequences of new rules and regulations. For example, compliance with The Health Insurance Portability and Accountability Act of 1996 (HIPAA) has been estimated to have added billions of dollars in administration costs.

The two major reforms suggested are to either adopt a single payer system to reduce transaction costs or to use improvements in information technology to decrease these costs. Critics of the first option agree that although a single payor system would decrease administration costs they would increase overall medical costs due to the removing disincentives for competitive pricing as well as the inhibitory effects of out of pocket expenditures. For example, the Congressional Budget office has suggested that a single payor system would reduce administrative costs by 7% but increase utilization by 12% thus resulting in a net increase in costs of 5% (Minnesota Office of the Legislative Auditor, 1995). Improvements in information technology such as the electronic medical record, paperless billing on the web, barcoding of prescriptions, etc. have significant startup costs but may eventually reduce overall costs. The key is to reduce the costs of information transfer between parties while protecting patient confidentiality. More studies on the return on investment of information technology are badly needed. Many have the experience that information technology innovations have produced more problems than remedies due to problems such as IT systems not being able to communicate with each other, problems in the design, and general expenses in maintaining and debugging the systems.

Integrative Health

Nicholas Cummings and his colleagues (Cummings et al., 1997; Cummings, O'Donohue, & Ferguson, 2003) have suggested that the current fractionated system results in unnecessary expense. The major focus has been on integrating behavioral health into primary care medicine. The issue seems to be that the current system either treats the body or the mind but does not treat both in any one setting. Many patients seems to prefer treatment in the medical setting but suffer from problems that this setting is not ideally suited to treat such as lifestyle problems (e.g., smoking, diet, and exercise), treatment adherence problems, and problems such as depression, anxiety and substance abuse. Some studies have revealed that the majority of primary care visits are driven by behavioral health problems (Katon, 1986). By integrating trained behavioral health specialists in these settings overall costs have been shown to be reduced significantly. Cummings (1997) treated 126,000 patients in Oahu and showed a 40% reduction in a sample of high utilizers. O'Donohue, Cummings, and Laygo (2004) colocated specially trained psychologists in primary care offices in Oahu and reduced medical utilization by 21%. Thus, integrating behavioral health into med/surgical healthcare seems to be a method in which patients can receive the care they need, become healthier and reduce expenditures.

Evidence Based Practice

A New England Journal of Medicine study of more than 400 indicators of quality care for 30 conditions determined that, on average, patients received recommended care only about half the time. A January 2003 study in the Journal of the American Medical Association found that only 11 percent of physician organizations had adopted clinical guidelines, trained physicians in their use and presented the information in patient charts, reminder systems or order-entry systems for each of four chronic conditions they treat: diabetes, asthma, congestive heart failure and depression.

In response to these and other problems the Institute of Medicine (IOM) (2001) has recommended some basic rules for the 21st Century health system:

Current Approach	New Rule
Care is based primarily on visits.	Care is based on continuous healing relationships.
Professional autonomy drives variability.	Care is customized according to patient needs and values.
Professionals control care.	The patient is the source of control.
Information is a record.	Knowledge is shared and information flows freely.
Decision making is based on training and experience.	Decision making is evidence-based.
Do no harm is an individual responsibility.	Safety is a system property.
Secrecy is necessary.	Transparency is necessary.
The system reacts to needs.	Needs are anticipated.
Cost reduction is sought.	Waste is continuously decreased.
Preference is given to professional roles over the system.	Cooperation among clinicians is a priority.

Table 1. The Institute of Medicine's New Rules for the 21st Century Healthcare System.
Source: Crossing the Quality Chasm: A New Health System for the 21st Century, 2001.

In addition it recommends a focus on redesigning primary care and care for those with chronic conditions, creating an information and communications technology infrastructure to support evidence based practice. A recent IOM report (2001) recommends that common conditions serve as a starting point for restructuring care delivery and, at the behest of the Agency for Health Care Research and Quality, the IOM (2003a) recommended 20 such priority areas for national action. These priority areas are as follows (not in any order of importance):

- Care coordination
- Self-management/health literacy
- Asthma–appropriate treatment for persons with mild/moderate persistent asthma
- Cancer screening that is evidence-based–focuses on colorectal and cervical cancer
- Children with special health care needs
- Diabetes–focus on appropriate management of early disease
- End of life with advanced organ system failure–focus on congestive heart failure and chronic obstructive pulmonary disease
- Frailty associated with old age–preventing falls and pressure ulcers, maximizing function, and developing advanced care plans
- Hypertension–focus on appropriate management of early disease
- Immunization–children and adults
- Ischemic heart disease–prevention, reduction of recurring events, and optimization of functional capacity
- Major depression–screening and treatment
- Medication management–preventing medication errors and overuse of antibiotics
- Nosocomial infections–prevention and surveillance
- Pain control in advanced cancer
- Pregnancy and childbirth–appropriate prenatal and intrapartum care
- Severe and persistent mental illness–focus on treatment in the public sector
- Stroke–early intervention and rehabilitation
- Tobacco dependence treatment in adults
- Obesity

The IOM report (2003a) also encourages the federal government to take full advantage of its influential position as purchaser, regulator and provider of healthcare services to determine quality for the healthcare sector. It recommends reforming health professions education to focus on evidence based practice and quality improvement. Authors of the IOM report (2001) underscore the importance of a dramatically improved information technology infrastructure to support a 21st Century health system. Building blocks for such a system include an electronic health record system and national standards. The IOM (2003b) identifies eight care delivery functions that are essential for such records to promote greater safety, quality and efficiency. These are:

- Health information and data
- Result management
- Order management
- Decision support
- Electronic communication and connectivity
- Patient support
- Administrative processes and reporting

One important innovator in this area is Brent James of Intermountain Health in Salt Lake City, Utah. Currently, eight medical conditions are addressed in primary care settings in James' model: diabetes, asthma, depression, congestive heart failure, chronic anticoagulation, lower respiratory infection, pediatric otitis media, and medical management of lower back pain. In each of those areas, evidence-based medicine is used to set practice norms. Thus, an integral part of this model is to pay healthcare professionals for their evidence based practice. James' model moves pay for performance from its current paradigm as a compliance model to a process model. James calls this idea "shared risk," as it incents based on shared savings. Savings that accrue from the implementation of quality improvement processes are split three equal ways. Shares go to the physicians who implement the processes, the healthcare services organization that employs the physicians (e.g., a hospital), and the health plan that covers the affected patients. At Intermountain Health Care Services, savings in overall costs from just a few dozen quality improvements have run into the tens of millions of dollars.

Interestingly, Wennberg has found that the unwanted variance that is produced by ignoring evidence based practice often results in more care, not less. Thus, bolstering the argument that present care is more expensive when it deviates from evidence based practice, "We found that no matter how preeminent the hospital, care varies widely. What was particularly interesting is that we found that quality is inversely correlated with the intensity of care. The better hospitals are using fewer resources and providing fewer hospitalizations and physician visits," says Wennberg (Sipkoff, 2004).

50 percent reduction in pneumonia costs

At Intermountain Health Care, the use of practice guidelines and protocols has reduced mortality rates, saved considerable amounts of money, shortened lengths of stay, and reduced medical complications.

Community-acquired pneumonia

Both inpatient and outpatient care

	1994 without guideline	1995 with guideline
Percent patients admitted	39%	29%
Average length of stay	6.4 days	4.3 days
Time to antibiotic	2.1 hours	1.5 hours
Average cost per case	$2,752	$1,424

Inpatient care only

	Without protocol	With protocol	Percent change	P
"Outlier" (complication) DRG at discharge	15.3%	11.6%	Down 24.7	<0.001
In-hospital mortality	7.2%	5.3%	Down 26.3	0.015
Relative resource units (RRUs) per case	55.9	49.0	Down 12.3	<0.001
Cost per case	$5,211	$4,729	Down 9.3	0.002

SOURCE: INTERMOUNTAIN HEALTH CARE

Table 2. Reductions in treatment costs, lengths of stay, medical complications, and mortality rates for persons with pneumonia at Intermountain Health Care.

Concluding Remarks

This chapter attempts to provide the big picture of healthcare in the United States. The system widely is viewed as in crisis and yet few understand the major dimensions of this crisis. This chapter attempts to discuss some of the historical trends, current status, and current controversies so that the reader can both place individual problems in a larger context as well as understand all of the major problems. Solutions to these problems are a priority and we hope that healthcare providers rather than politicians and lawyers participate more fully and knowledge-ably in the debates concerning how to improve the system.

References

American Medical Association. (1989). *The impaired physician: A special report.* Chicago, IL: Author.

American Medical Association Center for Health Policy Research. (1989). The administrative burden of health insurance on physicians. *SMS Report, 3*(2).

Anderson, G., & Knickman, J. R. (1984). Patterns of expenditures among high utilizers of medical care services. *Medical Care, 22,* 143-149.

Ash, A., Zhao, Y., Ellis, R. P., & Kramer, M. S. (2001). Finding future high-cost cases: comparing prior cost versus diagnosis-based methods. *Health Services Research, 36,* 194-206.

Berk, M. L., & Monheit, A. C. (2001). The concentration of health care expenditures, revisited. *Health Affairs, 20,* 9-18.

CBS News. (2000, July). *U.S. spending on mental illness drops.* Retrieved March 7, 2005, at http://www.cbsnews.com/stories/2000/07/18/national/main216465.shtml

Centers for Medicare and Medicaid Services (CMS). (2004c). Private health insurance. In *An overview of the U.S. healthcare system: Two decades of change, 1980-2000. The CMS chart series.* Retrieved January 24, 2005, at http://www.cms.hhs.gov/charts-/healthcaresystem/all.asp.

Centers for Medicare and Medicaid Services (CMS). (2004b). Public Programs: Medicare, Medicaid, SCHIP. In *An overview of the U.S. healthcare system: Two decades of change, 1980-2000. The CMS chart series.* Retrieved January 24, 2005, at http://www.cms.hhs.gov/charts-/healthcaresystem/all.asp.

Centers for Medicare and Medicaid Services (CMS). (2004d). Uninsured. In *An overview of the U.S. healthcare system: Two decades of change, 1980-2000. The CMS chart series.* Retrieved January 24, 2005, at http://www.cms.hhs.gov/charts-/healthcaresystem/all.asp.

Centers for Medicare and Medicaid Services (CMS). (2004a). U.S. healthcare system. In *An overview of the U.S. healthcare system: Two decades of change, 1980-2000. The CMS chart series.* Retrieved January 24, 2005, at http://www.cms.hhs.gov/charts-/healthcaresystem/all.asp.

Cummings, N. A. (1997). Behavioral health in primary care: dollars and sense. In N. A. Cummings, J. L. Cummings, & J. N. Johnson (Eds.), *Behavioral health in primary care: A guide for clinical integration* (pp. 3-31). Connecticut: Psychosocial Press.

Cummings N. A., Cummings, J. L., & Johnson, J. N. (Eds.). (1997). *Behavioral health in primary care: A guide for clinical integration.* Madison, CT: Psychosocial Press.

Cummings, N. A., O'Donohue, W. T., & Ferguson, K. E. (2003). *The impact of medical cost offset on practice and research: Making it work for you.* Reno, NV: Context Press.

Frank, R. G., Goldman H.H., & McGuire, T. G. (2001). Will parity in coverage result in better mental health care? *New England Journal of Medicine, 345*(23), 1701-1704.

Garis, R. I., & Farmer, K. C. (2002). Examining costs of chronic conditions in a Medicaid population. *Managed Care, 11*(8), 43-50.

Gilmore, G. J. (2005, January). DoD healthcare spending doubled in the past four years. *Military Money*. Retrieved March 6, 2005, at http://www.militarymoney.com/news/339.

Hayes, S. C., Barlow, D. H., & Nelson-Gray, R. O. (1999). *The scientist practitioner: Research and accountability in the age of managed care* (2nd ed.). Needham Heights, MA: Allyn and Bacon.

Henderson, J. W. (2005). *Health economics and policy* (3rd ed). Mason, OH: South-Western (Thompson Corporation).

Hennessey, K. D., & Barry, C. L. (n.d.). *Parity in the federal employees health benefits program: An overview*. Substance Abuse and Mental Health Administration. Retrieved March 6, 2005, at http://www.mentalhealth.samhsa.gov/publications/allpubs/SMA04-3938/Chapter14.asp

Institute of Medicine. (2001). *Crossing the quality chasm: A new health system for the 21st century*. Washington, DC: National Academy of Sciences.

Institute of Medicine. (2003b). *Key capabilities of an electronic health record system*. Washington DC: National Academy of Sciences.

Institute of Medicine. (2003a). *Priority areas for national action: Transforming health care quality*. Washington DC: National Academy of Sciences.

Insurance Finder. (2005). *About indemnity health insurance*. Retrieved February 20, 2005, at http://www.insurancefinder.com/healthinsurance/indemnity.html.

1st Insured Everything Insurance. (1999). *Medicare supplemental health insurance*. Retrieved March 5, 2005, at http://www.1stinsured.com/medicare_supplemental_insurance.htm.

Jordan, J. (2004). An early view of the impact of deregulation and managed care on hospital profitability and net worth. *The Journal of Healthcare Management, 46*(3), 161-171.

Katon, W. J. (1986). Panic disorder: epidemiology, diagnosis, and treatment in primary care. *The Journal of Clinical Psychiatry, 47*(suppl 21-30), 21-30.

Levit, K., Smith, C., Cowan, C., Sensing, A., & Catlin, A. (2004). A health spending rebound continues in 2002. *Health Affairs, 23*(1), 147-159.

Liptzin, B., Regier, D. A., & Goldberg, I. D. (1980). Utilization of health and mental health services in a large insured population. *American Journal of Psychiatry, 137*, 553-558.

Lynk, W. J., & Longley, C. S. (2002). The effect of physician-owned surgicenters on hospital outpatient surgery. *Health Affairs, 21*(4), 215-221.

Mark, T. L., Coffey, R. M., King, E., Harwood, H., McKusick, D., Genuardi, J., et al. (2000). Spending on mental health and substance abuse treatment, 1987-1997. *Health Affairs, 19*(4), 108-120.

Minnesota Office of the Legislative Auditor. (1995). *Health care administrative costs*. Executive Summary (95-02). Retrieved March 16, 2005, at http://www.auditor.leg.state.mn.us/ped/1995/hlthexec.htm.

O'Donohue, W. T., & Cucciare, M. A. (2005). The role of psychological factors in medical presentations. *Journal of Clinical Psychology in Medical Settings, 12*(1), 13-24.

O'Donohue, W., Cummings, N., & Laygo, R. (2004, July). *Results from the Hawaii Integrated Healthcare Demonstration Project.* Symposium presented at the Annual Meeting of the American Psychological Association (APA), Honolulu, HW: July 28 – August 1st.

Phelps, C. E. (1997). *Health economics* (2nd ed.). Reading, MA: Addison Wesley Longman, Inc.

Physicians Insurers of America. (2003, July). *The Weiss Ratings Report on medical malpractice caps: Propagating the myth that non-economic damage caps don't work.* Rockville: MD. Retrieved March 16, 2005, at http://www.thepiaa.org/text_files/WEISS070903.htm

Schilling, A. G. (2004, December 27). Open bar for health costs. *Forbes,* 192.

Sipkoff, M. (2004, December). A better case for quality: Share the savings! *Managed Care Magazine.* Retrieved March 16, 2005, at http://www.managedcaremag.com/archives/0412/0412.james.html.

Sowell, T. (2004). *Basic economics: A citizen's guide to the economy.* New York: Basic Books (Perseus Books Group).

Stossel, J. (2004). *Give me a break.* New York: Harper Collins.

U.S. Census Bureau. (2004). *Three-year-average median household income by state: 2001-2003.* Retrieved March 11, 2004, at http://www.census.gov/hhes/income/income03/statemhi.html.

Woolhandler, S., Campbell, T., & Himmelstein, D. U. (2003). Costs of health care administration in the United States and Canada. *New England Journal of Medicine, 349*(8), 768-775.

Wurman, R.S. (2004). *Understanding healthcare.* Newport, RI: TOP

Chapter 2

Resolving the Dilemmas in Mental Healthcare Delivery: Access, Stigma, Fragmentation, Conflicting Research, Politics and More

Nicholas A. Cummings
University of Nevada, Reno and
The Cummings Foundation for Behavioral Health, Inc.

If all economists were laid end to end, they still wouldn't reach a conclusion.
George Bernard Shaw

As we are reminded of George Bernard Shaw's statement over a century ago, this can be said doubly for healthcare economists. And if healthcare has bedeviled economists for decades, mental health is so baffling that economists try to avoid it entirely. Seldom is mental health mentioned in texts addressing healthcare in general, and even the Institute of Medicine (2001) in its landmark report, *Crossing the Quality Chasm: A New Health System for the 21st Century*, totally sidestepped the subject. The absence of mental health would suggest that either mental health is not important, or the IOM had left a gaping hole in their otherwise comprehensive study of our health system. This chapter will address a number of policies and events that have either promoted or inhibited the effective delivery of mental healthcare services, will also discuss the difficulty of interpreting and applying mental health data, and finally will touch on the political and economic debate that surrounds the financing of healthcare, and particularly mental healthcare.

The author's style in this chapter is somewhat reminiscent of the story of the two rams standing on the edge of a cliff and looking down at a flock of ewes grazing in the valley below. The younger ram suggested they run down and get a couple. The older and much wiser ram interjected that they should walk down and get them all. This author claims no particular wisdom, but rather would walk us through the too many issues confronting the mental healthcare delivery system in which he has been an activist participant for well over half a century. Since in mental healthcare delivery there are no straight lines from here to there, I apologize in advance for meandering, and also for proffering no easy solutions. Henry L. Menken is reputed to have said, and this author agrees, "For every complex issue there is a simple solution that is wrong" (Kennedy, 2004).

The Importance of Presidential Mental Health Commissions

As of this writing, President Bush's New Freedom Commission on Mental Health has rendered its final report (Hogan, 2003), stating that mental and emotional conditions are more prevalent than previously believed, and stressing the importance of access and even national screening to facilitate early detection and treatment. Many Americans believe that presidential mental health commissions are routine, like the ubiquitous energy commissions appointed by every president since Franklin D. Roosevelt. There have been only three presidential mental health commissions in our nation's history, and all in the last half century, and although it is too early to tell the outcome of President Bush's Commission, the first two resulted in great gains in the delivery of mental health services. The first such by President Kennedy (1961-1963) was not officially a commission, but a Task Force he brought together to design what later became our community mental health centers. Because of my early work in prepaid healthcare at Kaiser Permanente, I was invited and privileged to participate. Assassinated before he could see his innovative ideas come to fruition, the Community Mental Health Centers Act was eventually signed by his successor, President Johnson. This gave a tremendous boost to behavioral care, spreading these services across the land as it put psychologists and social workers in rural areas in significant numbers for the first time.

The second presidential mental health commission, and the first one bearing that title, was appointed by President Carter (1977-1980). Without giving herself the title of chair, the First Lady enthusiastically led this commission, participated in its meetings, and energized its members. She insisted that all facets of mental healthcare had to be addressed, and divided the members into a series of panels. Again I was privileged to serve, this time on the panel grappling with cost and financing of mental health care. Mrs. Carter took particular interest in our group, stating that unless the problems of cost and financing were resolved, not much else would happen. We rendered our commission report just two months before President Carter lost his reelection, abruptly ending the influence of this commission. But our work did result in the Mental Health Act of 1980, which mandated a minimum of 20 psychotherapy sessions in health maintenance organizations, and made psychotherapy and counseling integral parts of all health insurance.

The fact there have been only three presidential commissions does not necessarily suggest that mental health is a low priority in our nation, although at times it would seem so. Healthcare is considered a top priority in Washington, but other than the ill-fated Rodham Clinton Health Care Task Force (1993-1994), there has never been a presidential healthcare commission. This is because healthcare is mired in politics, and addressing it is regarded as political suicide. The demise of Mrs. Clinton's efforts has only underscored that belief, and presidents have restricted their efforts to high-sounding campaign speeches and state of the union addresses, all falling far short of implementation. Nonetheless, there has emerged significant healthcare legislation, such as the Hill Burton hospital construction act of the late 1950s, Medicare and Medicaid in 1965, the HMO enabling act of 1975, and recently President Bush's bipartisan drug benefit for seniors.

Several Stupid Stories: Lessons to be Learned

The railroad industry was America's 19th century success story, only to become a 20th century failure. Within an amazingly short time its steel rails had spanned the nation, and seemingly shrunk the continent as it made travel and shipment of goods rapid and affordable for the first time. By the middle of the 20th century, however, the once prosperous railroads began a precipitous decline into bankruptcy and had to be rescued by the federal government. Along had come air travel, air cargo, and trucking, all affordable and far more rapid than the cumbersome railroads. The railroads had made an irreversible mistake; believing they were in the "railroad business" rather than in the "transportation business," they missed the opportunity to own and operate the transportation systems that superceded them. Scrambling to survive, they finally began looking at technologies available to them, and later in the 20th century they developed container cargo and piggy-back shipping (loading and unloading large containers directly on ships or trucks, respectively), but it was too late. They lost their primacy forever. But through these technologies the railroads have learned how to survive. Fifty years ago two million Americans worked for the railroads. Thanks to new freight technology, the railroads now ship twice as much cargo and with only 150,000 employees.

Another 19th century miracle was the telegraph that had made instant communication to all parts of the nation possible for the first time. Rivaling the railroad companies for stupidity, the telegraph companies decided they were in the telegraph business, when in reality they were in the communication business. Seeing that the telegraph wires already spanning the continent could be easily modified to accommodate the telephone, Alexander Graham Bell attempted to sell his invention to the telegraph companies. The response was an emphatic rejection, and in essence saying it was in the telegraph business, and saw no future in the telephone. Where once they could have owned the telephone, Western Union is now an archaic little company through which one can wire money to a distant recipient.

Our stupid stories continue into the 20th century. The giant IBM did not comprehend that it was in the information business, not the mainframe business. This decision resulted in the myopic declaration that Americans would never want an electronic machine in their homes. Along came Steve Jobs and Michael Dell, the personal computer was soon an affordable reality, and the information age was in full swing as the PC became almost as common in every home as a television set. Down plunged IBM's stock. Similarly, Xerox pioneered efficient dry copiers and was inordinately successful for decades as it essentially had the copier market to itself. Not realizing it, too, was in the information business and not just the copier business, other companies like Ricoh, Sharp, and Kyocera transformed the simple copier into a computer, a scanner, a fax, and a host of other functions that reflected they knew they were in the information business. Xerox adapted too late and is now lagging in the industry.

Sadly, we in mental health are replicating this lack of foresight and understanding by insisting that we are in the mental health business, when in reality, we are a part of the healthcare industry. Primary care physicians (PCPs) know that the mind and the body are not separate entities, and they are providing 80% of the mental health services right in the primary care setting, including psychological advice, counseling and the dispensing of antidepressants and other psychotropic medications (Cummings, O'Donohue, Hayes, & Follette, 2001). Sadly compounding this stupidity, psychologists and social workers see themselves narrowly as the psychotherapy and counseling business, while psychiatrists regard themselves to be the mental health medication and hospitalization business.

Parity Legislation: Separate and Unequal

One of the nation's most successful legislative efforts has been the drive for parity. Mandating equal expenditures with physical health for mental health, parity laws have been enacted in 34 states and the federal government, a remarkable achievement were it not for the fact that less money is being spent on mental health today than before there were parity laws (Carnahan, 2002). The managed care companies and the health insurance industry, fearing runaway costs for mental health, put in place more draconian requirements to qualify for mental healthcare than for physical care. Yet the political battle to renew the federal parity law and to enact such laws in the remaining 16 states that do not have them continues with vigor. In the end it merely makes mental health advocates appear to be successful and to justify contributions from rank-and-file practitioners who are frightened by their dwindling practices.

Unfortunately, the drive for parity merely perpetuates the separation of mental health from physical health. Separate but equal did not work in education before the civil rights movement inasmuch as white schools were more "equal" than black schools. The idea that mental health is entitled to one-half of the nation's $1.4 trillion budget, especially when the physical healthcare system is providing 80% of the mental healthcare, rounds out our list of stupid stories. It will be only after mental health is an integral part of healthcare and is funded as part of healthcare that it will be appropriately funded.

Access and Stigma May Largely Be Self-Created Artifacts

As long as we maintain two separate silos, one labeled healthcare and the other mental healthcare, we are inadvertently restricting access. As stated, 80% of mental health is dispensed by PCPs, while only 10% of those referred to the separate mental health system ever cross the chasm of stigma, resistance and access by actually seeing a behavioral health specialist. PCPs are in the trenches with the patient, and behavioral care providers (BCPs) should be there in the primary care setting with them. Research in systems where BCPs are co-located with PCPs reveals that 85% to 90% of patients identified as needing psychological services will accept that help because the PCP can merely walk the patient the short distance down the hall to the office of the immediately available BCP (Strosahl, 2001). Called the "hallway handoff" in settings where primary and behavioral health services are integrated, the patient is receiving mental health services where she or he expects to receive them:

in the healthcare system, not a separate system in another location called "mental health," that has all sorts of resistances and stigmas attached to it.

The experience at Walter Reed Army Medical Center, one of our nation's healthcare showcases where presidents have received care, is illuminating. According to one report (James, 2004), the earlier problems until recently replicated those investigated and later corrected at Tripler Army Medical Center. In 1997 the following deficiencies were extant at Tripler: (1) psychiatry and psychology were away from the mainstream of the hospital, resulting (2) in a 50% to 60% no show rate attributed (3) to a stigma associated with going to the mental health part of the building. (4) Consultations were frequently lost or misplaced and (5) mental health staff members were not showing up for their assigned duty to see walk-in emergencies. (6) Psychiatrists were simply inefficient and ineffective managers, and (7) it took anywhere from three to eight weeks for a patient to be seen for medication evaluation. A plan was implemented that placed the mental health outpatient clinic in the middle of the family practice department (i.e., primary care setting) and the seven deficiencies were largely overcome. In 2003 the same plan became an initiative at the Walter Reed Army Medical Center where most, if not all of the seven deficiencies found at Tripler were manifest (James, 2004). The lesson to be learned, and as one researcher put it, even across the street is too far away.

Since the problems of access and stigma seem to essentially evaporate in the integrated behavioral health/primary care setting, the following finding should not be surprising. In American Psychological Association (APA) conducted focused groups, stigma was seen as a distant second in a list of impediments to seeking psychotherapy. Rather, the participants identified "it doesn't work" as by far the number one reason they would not undergo psychotherapy (Saunders, 2003). These embarrassing results were not widely disseminated; rather the APA later authorized a more structured, limited item poll, leaving out the choice that psychotherapy may not be effective as a reason for not seeking it. Responding to the available choices in this national poll, cost and lack of insurance coverage were the main barriers, while stigma continued to be less important in seeking treatment (Association for the Advancement of Psychology, 2004). Confirming the APA findings, the National Association of Addiction Treatment Providers (NAATP) found that 41.2% of those not seeking addiction treatment in 2003 stated they were not ready to give up their using, 32.2% pointed to cost or insurance barrier, while only 17.2% feared a stigma (NAATP, 2004).

As long as separate systems of health and mental health exist, stigma will continue to be a ready excuse for low utilization of mental health services. In a recent review (Corrigan, 2004), stigma is well conceptualized and its effects on the individual are convincingly presented. Less convincing is the argument presented that stigma is the primary reason why persons needing services do not seek them, or persons receiving services fail to adhere to the psychiatric regimen. Even President Bush's New Freedom Commission advocates anti-stigma programs as a way of improving the mental health system (Hogan, 2003). Whether, as some findings suggest, stigma is less significant than practitioners believe, or whether this stigma disappears when a patient feels a part of the *health* as opposed to the mental health system, making behavioral care an integral part of primary care would be an effective way of addressing these barriers.

Encouraging is that many authorities within the APA, which usually lags behind in delivery innovation, see the future role of the psychologist heavily in primary care and working closely with primary care physicians (Kerstine, 2004). Importantly the 2005 APA president has made the integration of psychology in primary care a major thrust of his administration (Levant, 2004).

The Evolution of Technology and Personnel in Mental Health

Mental healthcare seems painfully static at times, yet a historical perspective reveals a series of relatively frequent and often massive changes so that various periods within the past century are hardly recognizable today. In retrospect, some of these changes even constitute upheavals that resulted in the disaffection of large cadres of practitioners and their ideologies. A chronology of the more significant waves is summarized in Table 1, with dates given representing modal approximations of events that developed not discretely, but over a number of years.

Descriptive Psychiatry

In the 19th Century and immediately thereafter psychiatry was essentially descriptive, addressing mostly the severely mentally ill for whom mandated institutionalization and physical restraint were the primary treatments. It also saw discoveries, such as hypnosis, and it was absorbed by a number of oddities with which it tantalized its few adherents, such as multiple personalities, astasia abasia, sleep walking, and automatic writing, to name only a few. Psychology was in its earliest phase, establishing primitive laboratories, and conducting basic experiments on illusions, psychological aspects of the five senses, and the beginnings of learning theory. While the American Psychiatric Association (APA) was founded in 1850, the American Psychological Association did not come into being until 1892. Through its first president, G. Stanley Hall, psychology began a scientific look at education, while an initial interest in philosophy and religion was defined by its third president, William James, also known as the Father of American Psychology. Soon this interest in education and spirituality were superceded by the German psychophysicists, and the laboratory that sought to emulate the physical sciences characterized the majority of psychology for decades. Psychotherapy as we know it today simply did not exist.

Freudian Preeminence

Psychotherapy as we know it today is an outgrowth of the Freudian tradition, which after establishing a foothold in Europe, began to spread to the United States following the increased travel and communication that characterized the post World War I era. This interest spiked incredibly following World War II, and the degree to which Americans espoused psychoanalysis was reflected in movies, literature, music and the news media, as well as by a seemingly insatiable demand

	Personnel:	Technology:
1850-1920	Psychiatrists	Descriptive psychiatry
1920-1980	Psychoanalysts (MD and lay)	Psychoanalytic methodologies
1948-1950	Post WW II training stipends	V.A. and the new NIMH
1950	Psychologists	Migration to private practice
1965	All personnel	Community MH Centers Act
1975	Psychiatrists	Remedicalization begins
1960	Psychologists/social workers	Family therapy movement begins
1965	Psychiatry	Medicare enacted; psychiatrist only
1970	All personnel	Insurance coverage gains momentum
1975	Social workers	Migration to private practice
1978	Psychologists	Licensed in all 50 states
1979	Psychiatric nurse practitioners	Rapid emergence with Rx authority
1980	All personnel	Mental Health Act of 1981 (Carter)
1980	Psychologists/social workers	Brief therapy movement begins
1980	Psychologists	Cognitive revolution begins
1985	All practitioners	Managed behavioral healthcare begins
1990	Psychoanalytic therapists	Psychoanalysis begins rapid decline
1990	Psychologists/social workers	Family therapy loses prominence
1990	M.A.-level counselors	Migration to private practice
1995	Psychologists/social workers	Cognitive revolution is complete
1995	Psychologists	Included in Medicare
2000	All practitioners	Managed behavioral care 175 M lives
2000	Psychiatrists	Biomedical revolution is complete
2000	Psychoanalytic therapists	Psychoanalysis loses prominence
2003	All personnel	Bush MH Commission report complete
2003	All personnel	Momentum for primary/behavioral care
2004	Psychologists	Prescription authority in NM and LA

Table 1. Practitioners and Their Technologies. The significant waves in mental health beginning with the 19th Century through the early 21st Century, with approximate dates, Personnel and technologies that characterized each successive period.

for services. Psychoanalytic institutes proliferated, but Freudian therapy was not limited to those who traversed the long, arduous years of psychoanalytic training because the preponderance of psychiatrists, psychologists and social workers were conducting psychoanalytically oriented psychotherapy without such training. There were offshoots, with leaders such as Carl Jung, Alfred Adler, Melanie Klein and a number of others, and as time went on with the Neo-Freudians (e.g., Harry Stack Sullivan, Frieda Fromm Reichman) psychoanalysis became more interpersonal and ego oriented. Nonetheless, all of these offshoots were rooted in the principle of unconscious determinism, with the personality shaped by experiences in infancy and early childhood.

Psychoanalytic thought dominated treatment for most of a half century, and its rapid ascendancy was rivaled only by the swiftness of its demise. Criticized for its lack of a scientific foundation, and plagued by the interminable nature of psychoanalytic therapies, the death knell came when managed behavioral care organizations stopped paying for psychoanalytic treatment. Psychoanalytic institutes shrunk and even disappeared, and even the famed psychoanalytically-oriented Menninger Clinic closed its doors in the late 1990s. By the dawning of the 21st Century psychoanalysis was not only in decline, but also in disrepute.

The Cognitive Revolution

The beginning of the 21st Century marks the era of the cognitive revolution, with cognitive behavioral interventions supplanting psychoanalysis. Behaviorism, which rejects the Freudian concept of unconscious determinism, has always been congenial to the academic setting, so it has been around for at least 75 years. The original radical behaviorism, which even rejects cognition, dominated the early clinical psychology training programs, but it produced mostly academicians, with an almost indiscernible number of clinicians practicing outside university and government settings. The rising tide of cognitive behaviorism had overwhelmed radical behaviorism by the mid-1980s and is producing most of the currently minted psychological practitioners. It received unexpected impetus in the new thrust for scientifically validated therapies inasmuch as it is much more amenable to quantification than were the older interpersonal and psychoanalytic therapies, and it has the advantage of being university based where most of the psychology training is taking place. In its zeal to over-throw interpersonal therapies, however, it threw out the baby with the bathwater, resulting in a sterile and often inflexible treatment approach that neglects individual differences in its one-size-fits-all templates. For example, cognitive behavioral interventions for depression will receive a differing response depending on whether the depressed patient is an alcoholic, a borderline personality, bereaving, or simply a neurotic. Additionally, cognitive behavior therapy (CBT) has been less able to address the many negative behaviors and therapeutic resistance of Axis II patients.

A Possible Rapprochement May be Emerging

Thomas Kuhn (1996) has documented that scientists seldom if ever embrace new theories, and retire still believing in what was au current in their hey day. Mental health practitioners more than replicate this pattern, perpetuating psycho-religions, often fiercely. Psychotherapy progresses as the high priests of the psycho-religions die or retire. Presently, however, there may be occurring a surprising melding of CBT and interpersonal psychotherapies. It all began as innovators in behaviorism began dressing up interpersonal interventions in behavioral and cognitive nomenclature and injecting them into CBT and even into radical behaviorism. Such thrusts as Acceptance and Commitment Therapy are slipping through the back door effective interventions that have been extant in psychoanalysis for decades, and were taken to new effectiveness by gestalt, Ericksonian, systems, solution-focused, and other brief therapies, and they are being heralded as brilliant innovations by the historically-challenged behaviorists.

Beginning in the early 2000s this rapprochement has become more open, with articles boldly championing the utility of combining analytic and behavioral therapies (Callaghan, Gregg, Marx, Kohlenberg, & Gifford 2004). And if wonders will never cease, the usually behaviorist-derided "chairwork" (i.e., the gestalt intervention of having the patient talk to an empty chair) has suddenly been discovered to be a form of cognitive restructuring (Kellogg, 2004). If as may be happening, two psycho-religions actually merge and evolve to a greater effectiveness, it will be the first time in the history of psychotherapy.

The Biomedical Revolution

Overlapping the cognitive revolution, and ascending to equal if not even greater importance, is the biomedical revolution which substitutes medication for counseling. In the 1970s the psychiatric profession began what it called its "remedicalization," a gradual process of abandoning psychotherapy in favor of medication. In the ensuing years psychiatric residencies deemphasized and even discontinued psychotherapy training, while psychology became the preeminent psychotherapy profession, with social workers doing most of the actual therapy.

Several factors gave impetus to the biomedical revolution, principle among them being the discovery of more effective antidepressants and other psychotropic medications. HMOs and other managed behavioral care organizations saw these newer medical treatments to be cheaper and more manageable than behavioral interventions. The pharmacology industry began direct advertising to consumers, and patients, having seen the promotions on television, began requesting and even demanding medications. Soon depression became the common cold of psychiatry, with patients demanding antidepressants for normal mood fluctuations just as decades ago patients began demanding antibiotics for the common cold. The medical profession and the psychiatric profession in particular, encouraged this by redefining most, if not all behavioral difficulties to be of genetic or biological origin. Primary care physicians, having been unsuccessful in getting patients to accept psychological referrals, took advantage of the new medications and began prescribing them in lieu of arguing with reluctant patients who might otherwise benefit from psychotherapy (Cummings, 2005b). A startling example in the decline of referrals for psychotherapy is demonstrated in the current paucity of post-psychiatric hospitalization referrals. In 1990 almost 95% of discharged patients were referred for outpatient psychotherapy, but by 2000 the figure had declined to only 10% (Carnahan, 2002).

The National Institutes of Mental Health (NIMH) are rapidly moving toward biomedicine, with increasingly more funds allocated for biomedical than behavioral research. The largest mental health pressure group, the National Association for the Mentally Ill (NAMI), representing mostly relieved family members of mentally ill patients who are better managed on the new medications, strongly support the expansion of biomedicine in mental health.

EBTs and the End of Name-Dropping

The beginning of the 21st Century is characterized by the movement toward evidence-based treatments (EBTs), creating a schism between academic/science-based psychologists and those in full-time practice who insist clinical experience is as important as research evidence. The lines are being drawn, and although the battle will continue for some time, the psychological "name-dropping" that has been used as authority has rapidly faded. It was typical during the entire 20th Century to quote a psychotherapist of stature (e.g., Freud, Jung, Erickson, Perls) as evidence, rather than to cite research. That practice is losing credibility rapidly, and with it is fading authoritative leadership, defined as psychotherapy movements centered about individuals, or what this author has termed "psycho-religions."

Economic Factors

Although the transitions described above occurred over time, they eventuated in upheavals that saw the disappearance of descriptive psychiatry, then the fading of psychoanalysis as it gave way to the cognitive revolution, and finally the displacement of much cognitive therapy by the biomedical revolution. All of these resulted in severe economic hardship to the technologies that were successively disaffected, especially since each revolution looks back disdainfully on its immediate predecessor. At the present time there are two major competing technologies, cognitive behaviorism and biomedicine (i.e., dispensing psychotropic medications), each so critical of the other that they appear to be ideologies, or even "psycho-religions." A minority of cooler heads is paying attention to the research that points to one or the other as more effective with certain conditions, while still other conditions are best treated by a combination of behavioral counseling and medication (Antonuccio, Danton, & DeNelsky, 1999).

It is the position of this chapter that the patient is best served by the co-existence of cognitive behavioral interventions and psychotropic drugs. Two things need to happen. First, cognitive therapy must continue its modification to incorporate useful technologies (e.g., the defense mechanisms, techniques for overcoming resistance, basic pathology) that were thrown out in haste in the cognitive revolution. In turn, biomedicine must recognize its limitations that it now attempts to overcome by adding more and more medications (called a med cocktail) when previous medications do not work. It must also cease its scorn of "talk therapy" and accept that many conditions are not medical, but behavioral. Both have to recognize that the mind and the body are not separate, and behavioral/primary care is the wave of the future.

While the battle continues, third party payers are discovering that the new psychotropic medications are expensive and in perpetuity, while counseling can often achieve therapeutic goals with less total expenditure and in a fraction of the time. When psychotropic medications do not work, psychiatrists are prone to keep adding more medications, calling this a therapeutic cocktail for which chemical restraint, not therapy, is more often the end result. Interestingly, in spite of a growing backlash, psychologists have accelerated their effort to attain prescription authority, and by 2004 had succeeded in two states, New Mexico and Louisiana. This early success will undoubtedly gain momentum, and it remains to be seen whether future psychologists will retain their identity as behavioral therapists, or succumb to the expediency of the prescription pad.

The Brief Psychotherapy Movement and the Role of Third Party Reimbursement

Superimposed upon all the foregoing treatment waves, and beginning post World War II, has been the brief psychotherapy movement that was forced upon an uncongenial mental health establishment by economic realities. A firestorm erupted when Alexander and French (1946) published their blueprint for brief psychoanalytically oriented psychotherapy, even though their definition of brief was in excess of 150 sessions. Extensive research at Kaiser Permanente, the nation's first HMO, revealed that most patients received maximum benefit from brief psychotherapy, and less than 20% of patients required long term psychotherapy (Cummings & Follette, 1968; Cummings & VandenBos, 1981; Follette & Cummings, 1967). Following the Mental Health Act of 1980 when coverage for psychotherapy became an integral part of health insurance, most third party payers began imposing session limits, with 52 sessions (one year at once a week) being the most frequent benefit. As research demonstrated that with brief therapy most patients improved sufficiently within 18 sessions, and that without sessions limits a phenomenon known as "therapeutic drift" emerged (Lambert, 1992), 20 sessions became the modal benefit. In therapeutic drift patients who were not improving kept coming, while therapists allowed them to do so in the hope that something would happen, all in an atmosphere where a third party was paying the bill.

By the late 1980s brief psychotherapy had become the main form of outpatient psychotherapy (Budman & Gurman, 1988), so when managed behavioral care imposed even more stringent session limits, most psychotherapists were practicing a more or less form of brief psychotherapy. It was psychoanalysts and other long term psychotherapists who suddenly had the economic rug pulled out from under them, and had to rely on a dwindling number of affluent patients willing to pay out of pocket for unrestricted services. Although there was much research demonstrating the efficacy of short-term therapy, the practice of brief therapy followed its long-term predecessor into regarding clinical experience as paramount, resulting in a host of brief therapy psycho-religions. Family therapy (i.e., systems theory) erupted at the Ackerman Institute (New York) and the Mental Research Institute (Palo Alto), became part of the brief therapy movement, and swept across the country from each coast, only to eclipse by the 1990s. Parallel to it were the other movements such as those of Milton Erickson and the Gestalt Therapy of Frederick (Fritz) Perls whose techniques have permeated brief therapy even though their psycho-religions have lost pre-eminence.

The Futile Economics of Parity

The drive for parity, defined as equal healthcare benefits for both mental and physical illness, has been one of the most successful legislative campaigns in history of healthcare advocacy. By 2003 parity laws had been enacted in 34 states and the federal government, a dazzling political achievement rendered inert by economic factors. There is less money being spent on mental health after these parity laws than before their enactment. The third party payers, fearing a spiking of mental health costs, put in place more draconian hurdles to qualify for receiving behavioral care than physical care. Furthermore, prescribing psychotropic medication can be construed as mental healthcare when no behavioral interventions have been rendered. The end result is that these legislative campaigns give lobbyists a deceptive success to justify the financial contributions made by their constituents, while these same constituents, not realizing the end result is a negative, can believe progress is being made to bolster their sagging practices.

From an economic standpoint, it is folly to believe that any statute could force the allocation of half of the $1.4 trillion annual health budget from physical to mental health, especially since 80% of mental health is being delivered by non-psychiatric physicians and mostly in the primary care setting.

Who Is a Mental Health Practitioner? Everyone

The seemingly insatiable demand for psychotherapy that followed the post World War II era was squeezed by the relatively small number of psychiatrists in practice at the time. Most were elderly with European accents, and they practiced long term psychoanalysis that itself limited the availability of practitioners. Confronted by this reality, and believing that there would never be enough psychiatrists, the federal government undertook the large scale funding of training not only for psychiatrists, but also psychologists and social workers, and later even paraprofessionals. Psychologists and social workers had proven their effectiveness in the military, and the NIMH and the Veterans Administration (VA) hoped their newly minted non-medical psychotherapists would staff the under-served public institutions. It is a little remembered fact that the federal government befuddled for all time the definition of a psychotherapist, embracing and funding all disciplines and non-disciplines, as well as paraprofessionals who in time inevitably demanded recognition as professionals.

Chafing under the psychiatric domination of the public institutions, the newly trained psychologists were the first to enter the domain of independent practice. There was no licensure or public recognition of psychology, but the young psychologists solved these problems by affiliating with established psychiatrists who, unable to keep up with the demand for their services, were happy to have their help. In addition, they provided the valuable service of administering batteries of psychological tests, at that time deemed imperative before undertaking psycho-therapy. Organized psychiatry formally opposed state licensure of psychologists, but because of widespread public acceptance of psychologists, all fifty states had statutory recognition (licensure or certification) by 1979.

Social workers were next to mount their campaign for statutory recognition, but as of 2004 they have yet to attain this in all fifty states. Concurrently, master's level counselors, marriage and family therapists (MFTs), addiction counselors, and others have attained success in more or less states, with psychiatric nurse practitioners having joined psychiatry and psychology as a ubiquitous mental health profession. As might have been predicted, psychologists sought to prevent licensing of social workers and all the others that came after them, as social work, too, has with those that came after them. To complicate matters more, in states that have not enacted master's-level counselor licensure, one can practice as a "counselor' as long as the titles that have statutory recognition (i.e., psychiatrist, psychologist and social worker) are not used. The public has sought to address this confusion by adopting the all-encompassing term "therapist." So now, who is a therapist? Almost everyone is, or 650,000 individuals who have some kind of state statutory recognition, and by adding the unlicensed or uncertified, the total number might easily exceed one million, perhaps three or more times the number needed.

A perusal of rosters of practitioners licensed to do psychotherapy or counseling reveals that the ranks of social workers, marriage-family therapists, counselors, psychiatric nurse practitioners, and other master's level licensees far outweigh the number of doctoral level psychologists licensed to practice, and who are essentially offering their services as psychotherapists. Similarly, the networks of managed behavioral care companies list a plethora of master's level psychotherapists. This overwhelming number of non-doctoral psychotherapists firmly establishes the reimbursement scale for psychotherapy on a pre-doctoral level. If doctoral psychologists are to compete, they must offer services that cannot be performed by their master's level counterparts, and they must reflect doctoral level skills not attained by counselors and social workers.

As long as these turf wars continue among a glut of practitioners, and with no culture to separate the wheat from the chaff, mental health will be hampered by an oversupply of competing disciplines, psycho-religions, and an unprecedented variability in competence, along with near quackery and actual quackery. Doubtlessly the NIMH and VA did not anticipate this state of affairs when this author entered the independent practice of psychotherapy in 1948 under government auspices.

Chicken Little, Our Healthcare Sky Is Falling

Listening to the constant stream of reports in the media, one would conclude that the American health system is rapidly becoming unraveled. We are told that we spend more money than anyone else in the world, and have less to show for it than other developed countries. In spite of this barrage, Americans tend to believe they have the best health system in the world, and survey after survey reveals that we like the healthcare we receive (Barlett & Steele, 2004ab). The press would have healthcare reform a top priority, but as late as only four weeks before the 2004 presidential elections, only 4% of those polled thought such reform was a top priority (ABC News/Washington Post, 2004). When foreign potentates, or when ordinary people with seemingly impossible medical conditions seek care, they come to the United States. How can we be the best and the worst health system at the same time?

Polarization of the Experts

Increasingly the health dialogue is becoming polarized between those who favor universal healthcare and those who would continue the current free-market system, and each side tends to interpret events and statistics in keeping with its predetermined position. Under the premise that people will not eat squid but will relish calamari, the code words for government medicine are "universal healthcare" and "one payer system," while those who would continue the present system refer to it as "freedom of choice" or the "free market." The first proponents see the current system as wasteful, inefficient, and plagued with fraud and duplication, while resulting in over 45 million Americans being left without health coverage. Their opponents see universal healthcare as synonymous with high taxes, rationing, big government, and bureaucratic interference with free choice of physician and treatment. The latter belief is bolstered not only by the experiences of nationalized healthcare throughout the world, but also by a provision in the ill-fated Rodham Clinton plan, the last serious universal healthcare proposal. This would have punished any physician operating outside the government system with a $10,000 fine and 6 months in prison, with corresponding sanctions against patients utilizing them, thus eliminating free choice of physician.

Only three things can be said with certainty: (1) healthcare information is processed and then interpreted according to ideology, not veracity; (2) the debate is contentious and the voices strident; and (3) anyone charting a middle ground, or seeing both truth and error in each point of view, will be damned by both sides. Such may be the fate of this chapter.

Mental Health Weighs In

Most psychiatrists and psychologists favor universal healthcare and are often eager to join in sounding the alarm that Americans are under-served, while most physicians oppose it. There is a growing barrage of articles purporting to show that Americans are increasingly under stress and nothing is being done about it, thus supporting universal care. A recent example was the front-page lengthy story headlined and syndicated to hundreds of newspapers just before Labor Day, pointing to an alleged stress explosion in the workplace, with scores of mental health practitioners chiming in and lending credence (Schwartz, 2004). This article had three themes: (1) employees today are driven to work longer hours, (2) so that stress levels are soaring, (3) resulting in higher levels of job-related sickness and accidents. Seligman (2004) challenged the report, replete with quotes from experts, showing that this new crisis is based on nothing more than junk statistics. According to the Bureau of Labor Statistics (see Figure 1), workdays lost because of anxiety, stress, or neurotic disorders has significantly and steadily declined since it peaked in 1993.

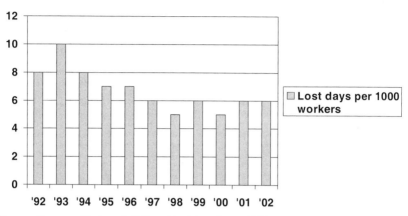

Source: Bureau of Labor statistics No data prior to 1992

Figure 1. Private sector workdays lost because of anxiety, stress, neurotic disorders.

More importantly, psychiatry and psychology are seeking to increase their revenue base by enlarging the pool of potential patients through expanding existing diagnoses to include more and more persons, and creating syndromes and disorders by grouping any collection of symptoms, so that treatment for these newly discovered conditions will be insurance reimbursable (Wright & Cummings, 2005). Perhaps the most startling example was seen when the American Psychiatric Association redefined attention deficit/hyperactivity disorder (ADD/ADHD) several years ago, and by doing so it literally quadrupled the number of potential patients who would qualify under that diagnosis (Cummings & Wiggins, 2001). Hopefully saner voices will prevail. In a rare and remarkably candid article, a past president of the APA who is also the current president of the APA's Division of Independent Practice, acknowledges psychology's dereliction in contributing to the costly system that was a "major catastrophe in the making" had not managed care come along. He calls for protecting the incomes of psychotherapists before they have to go out of business, but only by first supporting "efforts to protect and advance the public interest in a fair and equitable health care system (Fox, 2004, p. 158)."

Healthcare Research Is Difficult to Interpret

Medical and behavioral research performed under ideal conditions such as randomized clinical trials is indispensable, but it seldom translates as intended out of the laboratory and into the delivery system. Consider that it is only after the FDA has approved a drug for use that all of the limitations, including death and disfigurement, are discovered. The purity of the laboratory requires subjects (patients) with only the condition being examined, whereas in the real world there are few if any patients who do not have co-morbidities that require poly-pharmacy for which most possible interactions have never been investigated. Interpreting healthcare statistics is even more elusive, and more often results in inaccuracy.

The complexities of healthcare delivery are so vast that they lend themselves to inaccurate conclusions. There are seemingly myriads of examples, and only two will be presented here as illustrative of well-meaning, but erroneous conclusions. For two decades it was widely believed that the higher rate of breast cancer deaths among African American women were due to their seeking medical care much later in the development of such cancers than do white women. In 2004 it was discovered that African American women are more prone to carry a gene that prevents the production of the enzyme that blocks growth of breast cancer cells. Similarly, for over a decade it was believed that the relatively small number of heart catheterizations among African American men was due to the lack of adequate care accorded minorities. In 2004 it was discovered that the relevant death rate between white and African American male heart patients was the same, and that the higher rate of catheters accorded white males was due to defensive medicine, not adequate or necessary care.

In mental healthcare logicians and philosophers continue to be skeptical of the level of confidence that can be placed on experimental results obtained when measuring the efficacy of one treatment modality over another (Lakatos & Musgrave, 1978). As Meehl (1978, p. 822) stated, "Putting it crudely, if you have enough cases and your measures are not totally unreliable, the null hypothesis will always be falsified, regardless of the truth of the substantive theory." Dumont and Fitzpatrick add, "It is commonplace … that we normally research those problems that are most amenable to neat and easy solutions…. Thus, we attack the easiest problems first." They then quote this author, "…for every study that identifies a statistically significant benefit of treatment, there may be an equal number of studies that report a statistically significant benefit that is truly useless" (Dumont & Fitzpatrick, in press, p. 11).

The Negation of Supply and Demand by Mental Healthcare

This and several succeeding sections will additionally address economic issues, and the faint of heart may wish to skip them. However, in so doing, they will overlook the hot-button issues in healthcare and mental healthcare today. The first of these involves a look at the reasons why the economic laws of supply and demand do not operate, or only partially apply within healthcare.

The Provider Controls Both Supply and Demand

By determining both the treatment and its frequency, the provider determines both supply and demand. Physicians, being in control of the process, merely render more treatment, and particularly more costly procedures, to a declining number of available patients. In psychotherapy, a reduction in the number of referrals can be subverted by increasing the length of treatment (longer term psychotherapy) as well as its frequency (twice or three times a week instead of once a week). In other words, a dozen patients seen twice a week almost interminably are equivalent to scores of brief therapy referrals and will constitute a nearly fulltime private practice. Called "unconscious fiscal convenience" (Cummings, 2005ab), a skilled psychotherapist can inadvertently foster dependency and discourage and even prevent many patients from terminating. This will result in a perpetual caseload that needs only a few occasional referrals.

These mental health practices are called *demand creation* (Feldstein, 1996) by economists, and have been essentially eliminated by the time-limited psychotherapy required by third party payers. But other forms of demand creation are flourishing, such as inventing a syndrome for which the psychotherapist already has a treatment. Psychotherapy has a number of established treatments for depression, and by a new syndrome, seasonal affective disorder (SAD), the state of feeling "blue" in the gloom of winter, these established techniques could be applied to an entire new population. Stretching our credulity even further, NIMH identified "reverse SAD" that ostensibly afflicts persons during daylight savings time (Spencer, 2003). Psychology already had the treatment, but the new disorders were created, thus expanding the number of persons who could be regarded as patients and for whom insurance coverage could be provided. Systematically the definition of depression has been expanded to encompass the slight mood swings involved in daily living. Similarly, bereavement counseling techniques were transposed to the new "grief and crisis counseling" that is rushed to the scene of every disaster, despite evidence it is ineffective and even deleterious (McNally, 2003). Interventions developed by military psychologists for treating combat post traumatic stress syndrome (PTSD) were transported to civilian stress reactions, most of which do not begin to approach the trauma of combat. Cummings (2005a) delineated the process by which this demand is created, while Lilienfeld, Lynn and Lohr (2003) and Lilienfeld, Lohr, Lynn, and Fowler (2005) have addressed the proliferation of dubious diagnoses and their treatments that have been spawned in the era of the psychotherapist glut.

How the Patient Inadvertently Distorts Demand

Before 1942 and the advent of the third party payer system the doctor-patient relationship was simple and one that had endured for over two thousand years dating back to Hippocrates: the physician was pledged to treat the patient, first doing no harm, and the patient was obligated to follow the doctor's regimen and to pay the fee. If the doctor was not helpful, extravagant, or insisted on unnecessary services, the patient merely found another physician. Once the employer or the government began paying for healthcare, sixty years of studies demonstrate patients overly utilize care because it is free (Friedman, 2004; Gingrich, 2003; Sowell, 2003). For example, a patient with a minor knee injury might demand an MRI, refusing to wait the two weeks time in which minor injuries improve. If the patient were paying out of pocket for this costly procedure, the doctor's advice to wait would be readily heeded. In psychotherapy it is usually manifested in a different way. Called "therapeutic drift" (Cummings, 2005a), both patient and psychotherapist may continue treatment despite no improvement because a third party is footing the bill. Even with no progress, the patient can narcissistically enjoy having the semi-weekly full attention of a renown therapist for a full hour, all for free! This is called *artificial demand*, created by variables being in the wrong juxtaposition rather than by need (Feldstein, 1996). Various ways are being suggested to return decision-making and responsibility back to the doctors and their patients as will be discussed below.

A different type of artificial demand known as *misperceived demand* (Feldstein, 1996) is the medical/surgical over-utilization that occurs because of somatization, defined as translating psychological stress into physical symptoms. It is well-established that 60% to 70% of all patient visits to primary care are by patients who have no physical disease, or have a physical disease that is being exacerbated by psychological factors (see for example Cummings, O'Donohue, & Ferguson, 2002, for an extensive review and healthcare delivery solutions). Somatization is reduced by as much as 65% in healthcare settings in which behavioral health is part of primary care.

Managed Care

In the 1980s healthcare became the last major sector of our economy to industrialize, having lagged far behind the industrializations of manufacturing (1900s), energy (1930s), transportation (1950s), and retailing (1970s). The first manifestation of this industrialized healthcare was managed care, the corporate ownership of healthcare financing and delivery made possible by the elimination of laws limiting the corporate practice of medicine and by the application of antitrust laws to the health system, all of which took place in the 1970s. Within a decade managed care became the dominate force in healthcare delivery, and managed behavioral healthcare emerged as separate companies that managed that sector, and known as "carve-outs." By the mid-1990s 175 million Americans received their mental health through managed behavioral healthcare organizations (MBHOs). These carve-outs began as utilization review and other monitoring device entities, but soon copied American Biodyne which was the first national comprehensive managed behavioral healthcare company.

By the beginning of the 21st Century the MBHOs had lost much of their punch thanks to a backlash that initiated a host of laws and regulations limiting their management of behavioral care. By early in 2000 the MBHOs had become essentially monitoring, network management and payment centers, and in the transition a number of bankruptcies and near bankruptcies occurred. The largest MBHO, Magellan Behavioral Health, restructured and emerged from Chapter 11 financially sound. The industrialization of healthcare, as well as mental healthcare, continues, but with a much different morphology, and it will continue to evolve in the future. Once a sector industrializes, there is no returning to the cottage industry that preceded it.

Managed care, including managed behavioral care, did not manage care, but managed costs. Companies like American Biodyne that resulted in cost-efficiency through managing effective mental healthcare were impossible to replicate in a corporate, rather than health-driven environment. Not that doctors were doing a better job of managing costs, but only in a few instances (e.g. American Biodyne) was there a melding of best practices with Edwards Deming efficiencies. Managed care imploded from a self-created backlash. It (1) had forgotten that patients vote as well as complain to their members of Congress, and it (2) falsely believed employers were their ultimate customers, not the patients.

In the discussions of the implosion of managed behavioral health as implemented in the 1980s, neglected is the fact that managed care as originally conceived was never implemented. Managed care was conceptualized by the Jackson Hole Group beginning in the 1970s. It was so named because all their meetings were held in that town in Wyoming where the Federal Reserve Board also meets, and it was comprised of some of the nation's most prestigious health economists (e.g., Paul Elwood, Alain Enthoven). Summarized, it called for every employer to provide a choice of basic coverage at employer's expense, and a series of upscale plans, each at the employee's choice and costs, ranging from bronze to platinum. An employee would always have a choice of managed care and indemnity plans, priced accordingly. Full information on every choice was accorded employees, who could switch plans once a year. Integral to the Jackson Hole concept was that no employee would be forced to accept managed care over indemnity insurance. Very few employers ever implemented such a choice, which would have significantly lowered patient complaints, and might have spared the backlash. In one setting, Stanford University, where faculty and other employees have a choice between managed care and indemnity insurance, 76% choose the HMO (Enthoven, 2003).

Consumerism

Information that would enable a patient to choose the health plan with the best value for the premium dollar is integral to the consumer movement in America, and the CEO of the APA sees this as the next step in healthcare (Bradshaw, 2004ab). It is intended that the most efficient and effective health plans would also have the lowest premiums. Ideally the consumer has influenced health plans to become more effective and efficient, thus lowering the premium. The idea of an informed purchaser connecting with a low-cost health plan certainly sounds appropriate, but unfortunately consumerism would end health insurance as we know it. The fastest way for a health plan to lower costs is to eliminate potential enrollees that are sick or likely to become sick. It is fundamental in our present system that the 80% of insured who use little healthcare pay for the 20% who use most of the services, thus resulting in an equal premium for the sick and the healthy. Given full information there is little doubt that buyers would gravitate to health plans that cherry pick healthy enrollees and thus have lowered pay-out and a very low premiums. This leaves the 20% of Americans needing extensive services facing an astronomical premium, with enrollment in what could be termed "sick plans" rather than health plans, essentially ending third party payment.

The Cost of Healthcare and the 45 Million Uninsured

A perusal of the past fifteen years indicates that the cost of healthcare and the cost of automobiles have risen about the same proportionally. However, in 2004 healthcare costs are rising at a faster rate than automobile prices, whereas for the first half of the fifteen year period the opposite was true. The reason is that for a number of years managed care dramatically lowered the healthcare inflation spiral, but in the last five years the number of laws and regulations encumbering managed care have resulted in its inability to continue controlling costs. So for a number of years automobile inflation was exceeding healthcare inflation, but now the opposite is true. There are currently more government regulations that lead to healthcare cost increases than are now hampering the auto industry. The startling difference, however, whereas almost every American has at least one automobile, 45 million do not have health insurance. Everyone buys a car, even if it is a clunker, but it is expected that health insurance will be provided. How many Americans forego buying a car and begin riding the bus so they can pay for health insurance?

The 45 million uninsured have become a political football, but who are they? They are not the poor who are covered under Medicaid. The figure does include uncounted college students, and especially graduate students, who are too old to be covered by their parents' health plan, but for whom mom and dad are providing a healthcare safety net. It probably includes many undocumented (i.e., illegal) immigrants. But the majority is the young entrepreneurs who have started their own small business, and can not afford healthcare for themselves or their employees. These small businesses are providing 60% of the new jobs in America, and the solution is legislation that will encourage them to band together and buy healthcare at a "bulk price" as do large corporations. Such legislation is proposed, but politics that would rather perpetuate the issue than solve it are hampering the outcome; thus, the figure keeps growing annually from its original 40 million four years ago to estimates in 2004 that put it at a yet to be defined, and perhaps over-blown 45 million.

There is one other variable that is overlooked. Many of these small businesses are mom-and-pop operations, such as one or two married couples, several single women, or other such arrangements that have other than the owners only one or two employees, but often none at all. These entrepreneurs are usually in their early thirties and have less than a 5% risk of a catastrophic medical condition. As are most entrepreneurs, they are not risk aversive, and would rather take that risk in favor of using the money that would go to health insurance to grow their fledgling businesses.

Medical Savings Accounts

The overwhelming evidence that third party payment systems destroy the doctor-patient relationship, resulting in the patient abdicating responsibility for both healthcare costs and his or her own health (Gingrich, 2003; Sowell, 2003) has prompted Nobel Laureate Milton Friedman (2004) to strongly favor tax-free medical savings accounts. The non-spent portions of the medical savings account can be carried over into succeeding years and still enjoy the tax benefits accorded these accounts. Eventually a healthy individual could cash in some of the accrual. It rewards good health, it encourages a healthy life style, and since one's own money is being spent, the patient is prudent in the use of care and demanding in its quality. It restores the doctor-patient relationship extant for the over 2000 years that preceded health insurance. In mental health it would end therapeutic drift, unnecessarily prolonged psychotherapy, the proliferation of dubious diagnoses, and the reduction of the unskilled practitioner.

This all seems viable, but in time the medical savings account system would encounter some of the same difficulties eventually facing consumerism. Medical savings accounts are not suitable for the chronically ill or persons with pre-existing conditions, although they can be a boon to small businesses. In time the healthy would gravitate to the medical savings account system, leaving the sick to face ever-increasing premiums in what has become an expensive "sick plan" (Brock, 2004).

One must ask, however, if those who maintain a healthy life style must be punished by having to pay for those who continue to smoke, over-eat and maintain a sedentary life style? Or should they be rewarded? This issue will be addressed below.

Tort Reform

Frivolous lawsuits directly cost the health system $28 billion annually, but the indirect cost of defensive medicine is estimated to be another $60 to $100 billion dollars. This exceeds the amount of money that would be necessary to provide coverage to the 45 million uninsured. The health systems of other nations do not have to bear this burden, and many have totally eliminated frivolous lawsuits by simply outlawing contingency arrangements by which the plaintiff pays nothing, but the lawyers collect 50% of the judgment plus all their costs. A number of states have capped non-economic (i.e., pain and suffering) payments and in 2004 a number of such bills are pending, especially in states where doctors are rapidly exiting because of astronomical malpractice insurance costs. Patients are suffering because of a shortage of physicians in their states, and in Nevada a pregnant woman must travel to California for prenatal care. In Las Vegas both trauma centers closed in response to the bleak litigious environment in which trial lawyers advertise on large bill boards, and critical patients must be transported to the Los Angeles area. Similar plights confront patients in a number of other states suffering from run-away litigation awards. Vaccines are often in short supply, with the 2004 shortage of the flu vaccine only the latest example, with child vaccines perpetually in short supply, because American manufacturers avoid the litigious environment confronting the manufacture of vaccines. California experienced a mass exodus of physicians decades ago, solved the problem by a combination of both tort and insurance reform, and is now considered a Mecca for physicians and their patients.

It would seem that tort reform is an obvious solution, were it not that the subject has become mired in partisan politics. Trial lawyers spend millions of dollars defending their lucrative practices, and they have become one of the largest contributors to the Democratic Party, unfortunately making the matter a partisan Democrat versus Republican issue.

Medical Errors

Medical errors have become an enormous problem that can be virtually eliminated by (1) electronic record keeping and (2) by transparency of data. The first is resisted by a medical culture that likes cellular phones but dislikes electronic record keeping, and a health system that concentrates on the cost of instituting such a system and without looking at the magnitude of future cost savings.

No corporation would be successful today without the transparency of data that enable it to elicit and correct production errors immediately. This principle so integral to business is absent in the healthcare industry because transparency means lawsuits. Who would admit a medical error, even though this is the first step to eliminating an error-system, when such an admission will surely result in a deluge of lawsuits? Tort reform that will eliminate frivolous lawsuits while compensating victims of medical error, and also encouraging data transparency so as to substantially reduce future errors and its victims, is a challenge that must be faced with a bipartisan effort that is long overdue.

Universal Healthcare

From the foregoing one might prematurely conclude that universal healthcare would eliminate many of the problems of our market-driven system. Polls seem to show that the majority of Americans favor universal healthcare, but these polls are not conclusive in that the questions are usually framed so as to render the positive response, making any respondent not so disposed appear lacking in compassion. Where universal healthcare has been instituted, which is every industrialized nation except the United States, it works well in the beginning but then costs accelerate exponentially, unacceptably increasing the tax burden, so that controls and rationing must be instituted. The Province of Ontario (Canada) in 2004 had to end its system of free healthcare for all by instituting premiums along with the other controls and rationing that have been put in place over prior years (Mackie, 2004). Several years ago Ontario announced in the beginning of December that the healthcare budget had been exhausted, and no healthcare would be paid for until after the new budget came into effect the first of the year.

Again, taking the highly touted Canadian system of universal care as an example, it is now plagued with "a number of shortcoming, including the growing shortage of doctors and nurses, the lengthening of waits for cancer care and surgery, and the mounting cost of drugs for an aging population" (Krauss, 2004; p. 11). Additionally, the cost to the taxpayer has grown 40% since its enactment in 1975, while furthering the silent rationing of care that manifests itself in long waits. The system would be even more stressed were it not that so many Canadians, despairing waiting, cross into the United States and pay out-of-pocket for immediate care

Included in this volume is an updated reprint of a universal care financing proposal that evolved from a study initiated by the National Academies of Practice in 1994 (see Dörken chapter in this volume). It is intended to build in the kinds of safeguards and controls that would prevent draconian measures in the future that would be necessary to curb ever-accelerating costs. The study was conducted in response to the absence of financing considerations in the thousands of pages of the Rodham Clinton Healthcare Task Force report that was unable to grapple at all with cost and financing.

A Viable Healthcare Model: A Beginning

It is time we returned decision making in healthcare to the doctors and their patients, but under an accountable system where both are held responsible for their side of the doctor-patient equation. It would preserve the employer sponsored coverage as well as the existing coverage for the poor, veterans, and the elderly (e.g., Medicare, Medicaid, Veterans Administration, TriCare), but it restores the responsibility of the patient to use the system wisely, while the doctor provides effective quality care without excessive treatment. It presupposes the elimination of frivolous lawsuits that will encourage data transparency, thus reducing and eliminating medical errors. It is a return to small, manageable, integrated group practices in which doctor and patient know and respect each other, and the patients' psychological needs are being addressed along with their physical health. It is a responsible system, serving the patient while also respecting the doctor.

Employer and Payer Responsibility

An enrollee is guaranteed a prepaid basic health plan that is adequate, and is provided the information to make a choice among several plans offered. These are basic bronze plans, and totally at employer expense. Additionally, each potential enrollee is provided information on plans rated silver, gold, and platinum with successively higher premiums to the insured above the basic bronze plan offered by the employer or agency. Such upgraded plans are voluntary, but always at an added increment to the basic plan which is payable by the subscriber. Information on available health plans is kept current and the enrollee may make a change at a prescribed date annually.

Preventive services that include intensive health education, integration of behavioral health into primary care, training the patient to manage chronic disease and stress, and essentially create incentives for the patient assuming responsibility for his or her health are integral, covered services. Whereas prevention accounts for less than 5% of today's healthcare budget, it would be substantially increased. As an example of today's unworkable system, the physician is reimbursed for treating the consequences of diabetes (amputations, blindness, etc.) but is not reimbursed for services that would prevent these unfortunate and costly consequences.

Patient Responsibility

The patient has the responsibility of keeping appointments and following the medical and psychological regimen prescribed, and the doctor has the option of refusing to treat an intractable patient. This would rarely occur, but would have a sentinel effect on patient responsibility. A co-payment is required for every visit, as much as five dollars for most plans, but a modest one dollar for the indigent and elderly. As modest as this co-payment is, research has shown it decreases unnecessary utilization without curtailing the seeking of needed services (Cummings et al., 2002).

The patient is taught responsibility for maintaining a healthy life style, which includes nutrition, activity and attitude (Gingrich, 2003). These include eating healthy foods, avoiding over-eating, not smoking, moderate use of alcohol, and no recreational drugs. Activity not only includes regular exercise, but having a healthy social involvement, spirituality, and other endeavors that lead to contentment. Attitude means reduction of anger, elimination of stress, and maintaining a positive psychology. The person with a chronic illness is taught best how to manage that illness. Gingrich (2003) calls this health before healthcare (i.e., prevention is preferable to treatment). Incentives toward healthy life styles are provided throughout the health system, and if all else fails, he believes there are ways to mandate them.

Government Responsibility

The federal government could do much to make health insurance available (Forbes, 2004). For example, (1) by allowing individuals to deduct health insurance premiums just as corporations do, this would not only offset the cost of the premiums, it would create an incentive to purchase such insurance. (2) Enact legislation that has been pending in Congress that would permit consumers to buy health insurance policies offered anywhere in the United States. Currently one can only purchase policies approved by each state for sale in that state. This would establish a national standard and get around the excessive state regulations that enormously increase premiums. (3) New federal legislation allows employers to offer their employees tax-free Health Savings Accounts (Forbes, 2004). In these HSAs money for medical purposes can be deposited by either employer or employee free of tax, it can continue to grow tax free, and it can be spent for medical purposes tax free. If withdrawn for any other purpose, it is subject to taxation. Also, these HSAs can choose to have high deductibles, making health insurance policies infinitely cheaper, and reconnecting in a financially responsible manner the patient responsibility for one's own healthcare. HSAs have portability inasmuch as they are owned by the worker, not the employer, so the policy accompanies the employee no matter how frequently there is a change of jobs. If all of these incentives were in place, the 45 million uninsured would nearly disappear within a short time.

Morphology of Physician Practice

Primary care group basic practices will be divided into patient cohorts of 20,000 to 30,000 enrollees assigned to each group practice. Each primary care provider (PCP) shall be expected to carry a reasonable patient load, with a smaller patient load expected in upscale practices that are providing such so-called healthcare frills as same-day-appointments, longer appointment time with each patient, house-calls as may be appropriate, and other niceties not unessential and absent in basic care. By limiting the patient cohort for each group the advantages of small group practice are maintained. For each eight PCPs there is one behavioral care provider (BCP) with a minimum of two per setting so that one BCP is always available for the hallway handoff.

Where such small, cohesive group practices exist, electronic data keeping has been attained rapidly and with relatively moderate cost. Medical errors are significantly reduced and the paperwork that currently is drowning most doctors becomes more manageable.

The third party payer contracts with each group practice on a fee-for-service basis, and monitors each group practice and compares effective and efficient group practices with those less so. It enables the latter to learn from the more successful groups, but also takes into account those groups whose cohort may have a higher percentage of seriously ill patients. Groups are liable for medical errors, but tort reform has capped non-economic judgments and eliminated frivolous lawsuits. The third party payer may cancel or not renew a contract with a substandard group, but it is important that the financial structure is such that it will attract skilled physicians and thus upgrade each group.

It is intended that as much as 80% of behavioral care is performed within the primary care setting, thus greatly reducing the need for referrals to specialty care that is caring for the chronically mentally ill. The PCPs are encouraged to upgrade their skills to include the first tier of other specialties (e.g., minor surgery, routine dermatology, and even uncomplicated prenatal care), in keeping with the trend to expand the range of primary care. This would significantly reduce the cost by eliminating unnecessary specialty referrals.

The third party payer reimburses the physicians for preventive services, something that is lacking in today's system. The present system is short-changing those physicians conscientious enough to provide health education, patient training in management of chronic disease, and other preventive services that would eventually reduce healthcare costs significantly.

Finally, the health plan makes available business advice as well as courses in business, since the absence of business acumen has caused many a medical group practice to fail.

Summary and Conclusions

This chapter has attempted to walk the reader through the dense forest of healthcare complexities and in a succinct, straightforward and nonpartisan manner. With space limitations undoubtedly some topics have received too brief attention, and there are other topics that may not have been included. The author has also provided a beginning model for returning the health system to the doctors and patients, but with accountability for the doctor and responsible use for the patient. Mind/body dualism would end with behavioral care being an integral part of primary care. In struggling to steer a middle course, the effort will inevitably receive criticism from both sides, as healthcare has become highly politicized and ideological.

While grappling with the unexpected volumes of primary care patients manifesting emotional and psychological distress as first discovered in the newly nationalized post-World War II British system, the prescient Michael Balint (1957) predicted that to meet this exigency physicians would have to become more like psychologists, and psychologists would have to become more like physicians.

References

ABC News/Washington Post Poll (2004, October 4). Washington, DC: Author.

Alexander, F., & French, T. M. (1946). *Psychoanalytic therapy: Principles and applications.* New York, NY: Ronald Press.

Antonuccio, D. O., Danton, W. G., & DeNelsky, G. Y. (1999). Raising questions about antidepressants. *Psychotherapy and Psychosomatic Medicine, 68*(1), 3-14.

Association for the Advancement of Psychology (2004). APA poll: Most Americans have sought mental health treatment but cost, insurance still barriers. *AAP Advance,* Summer, p. 12.

Balint, M. (1957). *The doctor, his patient, and the illness.* New York, NY: International Universities Press.

Barlett, D. L., & Steele, J. B. (2004a). *Critical condition: How health care in America became big business – and bad medicine.* New York, NY: Doubleday.

Barlett, D. L., & Steele, J. B. (2004b, October 11). Health care can be cured: Here's how. *Time,* pp. 50-51.

Bradshaw, A. (2004a, January-February). What will follow managed care? "Consumerism" will guide change in health care, APA's CEO says. *National Psychologist, 13*(1).

Bradshaw, A. (2004b, January-February). What will follow managed care? National health is coming, predicts pioneer in managed care. *National Psychologist, 13*(1).

Brock, F. (2004, September 21). Weighing the risks in a health savings account. *New York Times,* pp. 17 and 20.

Budman, S. H., & Gurman, A. S. (1988). *Theory and practice of brief therapy.* New York, NY: Guilford Press.

Callaghan, G. M., Gregg, J. A., Marx, B., Kohlenberg, B. S., & Gifford, E. (2004). Fact: The utility of an integration of functional analytic psychotherapy and acceptance and commitment therapy to alleviate human suffering. *Psychotherapy: Theory, Research, Practice, Training, 41*(3), 195-207.

Carnahan, I. (2002, January 21). Asylum for the insane. *Forbes,* 33-34.

Corrigan, P. (2004). How stigma interferes with mental health care. *American Psychologist, 59*(7), 614-625.

Cummings, N. A. (2005a). Expanding a shrinking economic base: The right way, the wrong way, and the mental health way. In R.H. Wright & N.A. Cummings (Eds.), *Destructive trends in mental health: The well-intentioned road to harm.* New York, NY: Brunner-Routledge (Taylor and Francis).

Cummings, N. A. (2005b). Treatment and assessment take place in an economic context. In S. O. Lilienfeld & W. O'Donohue (Eds.), *The great ideas of clinical science: The 18 concepts every mental health researcher and practitioner should know.* New York, N.Y.: Brunner-Routledge (Taylor and Francis Group).

Cummings, N. A., & Follette, W. T. (1968). Psychiatric services and medical utilization in a prepaid health plan setting: Part II. *Medical Care 6*, 31-41.

Cummings, N. A., O'Donohue, W. T., & Ferguson, K. E. (2002). *The impact of medical Cost offset on practice and research: Making it work for you.* Foundation for Behavioral Health: Healthcare Utilization and Cost Series, Volume 5. Reno, NV: Context Press.

Cummings, N. A., O'Donohue, W., Hayes, S. C., & Follette, V. (Eds.) (2001). *Integrated behavioral healthcare: Positioning mental health practice with medical/surgical practice.* San Diego, CA: Academic Press.

Cummings, N. A., & VandenBos, G. R. (1981). The twenty years Kaiser Permanente experience with psychotherapy and medical utilization: Implications for national mental health policy and national health insurance. *Health Policy Quarterly, 1*(2), 159-175.

Cummings, N. A., & Wiggins, J. G. (2001). A collaborative primary care/behaviora lhealth model for use of psychotropic medication with children and adolescents. Report of a national retrospective study. *Issues in Interdisciplinary Care, 3*(2), 121-128.

Dumont, F. & Fitzpatrick, M. (In press). Fault lines in the great EST debate. *Journal of Contemporary Psychotherapy.*

Enthoven, A. (2003). Remarks to the World Health care Congress, Washington, DC.

Feldstein, P. J. (1996). *Health care economics* (5th ed.). Albany, NY: Delmar.

Follette, W. T., & Cummings, N. A. (1967). Psychiatric services and medical utilization in a prepaid health plan setting. *Medical Care, 5*, 25-35.

Forbes, S. (2004, September 20). Insuring health care coverage. *Forbes,* p. 33.

Fox, R. E. (2004). It's about money: Protecting and enhancing our incomes. *Independent Practitioner, 24*(4), 158-159.

Friedman, M. (2004, January 27). Keynote address to the World Health Care Congress, Washington, DC.

Gingrich, N. (2003). *Saving lives and saving money.* Washington, DC: Alexis de Tocqueville Institution.

Hogan, M. F. (2003). New Freedom Commission Report: The President's New Freedom Commission - Recommendations to transform mental health care in America. *Psychiatric Services, 54*, 1467-1474.

Institute of Medicine (2001). *Crossing the quality chasm: A new health system for the 21st century.* Washington, DC: National Academy of Sciences.

James, L. (2004). Personal communication, September 21.

Kellogg, S. (2004). Dialogical encounters: Contemporary perspectives on "chairwork" in psychotherapy. *Psychotherapy: Theory, Research, Practice, Training, 41*(3), 310-320.

Kennedy, E. (2004, October 9). Comments made on the U.S. Senate floor regarding healthcare. Washington, DC: C-Span Cable Network.

Kerstine, K. (2004). Health-care change is coming: What do we do? *Monitor on Psychology, 35*(9), 56-57.

Krauss, C. (2004), September 23). Canadian health care deal adds $14 billion to ailing fund. From the *New York Times Syndicate. San Francisco Chronicle,* p. A11.

Kuhn, T. (1996). *The structures of scientific revolutions.* Chicago, IL: University of Chicago Press.

Lakatos, I. & Musgrave, A. (Eds.) (1974). *Criticism and the growth of knowledge.* Cambridge: Cambridgr University Press.

Lambert, M.J. (1992). Psychotherapy outcome research: Implications for integrative and eclectic therapists. In J. C. Norcross & M. R. Goldfried (Eds.), *Handbook of psychotherapy integration* (pp. 94-129). New York, NY: Basic Books.

Levant, R.F. (2004). 21st century psychology: Toward a biosocial model. *Independent Practitioner, 24*(3), 128-139.

Lilienfeld, S.O., Lohr, J.M., Lynn, S.J., & Fowler, K. (2005). Pseudoscience, nonscience, and nonsense in contemporary clinical psychology. In R. H. Wright & N.A. Cummings (Eds.), *Destructive trends in mental health: The well-intentioned path to harm.* New York, NY: Brunner-Routledge (Taylor and Francis).

Lilienfeld, S. O., Lynn, S. J., & Lohr, J. M. (Eds.) (2003). *Science and pseudoscience in clinical psychology.* New York, NY: Guilford.

Mackie, R. (2004, June 10). Ontario budget will re-introduce health-care premiums. *Canada,* pp. 1 and 9.

McNally, R. J. (2003, September 12). As extensively quoted in S. Begley, Is trauma debriefing worse than letting victims heal naturally? *Wall Street Journal,* B1-2.

Meehl, P. E. (1978). Theoretical risks and tabular asterisks: Sir Karl, Sir Ronald, and the slow progress of soft psychology. *Journal of Consulting and Clinical Psychology, 46,* 806-834.

National Association of Addiction Treatment Providers (2004). 20.3 million needed Addiction treatment and did not get it in 2003. *NAATP Visions, 10,* September.

Saunders, T. R. (2003). Personal communication.

Seligman, D. (2004, October 18). New crisis – junk statistics. Forbes, 118-119.

Schwartz, J. (2004, September 3). Always on the job, employees pay with health: The stress explosion. *New York Times Syndicate, 1 and 13-14.*

Sowell, T. (2003). *Applied economics.* New York, NY: Basic Books.

Spencer, J. (2003, May 22). When blue skies bring on the blues: Research shows why some despair on sunny days and relish gloom of winter. *Wall Street Journal,* D1-2.

Strosahl, K. (2001). The integration of primary care and behavioral health: Type II changes in the era of managed care. In N. A. Cummings, W. O'Donohue, S. C. Hayes, & V. Follette (Eds.), *Integrated behavioral healthcare: Positioning mental health practice with medical/surgical practice,*(pp. 45-70). San Diego, CA: Academic Press.

Wright, R. H., & Cummings, N. A., (Eds.) (2005). *Destructive trends in mental health: The well-intentioned path to harm.* New York, NY: Brunner-Routledge (Taylor and Francis).

Chapter 3

The Financing and Organization of Universal Healthcare: The Recommendations of the National Academies of Practice As Revised and Updated by the Original Author in 2005

Herbert Dörken

Scientific Director, Cummings Foundation for
Behavioral Health, Reno, Nevada
Forward by Nicholas Cummings

Forward to the Dörken Report

In 1994 the National Academies of Practice recognized that the financing portion of President Clinton's Health Security proposal, emanating from the task force chaired by the First Lady, suffered from weak conceptualization. The NAP commissioned a blue-ribbon task force to study the problem, and its report was widely disseminated to Congress and the White House, creating a demand that required three reprints of the document. Known as the "Dörken Report" after its chair, Herbert Dörken, Ph.D., the 1994 version has been updated because the issue of universal healthcare is once again becoming the topic of political debate, while its cost and financing continue to bedevil its proponents.

The so-called Rodham-Clinton Task Force suffered its first political blow when the powerful Democrat Representative Dan Rostenkowski stated flatly that universal coverage would require significant new taxation, contradicting widely publicized, though fanciful suggestions that universal coverage could be financed by a levy on such items as gasoline, cigarettes and bullets. The latter prompted Jay Leno to quip on his late night TV show that "healthcare in America will be financed by chain-smoking drive-by shooters." Equally devastating, but far more serious, was Senator Daniel Patrick Moynihan's conclusion that the financing portion of the Clinton proposal was "pure fantasy." Without adequate financing there can be no universal coverage in spite of the polls showing the majority of Americans now favor the concept. Paradoxically, the polls also reveal distaste for both new taxes and increases in deficit spending, placing a conundrum before our policy makers. It is often easier to gloss over the difficult aspects of funding, but recognizing the importance of funding, the Cummings Foundation for Behavioral Health is reissuing this updated and once again timely report.

The issue of government sponsored universal coverage has been a controversial and often explosive topic for three-quarters of a century, culminating in the 21st Century with the United States being the only major industrialized nation without some form of universal healthcare. In the 1930s it was called socialized medicine, an appellation the American Medical Association (AMA) demonized, thus preventing the momentum of President Franklin D. Roosevelt's New Deal from incorporating it as one of his several government solutions to the Great Depression. The topic never went away, and a number of government measures designed to "fix" healthcare were adopted over the next decades. Principal among them was the Hill Burton Act in the late 1950s that ended the hospital shortage, the enactment of Medicare and Medicaid in 1960s, and the HMO Enabling Act in the 1970s that, coupled with the Diagnosis Related Groups (DRGs) enacted in the 1980s, set the stage for the growth of managed care in the 1980s and throughout the 1990s. The topic received a new thrust and a new name (National Health Insurance) when Senator Edward Kennedy became chair of the Senate Finance Subcommittee on Health (Kiesler, Cummings, & VandenBos, 1979). He held a series of hearings at which the author of this Foreword testified on behalf of the American Psychological Association (APA). Subsequently I was asked to work closely over the next three years as an adviser to Stanley Jones, Senator Kennedy's health staffer. Because of the momentum generated, I was persuaded that national healthcare was not only inevitable, but also imminent. Suddenly what seemed like an upheaval, pitting Democrat against Democrat in the Democratic-controlled Congress, Senator Russell Long became head of the Senate Finance Committee, and promptly ousted Senator Kennedy, replacing him with Senator Herman Talmadge. The thrust toward National Health Insurance died abruptly, seemingly over-night.

Universal coverage did not surface again as a serious proposal until the ill-fated Rodham-Clinton Task Force (1993-1995) that suffered from a number of problems other than its inability to grapple with funding. For one, the task force was shrouded in secrecy, prompting the AMA to file a lawsuit under the "sunshine laws" to force public disclosure of its membership. Once the approximately five hundred members (a precise count has never been established) were revealed, these were mostly government employees. Another flaw was the proposed severe penalties, fines plus prison, to be imposed on any physician or patient who dispensed or received healthcare outside the approved system. Undoubtedly fearing that government medicine could never compete with private care just as public schools can not compete with private education, Mrs. Clinton enraged the American public by essentially planning to remove the time-honored patient choice of doctor. The failure of the Clinton Plan was so pervasive that politicians since have been reluctant to proffer a substantive plan, even though recent presidential campaign rhetoric waxed loud, but predictably ethereal.

Perhaps realizing that most Americans favor universal coverage, and undoubtedly emboldened by the "mandate" handed it in the 2004 presidential election, the Bush administration is proposing a series of initiatives to strengthen what remains of private healthcare. It must be kept in mind that with the growth the past fifty years of Medicare, Medicaid, the Veterans Administration, TriCare (military dependents and retired military, Federal Employees Benefits Program, etc.), nearly 50% of healthcare is currently dispensed under government auspices. Additionally, the Congress continues to enact regulatory laws, along with their subsequent restrictions on private healthcare, all of which it exempts from its own government supported platinum healthcare plan. The Congress is loathe to subject itself to the kind of healthcare it proposes for the rest of us.

Health savings accounts (HSAs) are designed to restore the responsibility, decision-making and ownership of healthcare to the individual, while restoring the doctor-patient relationship that was destroyed with the intrusion of the third party payer, be it government or private health insurance. With tax-free medical savings accounts, the non-spent portions can be carried over into succeeding years and still enjoy the tax benefits accorded these accounts. Eventually a healthy individual could cash in on some of the accrual. It rewards good health, it encourages a healthy life-style, and since one's own money is being spent, the patient is prudent in the use of care and demanding in its quality. Critics would point out that medical savings accounts are not suitable for the chronically ill or persons with pre-existing conditions. In time the healthy would gravitate to medical savings accounts, leaving the sick to face ever-increasing premiums, or be the only ones forced into government-sponsored care.

HSAs are part of a broader scenario by the administration to make working people part of the wealth-acquisition system. Tandem to HSAs would be legislation pending in the Congress and introduced by Representative Paul Ryan (R-WI) and Senator John Sununu (R-NH) that would allow workers to shift what they now pay in payroll taxes (roughly the amount in the FICA box of the payroll stub without the presence of upper limits in income) into their personal "social security accounts." It is argued that personal accounts of 6.4% invested half in corporate bonds and half in stocks earning standard long-term market investment returns would provide roughly two-thirds more in benefits than what Social Security promises and cannot pay. As stated by a proponent, "Such vast, broad-based wealth ownership would transform America, economically, socially and politically. Capitalism works when people have capital. For the first time in history, the working poor will have access to wealth creation," (Gingrich, 2004, p. 36). Whether such far-reaching transformation can be enacted into law, and whether it would curtail the drive toward universal coverage, remains to be seen.

Healthcare reform is so paralyzed by politics and conflicting ideologies it reminds one of the 1930s when the route for the planned Pennsylvania Turnpike, the first of its kind, was stalled in debate. Every small town, recognizing the economic self-interest of having the route go down its main street, intensely lobbied the state. Yet it was this slow threading of traffic through every town and hamlet that necessitated the building of the turnpike in the first place. Finally, in exasperation, the state empowered an independent group of civil engineers to formulate the route. This independent panel ignored all politics and designed a thruway in keeping with the intent of moving traffic efficiently and rapidly from east to west. The route missed every town. In looking at healthcare today, an independent panel is needed to address the issue of the national health, ignoring if necessary ever special interest group. In disseminating the Dörken report, the NAP (and now the Cummings Foundation in this update) did not intend an all-special-interests-be-damned approach, but rather it reflects the need to provide a template as to what is best for the national health without regard to these special interests and political ideologies. This is why this report stresses what is realistic, what can and cannot be afforded, and delineates the best delivery system within these confines.

Dr. Dörken was chosen to chair the NAP Task Force on the Financing of Healthcare in America because of the breadth of his experience on issues of financing. Dr. Dörken has spent a lifetime researching, designing, and implementing health delivery systems in the United States and Canada. Funding and budgeting are both second-nature to him in contrast to most successful health professionals who would rather concentrate on actual practice problems. Yet because of his original training as a clinician and subsequent experience in the delivery of services, Dr. Dörken has a keen appreciation of what goes on in the trenches, and how this is translated to healthcare financing and delivery. Not your usual policy wonk, Dr. Dörken's thinking is concise, practical and workable. The report of his Task Force was the subject of the NAP's Fifth Interdisciplinary National Health Policy Forum in which First Lady, and now Senator Hillary Rodham Clinton was an invited guest. The original 1994 report was disseminated to the Congress and the White House as a policy of the National Academies of Practice (Cummings, 2002).

In addition to developing health services and major clinical research studies Dr. Dörken has found that amending current or formulating new law can enable an improved, broader, and more effective range of health services. In 1973 he participated in drafting HR 9440 (Waldie) which became Public Law 93-363 in 1974 amending the Federal Employees' Health Benefits Act to require direct recognition of clinical psychologists and optometrists in all federal employee health plans. And now thirty years later working collaboratively with the California Conference of Local Health Officers the system for adding or deleting diseases to be reported by California practitioners was updated and made more practical and signed as an urgency measure by California's new Governor Schwarzenegger on 8-23-04 (AB 1091 Negrete McLeod, Chapter 262). Lyme disease is now becoming laboratory reportable and West Nile disease and SAARS are also becoming reportable. Over the years Dr. Dörken has drafted and helped lobby into enactment 44 bills (1 federal, 8 Hawaii, 1 province of Alberta, 34 California). His view is that current laws and regulations regarding healthcare are to often outdated and thwart new developments.

With the permission and participation of its original author, the Cummings Foundation for Behavioral Health is pleased to publish this updated version of the Dörken Report.

Nicholas A. Cummings, Ph.D., Sc.D., Founding President (1981-1993) and Past President (1993-in perpetuity) National Academies of Practice, Washington, D.C.

Former President, American Psychological Association

President, Cummings Foundation for Behavioral Health, Reno, NV

Overview

As of the end of 2004 we have in this country centers of great and specialized excellence, but overall a non system of healthcare. There is a substantial public focus now on who has or does not have health insurance. That is only one aspect of our non system. Fundamental changes are needed to make a national healthcare system feasible.

During the so called World War II there were wage and price controls. To by pass those restrictions fringe benefits of employment were sought after since wages could not be increased. Health insurance coverage for the employed and often their families was the most popular and common benefit, COBRA stop gaps were established for those unemployed between jobs. With employment mobility in a changing job market, coverage changed and with escalating prices often ended on retirement. Would Medicare be sufficient?

Should the government provide your healthcare - federal, state, or municipal? Or should the choice not be made by each citizen/family? If we are to have a national plan, it makes no sense to have the licensing requirements for each health professional differ among states. We need a national uniform licensing standard. This would also assure mobility of all licensed health practitioners across states and phase out 50 such state bureaucracies.

In general, the public has little conception of the enormous cost of healthcare. The current gross domestic product of the USA is about $10 trillion and $1.4 trillion or 14% is the cost of healthcare. Military spending as a percentage of GDP was 3.2% in 1999 and education 7.3% in 2000, together 10.5%. It appears then that the cost of healthcare may exceed the cost of the defense and education combined! With a population in 2004 of 294,507,000 the per person cost in about $4414 per year. But the population includes the 45 or so million uninsured, 6.5% of the population. Estimated healthcare costs for 2005 are $1.8 trillion, up from $1.4 trillion in 2004 and estimated to rise to $3.4 trillion in 2013. If our population is 295 million in 2005 with $1.8 trillion costs that's $6100 per person and upward per year.

Great Britain has had a national health plan for over 4 decades and to keep it afloat the government has poured millions more into it periodically. At the outset it was an attraction for tourists from Europe who took advantage of free care while on holiday! We know our northern neighbor Canada has national hospital and health insurance. Its Prime Minister was just re-elected on his promise to fix Canadian healthcare. Twenty years ago Canada's federal government unified the various health insurance programs run by the provinces. Ottawa offered to pay 50% of the programs operating budgets provided the provincial plans accepted 5 basic principles including nationwide acceptance of each provincial plan, comprehensive coverage and no out of pocket costs (co-payments or deductibles) for insured services. Since then the federal share had dropped to as low as 14% forcing governments to attack their budget deficits, some hospitals were closed, physician fees were frozen or cut, nurses were laid off, etc. Thus relative to population Canada now has fewer hospitals and most are public rather than private while the reverse is true in the US. Another result of the fiscal shortfall is that Canada now has a shortage of physicians, particularly specialists and surgeons and has suffered a drain of doctors and nurses lured by higher pay and lower taxes in the United States. None the less Canadians appear to be healthier with a longer life span than Americans and lower infant mortality. Canadians in general think of their national health system as a mark of their national identity with pride. To the ailing $60 billion national healthcare systems the federal government agreed to send an additional $14 billion (23.3%) over 6 years with guarantees of 6% annual increases thru 2015, that's 6% more a year for 11 years (66% not compounded). The population of Canada which is larger in territory than the US has about 1/10th of our population. As one Senator commented, "What it does is put the patient (the healthcare system) on life support, but it does not put it on the road to full recovery as it is threatened by an aging population and the rising costs of technology and drugs." And if this is the survival cost to the Canadian government where do you suppose the money comes from? TAXES. In 2004 Canada's healthcare expenditures were 10% of national economic output. They have just added 23.3% plus a 66% guaranteed increase through 2015.

Do you want to pay more and more for your health insurance or do you want to have your taxes raised again and again? One answer is that there must be serious control over costs and coverage.

Why should individuals be limited in their choice of health plans to those developed by their employer or accessible in their state. A national plan should have national choices. Let the market determine them. If you reside in California or Nevada perhaps there is a plan at a better price or better coverage in Connecticut or some other state. State regulations or laws restricting choice need to be abolished and replaced with national standards.

If we are to have a national health plan it means that every citizen and legal permanent resident who is employed must pay to be covered an amount offset by tax deduction. There can be no employed uninsured. Those who receive government benefits must receive Medicare and Medicaid. Those here illegally have no eligibility for health coverage, emergency services, maternity services - nothing. Tourists, foreign workers, and students here on a valid visa must expect to pay for any care on a fee for service basis and must have a valid visa to gain such care or prepay to have health insurance coverage if their stay is more than a year as in the case of workers and students. Further if they cannot speak or understand English it is up to them when they seek healthcare that they bring an interpreter with them at their expense. There will be no mandate that the practitioner's healthcare must be rendered in the language of the patient or that the patient prefers. English only. All laws or regulations to the contrary must be voided.

All treatment decisions are to be made by a licensed healthcare practitioner based on personal examination/evaluation of the patient from which a treatment plan is evolved based on the patient's informed consent and on generally accepted standards of practice. When there is more than one standard of care as for breast cancer, prostate cancer, or Lyme disease the pros and cons and risks of each must be presented to the patient who has the ultimate right of choice. When there are unusual or potential major complications it is not unreasonable to gain a second opinion from another practitioner considered to have more expertise or experience with the condition to guide the patient's decision. Treatment decisions agreed upon by the patient and practitioner cannot be denied or altered by anyone who is not qualified to examine the patient and has not done so. The generic term "licensed practitioner" includes physicians (allopathic and osteopathic), dentists, podiatrists, psychologists, optometrists, nurse practitioners, physicians assistants, and school nurses. Also when treatment for a particular condition has been shown to be effective, action to limit visits or increase co-pay for that condition is not acceptable.

The outcome of any agreed treatment plan cannot be guaranteed. If the plan agreed to is considered legitimate and the care was appropriately delivered with due caution, and the risks noted beforehand, but the outcome was unfortunate there are no grounds for malpractice suits or awards unless it can be determined that the treatment was delivered in an incompetent manner or was not the treatment agreed to. In such cases the cost of remedial care is charged to the erring practitioner and any claim for pain and suffering as a malpractice award cannot exceed $250,000. Fraud, which is the submission of claims for services not provided will lead to loss of the practitioners license to practice not simply in the state of residence but anywhere in the USA. The same applies to attorneys who pursue claims for services they have not rendered.

Many practitioners continue to live and work in fairly close proximity to the professional school they graduated from. Such maldistribution, however, thwarts the implementation and delivery of a national health plan. In most communities of the country it is unlikely that there will be renowned treatment centers, perhaps not even a hospital, but within each geographic area with clusters of residents and some public schools within a radius of 60 to 100 miles in which there are a thousand people, efforts and resources should be focused on the development of community health centers served by multidisciplinary practitioners who can provide family and emergency care. In such rural or sparse areas there may need to be a fee differential attractive to practitioners.

Also for those practitioners whose education was publicly funded or based on training grants repayment by practice at such centers should be encouraged if not required.

A major virtue of a national health plan is that the coverage is portable. It is not dependent on a particular employment. Small businesses with 1-49 employees are 94.7% of all employers and 41.5% of the workforce in 1999. Many if not most cannot afford to pay healthcare for their workforce. If we are seeking to promote personal responsibility it does not follow that we should continue to expect someone else to pay for one's healthcare, either an employer or the government. Rather the patient/family should prepay/buy their coverage, but the income tax system should be amended to provide tax credits for the purchase of health insurance. We should expand the use and availability of Medical Savings Accounts (MSA) whereby individual/families can pre-save to pay tax free towards the costs of future healthcare. Having the cost born by the consumer will generally exert some control on utilization.

Holding the same job for one's working life is increasingly uncommon in our mobile and changing society whereas a profession or religious or academic affiliation tends to be permanent. Therefore we should encourage the formation of Affinity Health Plans, since they will engender stable and identified groups for health policies.

Too often younger people feeling fit claim they do not need health insurance. One unexpected major accident or one sudden serious illness abruptly changes that. In a national health plan everybody must obtain and pay for their health insurance. Simply transferring the cost to employers or the government does not make it free. At the very least the base policy should derive from an MSA to be used toward a major deductible but backed then by catastrophic policy coverage.

While there are organized systems of care today such as Kaiser Permanente and the Veterans Administration which have an incentive to keep their clients healthy and thereby lower costs, there is a big gap in the adoption of information technology among independent physicians, even in small groups since these lack the economy of scale to benefit from modern technology (Kiesler, Cummings, & VandenBos, 1979). However, this may be changing as innovative primary care groups of typically 6 to 14 physicians engaged in staff model practice are beginning to appear across the country. One such, LifeScape, is illustrative. A number of former Scottsdale Mayo Clinic primary care physicians launched a cutting-edge practice encompass-ing all modern technologies that include not only electronically kept medical records that can be transmitted electronically as required, but also computer printed prescription that can be e-mailed to any pharmacy. This and other innovations are paid for by an annual upfront fee of $100 per enrollee which covers all administra-tive costs for the group, after which LifeScape accepts payment from the patient's third-party payor, including Medicare. This modest fee also makes possible guaranteed same day appointments, 24 hour consultation, and other healthcare amenties not found in the usual primary care practice. LifeScape meticuloussly follows the Mayo tradition of beautifully designed and appointed facilities with a number of conveniences, such as children's play areas featurning large screen age-appropriate educational videos. The staff not only reflects the epitome of competence and professionalism, it dresses accordingly rather than in the slovely fashion found in most healthcare facilities. Courtesy and customer service abound, all made possible by an upfront annual fee that amounts to foregoing one dinner at a moderately priced restaurant. This fee also enables LifeScape to have a reduced physician-to-patient ratio, resulting in longer and more attentive visits which stress family care, lifestyle changes and preventive medicine, and also include attention to the behavioral problems that lead to somatization. Everything is available to the patient on the premises, including convenient full-scale laboratory services.

Solo practitioners are at a serious disadvantage today. They cannot provide care on a 7 day, 24 hr/day basis. Some have formed small group practices partly to diversify, partly to cover "on-call", but mainly to have office staff to schedule booking and to complete third party billing claims (Gingrich, 2004). Even so, they do not have the resources of scale to generate outcome data and are hard pressed to have specialty resources in depth beyond having staff membership in a local or nearby hospital. They can however, develop the personal relationship that most patients desire.

The American healthcare system is confronting a crisis. According to the Institute of Medicine (2001) "the system is incapable of meeting the present let alone the future needs of the American public." One significant weakness is too often an isolated training and practice orientation of each of the health professions. What we need is an interdisciplinary focus and involvement in training and in healthcare delivery.

This proposed plan of prepaid healthcare for all US citizens would have multiple funding sources. The uniform comprehensive benefit (UCB) would be delivered mainly by managed competing healthcare organizations subject to community rating. To facilitate universal access and care, all health professionals licensed for independent practice could be recognized providers. All citizens would have a fake-proof, signed, photo healthcare identification card (HIDC) of eligibility for all services within the UCB and a personal current medical care chip electronically transmissible to a new treating physician in the event of an accident or emergency.

The UCB will include specified services that have clearly been shown to be both clinically and cost effective. Emphasis will be placed on the prevention of disease and disability, public education toward healthy life styles, early intervention for illness or injury and primary care. Preference will be given to the least intrusive means of healthcare delivery considered effective. All persons, or their guardian or conservator, have the right to refuse treatment.

With universal access, the National Health Plan (NHP) would subsume the aegis for most civilian healthcare. Healthcare would no longer be dependent on employment status, would be available throughout the nation, would be provided on a no-fault basis and, to the extent feasible and cost effective, would be delivered by private rather than public services. With benefit standardization, all eligible people would choose among competing plans. Those choosing a managed or fee for service plan within the annually established average pre-payment cost would have no deductibles or co-payments. Those electing plans exceeding the limit would be responsible for the cost difference and not have a tax advantage for this difference.

Both professional and facility provider rates would be redetermined annually in advance for all care on a fee for service basis. Capitation rates would also be redetermined annually. Rates would be the same within a region for like care for all eligible persons the rates would vary by age. Healthcare organizations would be encouraged to contract with local providers and provider groups where cost effective for all care within the UCB. All competing plans must have the resources to assure access to quality multi-disciplinary care in order to be recognized.

A common data system will be developed and used by all competing plans to enable comparison of utilization and differences by region and by major age groups, derive provider profiles and conduct outcome and other studies. A set proportion of the healthcare fund will be allocated annually to such applied research and other studies which hold promise of furthering quality improvement and cost effectiveness.

Before we even attempt to deliver services under a National Health Plan we should first address and resolve fundamental aspects of the infrastructure. There are numerous aspects of public and professional attitudes which can facilitate or seriously hinder a NHP. There are also many steps which can be taken to effect major savings in healthcare costs today. These steps should be initiated in order to lay a solid foundation for the introduction of the NHP. In essence, these should be the first two phases and they are detailed in the following two sections.

Public and Professional Attitudes

For us to be serious in our objective to have a national health plan, it will require some major changes, or at least consensus in the broad public attitude of Americans (Cummings, 1992). This is a fundamental necessary first step. Here are some of the parameters:

1. *Individualism.* Our historical commitment to individual freedom and rights is in conflict with the common good. We have superb resources to care for an individual but we fail to address the health conditions of our larger society. We are past due in addressing our national health problems.
2. *Redistribution.* If we are to have a national healthcare plan we must first recognize and accept that it will involve a measure of economic redistribution from those who now have healthcare to the 45 million who in 2004 did not. It will also require some equalization in the distribution of professional resources from the present serious maldistribution.
3. *Finite Resources.* We must realize that our resources are finite. We do not have unlimited funds for healthcare, we do not have unlimited professional resources and we still have serious limitations in our knowledge of human diseases, human behavior and human genetics. Current healthcare is far from infallible.

We must realize that all people cannot have everything in healthcare, that all people will not receive the very best, and that national priorities will have to be set. And we can not have everything for nothing. A NHP will not be free. Indeed, the Institute of Medicine in 1992 released Guidelines for clinical practice which found that 45% of medical practice was based on consensus without evidence, the bulk of medical practice is about managing uncertainty in the absence of definitive research. At the time only 4% of total medical services provided were based on strong scientific evidence. The demand of pure managed care corporations for strong scientific evidence for the treatment of some diseases or conditions which are not yet broadly recognized may simply be the easiest way of denying for the care rendered.

4. *NIMBY Paralysis*. Many people are for things until they realize that it affects them and then they stonewall it. It's great but Not in My Back Yard. They don't want to change their circumstances, certainly not their costs or their convenience. I've got mine and you −tough luck!

5. *Prevention*. The primary focus of a national health plan must be on health enhancement, health education, illness prevention, vector and disease control, and on strengthening our public health services after decades of disregard.

6. *Preparatory Savings*. Before we commence any national healthcare delivery we must first put the major sources of cost reduction into place. We must streamline both the acquisition of funds and their distribution delivery sites. The more hands that money passes through the more rubs off. Fraud must be eliminated under penalty of loss of licensure. Our historical over-utilization of hospitals for service delivery and training sites must be curbed. Professional training and services must be multidisciplinary and community based where the problems are. We must accept and appropriately deal with the fact that 60% of all physician visits present with problems that are essentially psychological rather than medical.

7. *Turf Wars*. The interprofessional disputes over turf under the guise of quality of care are motivated by striving for power and money and efforts to acquire or enhance a monopoly. There is a substantial overlap in the licensed scope of practice of many health professions. It is time to recognize and publicly accept this fact. Interprofessional collaboration can be a major asset in improved quality of care. Further, as each science-based health profession is encouraged to develop new knowledge and procedures this will advance the quality of healthcare for everyone.

8. *Single Collector*. The federal government is in the business of collecting revenue and does so efficiently. To the extent that employees will be involved in the financing of their healthcare it can be federally acquired at source far more efficiently than by any other means. Likewise, for any special taxes that might be involved.

9. *Public Trust*. The funds that are collected for health- care must be assembled and permanently transferred to a National Healthcare Trust Fund to be

administered outside the federal bureaucracy but by a non-partisan public agency and no such funds can be "borrowed" by congress or left with paper IOU's as currently happens to the Social Security Trust Fund.

10. *Professional Determination.* The Uniform Comprehensive Benefit (UCB) must be determined by a multidisciplinary health professions body in accord with the state of our knowledge, their science-based conviction of what works and what is futile or unnecessary, all subject to regular review to accommodate new developments. What is critical is that the benefit determination remain fundamentally under the decision of health professional expertise. It is to be emphasized that the UCB is standardized, that is, the same across all health plans.

11. *Relicensure.* Not every professional is optimally competent, in fact, statistically, 50% in any profession are below average. Consider that in 1989 the "American Medical Association estimated that 7,000-10,000 currently practicing physicians in California are so severely impaired that they cannot safely practice medicine (AMA, 1989)."
Licensed once, licensed forever is no longer an acceptable policy. All practitioners, in rotation, should be relicensed, say, every six years when designated peers can review the nature, quality and focus of their practice, their continuing education and personal stability and competence when licensing is nationally based so too will be the periodic review.

12. *Cost Control and Quality.* The Centers for Medicare and Medicaid estimate that healthcare costs for 2005 will be approximately $1.8 trillion (up from $1.4 trillion from 2004). Furthermore, these healthcare costs are expected to increase to $3.4 by 2013. The concepts of cost control and quality are not antagonists but can be synergists. It is time to use not only the expertise of science but healthcare management, the economics of scale, and efficiencies in distribution. The new technologies of the information superhighway video and teleconferencing can bring sophisticated expertise to rural and other areas far more effectively than presence in person.

13. *Law Changes.* Many constructive changes can readily be identified and made. All plans to be approved must comply with community rating. There can be no denial of coverage based on a preexisting condition. Eligibility and choice of plan must be nondiscriminatory for all citizens and legal residents. All state laws which preclude or hinder the delivery of managed care are to be preempted. Professional conflicts of interest can be prohibited, e.g., you cannot refer to a facility or lab in which you have a proprietary interest. Litigation in civil damages can be replaced by binding arbitration and professional services can be provided on a no fault basis. Caps can be placed on damages. All states can adopt provisions for living wills so that patients can decide when there is no benefit to initiate or continue treatment when the short term outcome is futile, painful and degrading, and whereby those with power of attorney can decide there is no point in keeping brain dead persons alive. Patients and significant

others should in the main make these decisions, it is their life. Anti-trust laws need to be moderated to enable the development of managed care enterprises where the clear objective is quality healthcare for the public and to assure that there is ample competition in the community or region.

14. *Price Consciousness*. It is most effective to make consumers price conscious in their choice of health plan on enrollment and annual re-enrollment or change when they must prepay its cost. Whether they are willing to pay more than the regional average of competing plans is a personal choice. Whether they want a point of service provision in a managed care plan or a fee for service rather than a capitated plan even if it costs more than the average plan must be honored. So too must they have freedom of choice of provider within each plan or more globally if that is the choice they selected. But to eliminate the enormous paperwork, hassle and processing cost of deductions and co-payments, these should be eliminated.

15. *Personal Responsibility*. All people must take personal responsibility for their health. Those who persist in high risk behavior known to be injurious to health must also pay the price. For example, a surcharge would be placed on the health plan cost of cigarette smokers; persons who are injured in an automobile or motor cycle accident because they failed to wear seat belts or a helmet; or persons who injure themselves or others while driving under the influence of alcohol or drugs. Other clearly high risk, unwise, unnecessary and unhealthy behaviors such as obesity could also be identified and a surcharge could be invoked.

16. *Federalism*. A national health plan is a federal plan in the collection of funds, the determination of benefits and the approval of plans. It is not acceptable to generate 50 state bureaucracies with 50 different sets of criteria. A national trust can recognize regional alliances and functional agencies with a record of successful negotiation of health plan benefits. The Federal Employee Health Benefits Plan does this now.

17. *Public Education*. Serious and systematic efforts must be made in the schools, on the job and in public media to educate the public to the health hazards of high risk behavior, not just smoking. Plan surcharges could also be placed on those who require treatment of injuries due to driving while drunk, without seat belts, or on motorcycles without a helmet. Students and employees should take risk avoidance and public health exams and be required to study until they have passing knowledge.

All of these conditions currently are faced with varying degrees of public resistance, a resistance which both drives up costs and hinders the quality of healthcare. The public attitude should be addressed first and the identified sources of savings and potential savings next. Then the country will be better prepared for the introduction of a national health plan.

Savings

While a National Health Plan could achieve various economies of scale as in the adoption of drug formularies, and purchase of generic drugs and supplies, and in the adoption of uniform provider rates, it should achieve even more major cost reductions that seldom enter the public debate.

Major sources of cost reduction are:

1. *Administration.* Common Cause (1993) cited the cost to administer Medicare as 1.4% of benefits paid in contrast to 17% under private health insurance. The most striking difference in the cost of healthcare in Canada and the USA is that administrative costs overall are 12% less in Canada.
2. *Hospitalization.* There is overall excess hospital capacity and commonly a private insurance benefit structure favoring hospitalization. Of the 925,000 hospital beds in the country, 310,000 are idle on any day. We have about 3.8 beds per 1,000 of population and only need about 1.8 per 1,000. Physicians and nurses, in particular, are primarily trained in hospitals rather than in local outpatient settings. Health maintenance organizations and some managed care plans have achieved lower costs by controlling and sharply reducing the extent of hospitalization. Where feasible, excess hospital capacity should be converted to other use or closed.
3. *Fraud.* The Government Accounting Office alleges that 10% of Medicare costs are attributable to fraud and are rising. The California State Insurance Fund (worker's compensation) reports 20% of cost due to fraud and rising. There are three links in a fraud chain, one essential: always a questionable practitioner, often a questionable lawyer and usually a malcontent person/ patient who does not want to work or is greedy. Remove the questionable practitioner and the fraud chain is broken. Loss of license to practice anywhere in the USA is the penalty to pay for practitioners engaging in fraud. The same would apply to an attorney. Patients must repay double the healthcare cost received on the basis of their fraud.
4. *Somatization.* In 1976, the AMA testified to the US Senate Health Committee that 60-70% of patients waiting to see a physician either have no physical disease but are somatizing stress, or stress is impeding treatment of a physical condition. The Kaiser Permanente Health Plan in northern California discovered in the sixties on review of patient records that 60% of visits were by patients who had no discernable physical disease. The physician CEO of Kaiser, in an invited address in 1993 to a professional audience, restated the 60% while noting the importance of psychological factors in healthcare. There is a wide and growing research literature documenting the fact that psychological intervention can reduce total healthcare costs even among patients with a chronic medical disease. It is essential then for reasons of cost and quality of care that psycho-social practitioners, as collegial practitioners, be integrated into mainstream medical care as primary healthcare. The basic or

general healthcare services of all health professions, as distinct from their specialized services, should be defined within primary care.

Add these up and what is achieved? Administrative streamlining 10-12%; reduced hospitalization, 20% not unrealistic; sharply reduce fraud, 8-10%; and integrate medical/psychological care, easily 10%. These four sources of cost reduction would together achieve a savings of 50%, that's half the cost of today's healthcare.

Additional savings and/or cost control:

5. *Uniform Comprehensive Benefit.* By limiting coverage to services that have been agreed to be professionally necessary and clinically and cost effective, there will be a reduction in services rendered of no established benefit and consequent reduction in healthcare costs.

6. *Rate Setting.* Rates must be sufficient to sustain provider cooperation and interest. Hence, in the short run this is not likely to yield reduced costs. But in the long run, moderation in rate increases can be achieved. There can also be incentives to primary and rural care practitioners to achieve a more equitable distribution of needed services.

7. *Multidisciplinary Participation.* By recognition and broad utilization of all health professions licensed for independent practice, achieve more constructive use of existing professional resources, broader consumer choice and more optimum interdisciplinary cooperation. A modest cost savings is likely.

8. *Minimal Paperwork.* Minimizing paperwork will reduce both administration and practitioner costs thereby enhancing net practitioner income while reducing practitioner resistance. Provision would be made for electronic billing and prompt paperless transfer of provider payment. All providers (by profession and facility) would have a provider number. The elimination of deductibles and co-payments would eliminate paperwork for patients.

9. *Deductibles and Co-payments.* Traditionally, these have been higher for outpatient care thereby promoting hospital use. Their removal will facilitate use of the least intrusive treatment and remove all such billing costs. Choice of plan requiring out-of-pocket expense at the point of selection is a more effective restraint on cost. It will be evident to the patient on prepayment for the plan chosen that it is neither free nor without limits.

10. *Immigration Control.* Removal of immigrant healthcare costs from states could both reduce state costs while focusing federal attention on necessary reform. In 1992-93, there were 322,400 known illegal aliens receiving Medicaid benefits in California at a cost of $899,400,000. The volume is increasing annually. It is alleged that 50% of the mothers of all babies now being born in Los Angeles are illegals. Federal law should be made to change automatic citizenship for offspring born to illegals. No illegal resident is entitled to any healthcare, other than lifesaving emergency care, after which they are subject to deportation.

Neither do they have any means of establishing eligibility while illegal. (See overview above).

11. *Tort Reform.* This is essential to gain reduction in malpractice costs only partly attributable to defensive medicine. It is also essential to replace contingency-based litigation with binding arbitration in civil disputes, to eliminate double recovery of economic damages, set a two-year statute of limitations (repose) in these cases and cap non-economic damages at $250,000.

While the extent of cost reduction which could be achieved by changes 5-9 is less certain, it appears that they could assure, in combination with the first four and the last two, that direct health costs could be more than cut in half. This should be more than sufficient to achieve universal coverage at less than the cost of present healthcare. Global budgeting is intentionally not recommended as it is a too convenient cap which can lead to the rationing of healthcare while avoiding the difficult process of achieving further systemic change. In any event, these "savings" should be in place preparatory to and before the initiation of nationalized healthcare services delivery.

Principles

1. *Universal Coverage.* All US citizens and permanent legal residents are covered. Not covered are:
   a) illegal aliens;
   b) tourists, students and others on temporary residency and persons admitted on a work permit basis, unless temporary coverage has been pre-purchased prior to or at entry, or on the basis of intergovernmental agreement between the USA and country of the alien's citizenship. Tourists with a valid visa may obtain services but only on a fee for service basis. Workers and students with valid visas expected to reside 6 months or longer must have a prepaid health plan otherwise they can have only fee for service care and none at all if their visa is no longer valid.
   c) US born children of illegal aliens (nor should such children have US citizenship at birth such federal law must be voided):
   d) federally admitted or non-deported immigrants without guaranteed employment, who are a direct federal responsibility for any health or welfare benefits.

2. *National Scope.* The Uniform Comprehensive Benefit (UCB) will supersede all of the following:
   a) employer (private and public) provided health coverage for employees, dependents and retirees, including coverage previously negotiated by unions and employer self-insured care;
   b) small employer or individually purchased coverage (whether self-employed, retired or unemployed), all to be allocated regionally to group umbrella coverage;

c) citizens receiving public welfare (state Medicaid);

d) Medicare Part A beneficiaries;

e) Medicare beneficiaries voluntarily enrolled under Part B;

f) healthcare currently mandated under Worker's Compensation (state or federal) consequent to occupational injury (but not including income replacement, disability benefits or settlements, vocational rehabilitation or damages, or necessary care beyond the UCB);

g) healthcare under automobile insurance (but not including disability settlements or income or non-healthcare expense replacement) would be eliminated;

h) all TriCare (formerly CHAMPUS beneficiaries) including dependents of active duty personnel and retired military and their dependents to have choice of plan federally paid (active duty healthcare remains a military responsibility);

i) Indian Health Services and other federal health programs provided to ambulatory US residents.

NOT included are:

i) veterans, for war or military related injury, disability or disease, who remain a federal responsibility;

ii) all imprisoned persons, state or federal, their healthcare remaining a responsibility of the respective governmental entity;

iii) persons institutionalized with chronic or contagious disease who remain the responsibility of their state. States may transfer direction, with funding, to political subdivisions, and may privatize the care by contracting with competing healthcare organizations.

3. *Multidisciplinary.* All professionals licensed to independently provide healthcare shall be broadly recognized within:

a) their licensed scope of practice;

b) any restraints placed on their license;

c) their demonstrated personal competence;

d) the Uniform Comprehensive Benefit;

e) pre-negotiated rates; and

f) standardized procedures and treatment guidelines;

g) integration of mental health within primary care so as to address broad somatization issues.

To the extent that scope of practice overlaps among professions, choice of provider should not be predicated by profession. When the skills of two or more professions are needed, their interdisciplinary collaboration should be on a collegial basis.

4. *Primary Care.* In all stages of organization, development, professional training, and the delivery of direct healthcare services, emphasis will be placed on prevention and primary rather than specialist care. However, the common definition of "primary care" limiting it to the services of four medical specialties (pediatrics,

internal medicine, obstetrics/gynecology and family medicine), misses the fundamental distinction. It is not who does it but what they do. Each of the health professions licensed to independently diagnose, treat and prescribe a treatment plan can and do provide basic or "general healthcare" as distinct from their more specialized services. Primary care must be redefined as general healthcare and, to that extent, recognize such services by all the health professions including behavioral care in as much as psychological issues are a factor in every medical diagnosis. Emphasis will also be placed on restoring functional capacity to the extent it is clinically and economically reasonable, including eyesight, hearing, locomotion and mental health. However, it is the right of any patient to refuse treatment.

5. *Managed Competition.* Plans are to compete on quality of care, access, efficiency and price. Large purchasing pools are to achieve economies of scale. All state laws which preclude or restrict managed competition are preempted. Within each region, to the extent possible, there shall be at least three and preferably more competing plans. Consumers selecting a plan which costs more than the average of the competing plans will lose the tax advantage for the difference as it would be taxable income or an out-of-pocket cost.

6. *Trust Fund.* All funding for included healthcare will be transferred to an independent non-partisan National Healthcare Trust Fund (NHTF). These funds may be expended only for approved health plans, necessary administration and development costs and authorized applied health research. It is intended that the revenues and services costs be in balance. The NHTF will be publicly administered and publicly accountable, but may approve both for-profit or non-profit plans based on quality of care. Any surplus or reserve accounts may only be invested in government obligations having guaranteed principal and do not revert to the General Fund.[1]

7. *Single Collector/Multiple Source Funding.* Given that there is to be universal healthcare with a common UCB, the funding from all relevant sources would be transferred to the NHTF. This would include employer payment for Worker's Compensation healthcare coverage, employee payroll payments for healthcare, allocations from Medicaid coverage, federal government transfers for Medicare and TriCare beneficiaries and so on. Illustrative major current healthcare funding is briefly detailed in the next section, followed by recommended financing to support a National Health Plan and sources of projected savings. Exact amounts will need to be actuarially determined. To cover persons currently under or uninsured will require some social transfer of assets.

8. *Provider Driven Benefit Determination.* The healthcare conditions to be covered and the procedures/services to be recognized will be determined by an Expert

---

[1] Nor can any trust funds be "borrowed" by any member or committee of Congress or otherwise diverted from their intended purpose.

Multidisciplinary Panel (EMP) of 18 members in which all the major primary health care professionals will be represented, including osteopathic medicine, dentistry, optometry, podiatric medicine, pharmacy, social work, medicine (4, family practice; internal medicine, pediatrics, obstetrics & gynecology), psychology (2, clinical psychology, health psychology), nursing (3, nurse practitioner, nurse midwife, school nurse), plus a healthcare economist, an outcome research scientist and a demographer. Once adopted, the UCB will be annually reviewed for possible expansion or change. The EMP will also develop guidelines for the professional resources necessary to deliver the UCB. Except for the initial appointments when "one-third" of members are appointed to five, four and three year terms, succeeding appointees will serve three years. It is intended that benefit determination and delivery will be professionally driven. The EMP is to assure consumer input and may seek specialty or other professional input.

9. *Regional Planning.* Each Statewide Office of Regional Planning (SORP) would oversee the phaseout of excess health facility capacity, the approval of necessary renovation or new construction and the development of community treatment centers were needed and the sharing and limits on purchase of very costly technology. To provide an incentive to effect some provider redistribution to areas of professional shortage the SORP (which may be state contracted) may authorize a modest fee or capitation surcharge for particular communities beyond rates established for the region on concurrence of the NHTF. If their professional staff meet established professional standards and their services would fill a community need, school based clinics and community health centers can be recognized providers. Reasonable access to necessary care is an essential consideration of regional planning. SORPs shall promote managed cooperation among providers and resources in rural areas.

10. *Single Source Funding.* Each capitation or fee for service plan approved by the NHTF will draw its revenue from this Fund, prepaid monthly based on plan enrollment. With each succeeding revenue period, NHTF payment would be reconciled with any changes in enrollment.

11. *Healthcare Identification Card.* Each enrolled resident will have a fake-proof, signed, photo Healthcare Identification Card. These cards are to be smart cards with minimum uniform data sets, including vital health status information.

12. *Providers.* So that there will be a data base for study of utilization, inter-regional differences in care and outcome, providers must complete a record of service on a common data form with a minimum data set for all services rendered.

13. *Quality Assurance.* Professional incompetence whether due to ignorance, loss of ability or impairment associated with abuse of alcohol or drugs or mental disorder, or chronic illness, will be subject to arbitration by small Regional Peer Panels (RPP), with public representation, selected by the SORP. An adverse judgment can lead to prompt suspension or loss of license. Sexual misconduct with a patient is automatic grounds for loss of license. Treatment guidelines

where not followed, or common use of atypical procedures may require justification to such a peer panel, and may increase the risk of malpractice liability. All practitioners will be subject to continuing education and periodic relicensure.

14. *Comprehensiveness.* The UCB will be limited to procedures and treatments that have been shown to be clinically and cost effective and professionally necessary as determined by the Expert Multidisciplinary Panel. An Oregon-type model will be adopted and semi-annually reviewed for refinement. The benefit will be generous and will include mental health services and prescribed drugs. The Oregon model ranks procedures by their degree of known effectiveness (most to least) and their usual cost (least to most) and then by likely frequency to derive a cumulative ranked gradient of estimated cost with a cut-off established for procedures which are likely to exceed the fiscal resources available. Procedures of little promise and low priority will not be funded, also procedures that in a given case are judged professionally to be futile or unnecessary.

15. *Geographic Uniform Rates.* Except for authorized provider supplements to attract services to underserved areas, provider fees by profession and procedure will be uniform throughout each region. There will be national annually approved geographic weights which adjust fees by regions to account for inter-regional economic differences. Balance billing for fees in excess of the set rate or for co-payments or deductibles would be eliminated. The intent is to not only make costs more predictable, but to eliminate cost shifting and needless paperwork. Universal and UCB coverage with consumer choice of plan will also eliminate both "adverse selection" and "cherry picking".

16. *Community Rating.* Within a community, each plan must adhere to a uniform price for all its plan members within actuarially determined age differentials. For like procedure delivered by like profession, on a fee for service basis, the allowed rate will be uniform throughout the community. Since all plans will be in quality of care and price competition, the cost of plan membership may differ between plans.

17. *Uniform Standards.* Standards of licensure and accreditation are to be established nationally across each profession and for each type of health facility subject to state-wide implementation and regular review.

18. *Consumer Choice.* On each annual open enrollment, consumers will have their choice among competing plans available in their community. All plans must include some coverage for out-of area services within the US for people traveling on business or pleasure. Persons who during the year move permanently outside their plan area will be eligible for re-enrollment in the most comparable plan in their new community. Within each plan people will have freedom of choice of plan providers.

19. *Open Annual Enrollment.* There will be annual open enrollment to all competing plans and no person eligible for prepaid healthcare in the community in which services are to be offered can be precluded from choice of available plan.

20. *Non Discrimination.* There shall be no discrimination in the quality of or access to healthcare for any eligible person by practitioner, facility or health plan based upon occupation, personal assets, age, sex, race, religion, national origin, pre-existing or current health condition, for any service recognized under the UCB for U.S. citizens and legal residents.

21. *Benefit Limits.* With universal coverage, the demand for healthcare will increase. Within the professional and fiscal resources available, the Expert Multidisciplinary Panel will determine which services are to be included within the UCB (Oregon model) such that the most effective comprehensive range of services will be available to people who will benefit from them. Emphasis will be on restoration of functional capacity where practical and improvement of the general health of the public. However, anyone paying out of pocket has a choice of any or all services available.

22. *Non-Duplication.* There will be no duplication of benefits and no double payment for services rendered. Those with a Healthcare ID Card may receive all necessary care within the UCB under their plan but no cash for services rendered or not rendered.

23. *Fraud Control.* Service claims filed for injury or illness that are non-existent, for patients who have since died, for services not rendered, for excessive services, or for more complex services than rendered each constitute healthcare fraud. Fraud constitutes grounds for loss of license and is to be aggressively and promptly investigated and eliminated. Final determination will be made by Regional Peer Panels, having counsel and some public representation, and not by state professional licensing boards. Loss of licensure for fraud will apply nationwide. Panel members who have acted in good faith are immune from liability for panel decisions and all RPP meetings are closed and confidential. Collusion to commit fraud is a federal offense warranting loss of license, imprisonment and fine.

24. *No Fault.* All healthcare will be delivered on a no fault basis. Civil disputes based on clear evidence of provider impairment or negligence, incorrect treatment or unwarranted treatment will be resolved by binding arbitration. Damages in such cases for pain and suffering shall be limited to a maximum $250,000. Damages in such cases for impairment of ability to work or function, loss of income, or death will be actuarially determined based on the patient's responsibilities, occupational standing and age, but cannot exceed $2,000,000. The intent is to eliminate litigation from civil dispute, insofar as possible, and to reduce the cost of professional liability (malpractice) insurance. Tort reform is essential to cost control and federal law and standards must preempt all state laws in these respects.

25. *Tax Deduction.* For employers who prepay the UCB costs for their employees, dependents and retirees through payment equal to a percent of payroll or pension, such costs are a tax deductible business expense. To the extent that persons pay for their own or their dependents' UCB costs, whether by payroll

or annuity withholdings, by quarterly income estimates, or prepaid in cash, such costs are deductible from taxable income.

26. *Professional Training.* All governmental support to universities and professional schools for the training of health- care professionals shall be consistent with an emphasis on primary care. All students, in all health professions, as a condition of accepting governmental support for professional training will be bound by a return in service contract to practice in locations where their services are needed. Currently 70% of the 600,000 US physicians are specialists, whereas perhaps 70% of the population needs primary care. Geographic mal-distribution is evident in all professions.

27. *Opt-Out.* Individuals who opt-out of the National Healthcare Plan will not receive a HIDC, will not be entitled to UCB services, and must post evidence of their financial ability to pay for such care as they may need. However, they will not be subject to any assessments on income for the prepayment of healthcare. Professionals who opt out of the plan will not be able to bill eligible patients for any service/procedure covered under the UCB. Employers who elect to be self-insured must post evidence of their ability to pay for all needed healthcare within the UCB for their employees, retirees and dependents.

28. *Sin Taxes.* Over-indulgence in certain foods, alcohol and tobacco products and certain high-risk behaviors such as purchase of hand guns and their ammunition are agreed health hazards. To the extent they are taxed, it should be toward general revenue and not for the support of healthcare. As more healthy lifestyles are adopted, these "sins" will be a dwindling revenue resource.

29. *External Evaluation.* All health plans will be subject to periodic external review for quality and appropriateness of care and for clinical and cost effectiveness by the Statewide Office of Regional Planning. Selection for review will be responsive to community complaints.

30. *Confidentiality.* There shall be respect for patient confidentiality and for individual dignity by all providers within the healthcare system. Communications among professionals and between professionals and patients regarding their care are considered privileged and are otherwise accessible only to courts under felony proceedings, or to the police or victims under duty to warn state laws.

31. *Healthcare.* Healthcare shall be delivered on the basis of informed consent by the patient.

32. *Phase-In.* The National Health Plan will be phased in over five years. It will be adopted in 2010 and $1 billion transferred from general federal revenue to the National Healthcare Trust Fund (NHTF). The Administration, subject to the advice and confirmation of the Senate, will appoint the expert officers of the independent non-partisan NHTF so that it may commence organization and operation January 2011. It will be publicly administered and accountable. The Expert Multidisciplinary Panel (EMP) of 18 members charged with formulating the Uniform Comprehensive Benefit (UCB) will also be appointed by the Administration, subject to the advice and confirmation of the Senate, so

that it may commence organization and operation January 2011. All members of the EMP will have nationally recognized expertise within their own professions. The EMP will be funded by the NHTF and will have two initial concurrent responsibilities. First, provide leadership and consultation to Statewide Offices of Regional Planning (SORP) for the implementation of health education programs for delivery in the schools, the work place and the public media. Second, from the outset commence formulation and plans for delivery of illness, injury and disease prevention programs known to be widely effective (e.g., immunization of children). Both services are to be underway by January 2012.

During the period 2005 to 2006, to gain direct information on the potential advantages and disadvantages of particular aspects of established universal health plans, the EMP will have selected members study the health services in two Canadian provinces such as British Columbia and Ontario, and then study the healthcare services in Hawaii under that state's Prepaid Healthcare Act, and study the universal plan in the United Kingdom. Attention will be given to the delivery of health services in each of these four systems in rural and remote areas and in inner cities.

The EMP will then formulate the Uniform Comprehensive Benefit (UCB) in 2009. Emphasis will be placed on assessment, early intervention, ambulatory primary care and least intrusive care. Only services/procedures known to be clinically and cost effective, and professionally necessary, will be included in the initial draft and there will be actuarial determination of its likely cost. The basic objective is optimum improvement in the general health of the public. During 2010, the EMP will monitor the conduct of pilot healthcare projects in four states selected by the NHTF, incorporating such information as well as that from their prior studies, as pertinent, into the UCB.

The UCB will then be implemented nationwide in 2011. Employer and employee withholding and payments, government fund transfers, and other authorized support will also be collected and transferred to the NHTF from by January 2011.

During 2012, the EMP will monitor the implementation of the UCB and take note of problems which arise and other services which may have proven to be effective or needed and refine/ reformulate the UCB as experience and resources warrant for implementation in 2013. By January 2015, the full-scale national health plan is to be operational. It will then be subject to biennial review for possible improvement.

33. *Elective Additional Coverage.* Once the Uniform Comprehensive Benefit is established, any health plan or insurer may offer additional coverage in the private sector provided it follows community rating and allows open enrollment. Such coverage when employer provided constitutes income to the employee for tax purposes. When purchased by an individual, the cost of elective coverage is not deductible from income for tax purposes.

Funding

Civilian healthcare coverage, or lack of it, now varies widely by employment, income, occupation, health status and age. About 45 million Americans are without healthcare coverage some part of the year, and one in four Americans will lose their healthcare coverage in the next two years for some period of time, approximately 63 million.

Current funding sources are:

1. *Medicare.* Limited to almost all Americans aged 65 and over and the chronically disabled, is a national health insurance plan. According to the 2000 census this age group was 12.4% of the national population but is an increasing proportion of it. Those 45-64 (now 49-68) were 22% of the census population and are beginning to expand the number of Medicare eligibilities.

    Part A, hospital services, paid by a 2.9% tax on all wages without limit. (1.45% employer, 1.45% employee); on a wage of $40,000, $508 by employee. Deductible for 60 days each hospitalization in 2005, $876.

    Part B, "physician" services, voluntary enrollment, deducted from Social Security income or paid by individual or employer. The 2005 per person monthly cost $78.20 ($1876.80 annually per couple), plus the per person $100 annual deductible. Medicare pays only 80% of authorized rate. Many people have "MediGap" insurance to cover the deductibles, co-pays and some excluded services such as out-patient prescription drugs.

2. *Workers Compensation.* With some differences in benefits among federal and state laws, healthcare coverage necessary for all job injured workers is mandated. In California, W/C premium costs have become so excessive that the legislature was forced into benefit restraint with more likely in 2005. Employers who do not provide general healthcare coverage experience higher W/C healthcare costs (cost shifting). One legislative proposal sought 35% W/C premium surcharge to offset.

3. *Medicaid.* Based on 50:50 federal/state matching funds (can be up to 75:25 in states with low economic index). Covers state plan healthcare costs of those on public welfare. Federal law mandates five services. States may add optional services (about 12) in their plan under federal match. Thus, there is wide variation among states in benefit scope, sufficient to induce some interstate migration.

    In 2000, California spent approximately $9 billion in Medicaid services, an average of $2,068 per Medicaid enrollee. Average Medicaid cost in Hawaii in 2003 per eligible child was $1,638, and $3,474 per eligible adult. Finally, total Medicaid costs in Michigan in 1996 was estimated to be over $5.3 billion for approximately 1.1 million eligible individuals, an average of $4800 per eligible person.

4. *TriCare.* Secondary benefit for military related dependents and retirees (about 5.8 million) not enrolled in Medicare. Care received cost $2.9 billion in FY 1992, or $497 per eligible (40% of eligibles used no TriCare services). Comprehensive benefit with $150 deductible/person, $300 per family in 1993, plus 20 or 25% co-pay (active dependent or retiree).

5. *Employers.* Major corporations typically provide healthcare coverage for employees, dependents and retirees. Working poor and migratory workers are typically without coverage, also many self-employed and many small business employees. Major employers are increasingly adopting managed care plans, increasing deductibles and co-pays, and curbing benefits to retirees. The increasing requests of employers for employees to pay a higher proportion of their plan cost has led to a number of union strikes.

The University of California 2005 contribution for high options university approved health plan for an adult couple in Medicare is $590/month, $7,080/year. Plus the couple can pay up to $300 in deductibles and up to $2,000 for out-patient prescription drug co-payments plus the entire cost of enrollment in part B of Medicare ($78.20 x 2 x 12 = $1,877). Thus without any hospital stay their monthly healthcare costs (university and personal) for a Medicare couple even with this high option coverage can readily exceed $900/month. With each open general enrollment there has been growth among the managed care plans having premiums that are fully covered plus some or all of the part B Medicare cost.

6. *Employee.* Hawaii, the only state with mandated employer coverage of employees (with certain exceptions) under its 1974 Prepaid Healthcare Act, requires all covered workers to pay 1.5% of wages toward healthcare.

Recommended Financing

The universal UCB would include the fiscal participation of employers, employees, retirees and government transfers to the NHTF.

1. *Medicare.* Increase the tax rate from 2.9% to 4% of wages. In addition, persons receiving a pension, Social Security payments, withdrawals from tax sheltered retirement plans or annuities to a combined limit of $200,000 per family, $100,000 per person would pay a healthcare charge of 2% on this income. In exchange, the Part A deductible and co-payments would be removed, and by incorporation into the increased payment, the voluntary aspect and contribution to Part B services would be eliminated and long term care added, including case management and home or hospice care.

2. *Medicaid.* Shift the responsibility and cost for the UCB from states to the federal government. Benefits will then be uniform across all states instead of having 50 variants and state bureaucracies. States would no longer receive a federal medicaid match, while the "state match" would become a federal expense from general revenue transferred to the NHFT. States which provide healthcare

benefits to welfare recipients beyond the UCB do so at 100% state expense. The healthcare of persons in state prisons or other state institutions is a state expense. Welfare beneficiaries meeting federal/state plan eligibility requirements will have a choice of enrollment in competing managed care plans. Local government health services necessary in underserved areas will be sustained as appropriate, based on statewide plans and fund transfer.

3. *Worker's Compensation.* Reduce the cost of Worker's Compensation insurance by removing healthcare costs to the extent of UCB coverage but not other aspects such as wage replacement, disability settlements or vocational rehabilitation. Strengthen enforcement of occupational safety and health conditions toward elimination of occupational disease. All fines and cash settlements beyond the cost of enforcement and awards to workers are transferred to the National Healthcare Trust Fund.

4. *TriCare.* The Department of Defense, as a benefit of military service, may determine that persons eligible for these services should receive broader coverage than under the UCB. That would be a federal expense. Since these federally paid healthcare services are primary for all eligibles not having other healthcare coverage (secondary for those who do) and in 2003 cost on average of approximately $625 per eligible per year, then a like amount per eligible (adjusted for future cost change) should be transferred from the DOD budget to the National Healthcare Trust Fund.

5. *Employers.* Since the advancement of fringe benefits during World War II under wage and price controls, employer payment for healthcare plan costs became increasingly popular while wages remained frozen. Major employers in 2004 still commonly pay for the employee's health plan, but with rising costs are increasingly demanding that employees assume part of this cost.

To the extent that employers pay employee health plan costs whether they are full-time, part-time, seasonal, intermittent, or hourly employees or retirees as included (but not independent contractors) their company payroll payments for healthcare will be transferred to the National Healthcare Trust Fund monthly and are an allowed deduction to the company as a business expense. Where two workers are married, even if employed by different companies, the payroll determination for their family plan will be based on the highest wage worker. There will be no duplication of coverage.

6. *Employees.* Legislation must be enacted so that to the extent employees, including the self-employed, pay part or all of their health plan expense that amount is to be an income tax credit but this credit cannot exceed their tax owed. If they pay no income tax there is no tax credit.

7. *Self-employed.* While they may choose and pay for any health plan on the market to suit their needs, they may well find a Medical Savings Account (MSA) backed by a high deductible catastrophic health insurance plan to be an ideal choice. The money in their MSA, which can be added to yearly, is tax sheltered and can be used to cover minor medical expenses and as it grows could well cover their annual deductible of say $1000 to $2000 or $3000. Any medical expense

beyond that is covered by the catastrophic plan. The catastrophic insurance premium of all such accounts would be transferred to the NHTF to pay the insurer.

According to the 2002 census bureau report there were more than 17.6 million Americans who work for and by themselves, a 3.2% increase over the previous year.

The recommended sources of financing are intended as a workable scheme to be fine-tuned by actuarial data. There will be no health insurance premiums for services within the UCB, including long term care. Insurers may offer coverage for services beyond the UCB, for disability income insurance, personal liability, life insurance and other insurance products.

System Change

The adoption of a prepaid National Health Plan with Uniform Comprehensive Benefit would not only change the financing of healthcare, and the delivery of services, but would significantly expand the economic marketplace for healthcare. System change would:

1. eliminate cost shifting between private and public care;
2. eliminate welfare interstate migration in search of higher benefits;
3. eliminate the need for TriCare or other overlapping healthcare coverage systems;
4. remove the substantial healthcare costs from Workers' Compensation;
5. eliminate healthcare from automobile/vehicle health insurance;
6. free employees from "job-lock" so that they may pursue other opportunities;
7. assure that persons laid off continue to have healthcare access to sustain their health and facilitate their reemployment;
8. eliminate pre-existing conditions and adverse selection as factors precluding coverage;
9. assure the self-employed, the migratory worker, the working poor, employees of small business, the unemployed and retirees of healthcare coverage;
10. prevent financial ruination of those who experience catastrophic healthcare costs, including long term care;
11. enable rational planning to effect better distribution of healthcare resources, personnel and facilities;
12. enable economies of scale in the purchase of supplies and negotiation of rates;
13. facilitate the acquisition of reliable and comprehensive data bases for the conduct of utilization, outcome and other applied research necessary to improving the quality of healthcare, its cost-effectiveness and the effectiveness of health practitioners;

14. standardization of provider service claim forms, reduce need for marketing and advertising, and reduce the cost of administration and overhead among the competing managed care plans;
15. achieve a more equitable distribution of healthcare cost over a national base;
16. reduce the cost of professional malpractice insurance and generally remove litigation as a healthcare cost in time and money; by delivery of healthcare on a no-fault basis and use of arbitration in any disputes (except felony charges) under Tort Reform;
17. reduce healthcare costs and raise the quality of practice by aggressive pursuit and virtual elimination of fraud among providers and remove from practice of licenses when indicted.

Roles of Participants in National Healthcare Plan

Federal Administration

1. Establish the National Healthcare Trust Fund as a publicly run, publicly accountable Trust;
2. Establish the Expert Multidisciplinary Committee of 18. It is intended that the EMC will formulate the UCB and that this professionally determined benefit package will be subject to regular EMC review and will always be professionally driven;
3. When the UCB becomes available transfer all employer payments to the National Healthcare Plan to the Trust;
4. Likewise, transfer all employee payments for healthcare to the Trust;
5. Likewise, transfer all self employed quarterly health costs estimates to the Trust;
6. Transfer all Medicare taxes (employer and employee) to the Trust;
7. Transfer all Medicaid funding for those on public welfare to the Trust on the basis of x dollars per eligible from general revenue;
8. Transfer a set amount to the Trust for each dependent of active duty military personnel and for retired military and their dependents from the Department of Defense budget;
9. Make like transfer from general revenue on a per person basis for all other federal health programs, such as Indian Health Services, sufficient to fund the UCB;
10. Increase the monitoring and enforcement of Occupational Safety and Health Standards;
11. Enforce the Clean Air Act and the systematic elimination of water pollution and the containment of toxic waste. Contract with private or public agents with the expertise to expedite the control of pollution and toxic waste;
12. Annually authorize and fund the support of peer reviewed applied research in healthcare on treatment effectiveness, treatment

guidelines, rate setting and other operational problems;

13. Enact legislation preempting all state/local laws that preclude or restrict the use of managed care or other forms of useful organized care;
14. Transfer funding to the Trust to support students in professional training who enter binding return in service contracts to communities of professional shortage;
15. Fund pilot projects in 2010 in four states that exemplify diversity in healthcare delivery, including Oregon and Hawaii, to gain data on the advantages of their different modes of health service delivery.

National Healthcare Trust Fund (NHTF)

1. Fund the Expert Multidisciplinary Committee;
2. Based on revenue received, adopt budgeting and planning to support universal healthcare for all US citizens and legal residents;
3. On a community rating basis, fund approved competing healthcare plans on a prepaid basis across the country which have the resources to guarantee delivery of the UCB and provide assurance that healthcare will be professionally driven and/or contract with various agencies;
4. Implement a uniform national data base management information system on services rendered and their cost, enabling empirically based determination of current utilization and projections of future utilization, review of regional and age differences in use and professional participation, the cost effectiveness of services, and other studies to assist in strategic planning and distribution of resources;
5. Annually negotiate provider rates by profession and region, drug formulary costs, major supplies and health facility budgets;
6. Select four mainland states to pilot or test innovative models such as the Kaiser Permanente Plan on the West Coast, and from this experience modify national planning as needed before nationwide implementation;
7. Study the Hawaii Prepaid Healthcare Act implemented since 1974, the first state with employer mandated coverage, identifying experience cogent to implementation of the National Healthcare Plan;
8. Similarly, study the health services in two Canadian provinces such as British Columbia and Ontario to ascertain, in particular, solutions for the delivery of healthcare in rural and remote areas and in inner cities and to indigenous people. Study the United Kingdom plan for methods, principles and service delivery potentially beneficially applicable to the USA.

Expert Multidisciplinary Panel (EMP)

1. Elect own tri-annual rotating chair;
2. Formulate and oversee implementation of health education strategy;
3. Formulate and oversee implementation of disease prevention services;

4. Giving priority to services that are clinically and cost effective, based on hard data, plus multidisciplinary judgment, formulate a UCB in which services are ranked;
5. Appoint no more than 10 consultants on a temporary (up to annual) basis for assistance and information on health education, prevention services or development of the UCB;
6. Fit the UCB to expected revenue;
7. All competing managed care plans and other entities which compete to be service providers must bid on the basis of agreeing to provide the full UCB as appropriate;
8. The competing plans may be for profit or not for profit, private or public;
9. In coordination with the National Healthcare Trust Fund, redetermine the UCB periodically, based on experience, new data, innovations in healthcare delivery, changes in expected purchasing power, and changes in expected fiscal resources.

Managed Competition Plans

1. As approved and funded by the NHTF, oversee delivery of the UCB;
2. Consistent within plan, providers can be paid on a fee for service basis, salary, case rate or capitation. Where FFS, rates cannot exceed those negotiated by the Trust for each profession;
3. Pay hospitals and health facilities according to negotiated local contracts on DRG, or per diem basis;
4. Issue individual Healthcare Identification Cards to all members. The fake-proof smart card shows full patient name, date of birth, photo and signature. It is encoded with plan and patient numbers, and Social Security number and will include vital health status information. The card is electronically entered with each service;
5. Establish non-discriminatory standards for all qualified, interested practitioners, all recognized professions;
6. Practitioner participation requires in-service orientation, selected continuing education, intermittent but infrequent audit review by peers regarding quality of care and adherence to treatment guidelines, and rotating relicensure;
7. Professionals who are owners of health facilities, laboratories or specialized services used by a plan, to avoid conflict of interest, cannot be practitioners in that plan unless aforementioned facilities are nonprofit;
8. No payment to patients for healthcare rendered;
9. No payment to providers for referrals;
10. Each plan to have risk reinsurance to guarantee fiscal solvency and plan cannot speculate with any reserve funds.

Statewide Office of Regional Planning (SORP)

1. Funded by state from general revenue (states will no longer have Medicaid health costs);
2. Review the occupancy of health facilities and project how this may change with universal coverage;
3. Oversee the phase-out of excess capacity or development of new resources as needed, including underserved areas;
4. Exercise control over the purchase, distribution and duplication of costly technology;
5. Monitor provider location and identify areas of professional shortage to qualify for fulfillment of professional training return in service contracts;
6. Authorize modest fee or capitation surcharges for professionals in severe shortage areas on agreement with the NHTF;
7. Appoint small Regional Peer Panels (with a public member) independent of the national licensing board to review and arbitrate with dispatch on complaints of professional incompetence/ misfeasance, or sexual abuse of patients. Adverse finding can institute probation, suspension or loss of license;
8. Examine cases of reported or suspected fraud. When a practitioner is found guilty, this adverse finding can institute placement on probation, suspension or loss of license and/or fine dependent of the extent of fraud. Where the fraud involves collusion between practitioners or with others, it is a federal offense and there is not only loss of license but fine and imprisonment in relation to the extent of fraud;
9. Generate provider profiles for audit review by peer panel;
10. Conduct periodic review of the quality of service rendered by each health plan;
11. Under guidelines of Expert Multidisciplinary Panel, oversee implementation of health education and disease prevention and management programs.

Implications of a National Health Plan for Practitioners

Unless you are practicing in remarkable isolation you know that managed and competitive healthcare is here and that it has replaced the majority of traditional indemnity health insurance plans. The industrialization of healthcare that is before us and progressing was both predictable and predicted. Think of healthcare not only as a public good but as a public need. In that sense, in an economic society, its purpose has elements in common with utilities, banking or agriculture. Because healthcare is so important to the well being of the country and requires such massive capital expenditure, it is remarkable that it has not been more organized long ago.

The managed competition movement in healthcare is the consequence of two forces. First, federal law, policy and funding have promoted these developments. Recall that the Health Maintenance Organization Act of 1973 (PL 93-202) preempted all state laws precluding the development of managed systems of care. "No state may establish or enforce any law which prevents a health maintenance organization ..." Hundreds of millions of federal dollars were provided as seed money. Then there were laws creating professional standards review organizations (PSRO) broadly implementing the concept of peer review to better assure the quality of care. The Agency for Healthcare Policy and Research was created and given as a major mission, the development of data based treatment guidelines. The concept of Resource Based Relative Value Schedules has also been implemented in recent years, intended both to effect a shift from specialty to primary care and to preserve fee-for-service practice as one viable choice in service delivery. Medicare, of course, is a national health insurance program. Progressively, over the past decade in particular, the range of health professions recognized as providers has been expanding. All these professions are now required to report to Medicare using CPT-4 (current procedure terminology). Other legislation could be cited, but, clearly, Congress has been determined to effect major changes in the manner in which healthcare services are delivered and paid for.

The funds expended on healthcare today exceed the budget for several major federal departments combined, and have risen to consume 14.6% of our Gross Domestic Product. Stated otherwise one dollar in every seven in the U. S. is expended on healthcare. That cash flow volume has attracted many entrepreneurial corporations for good reason. The realization of the extent to which our national economy is consumed by healthcare without universal coverage awakens us to the dimension and shortfalls of our current non-system, the many parties involved, and their competing and political interests.

There is enormous potential to improve the quality of care while reducing its costs by identifying what works. We can eliminate procedures/methods/ substances that are without proven benefit for specific conditions (ineffective care). We can, based on peer review and treatment guidelines, eliminate unnecessary care (over-utilization). And alerted to the problem, we can devise strategies to eliminate misrepresentation (conflict of interest, fraud and collusion).

Managed care programs simply, by their scope and volume, can generate data on healthcare utilization and outcome that is impossible in a solo private practice. They can also marshal a range of professional expertise in both scope and depth that is simply not accessible to an individual practitioner. And, of course, they can deliver services at varying levels of intensity twenty-four hours a day, seven days a week, year round.

Healthcare has industrialized no less than merchandising, marketing, manufac-turing, agriculture and investing. In the main, the growth and initiation of healthcare enterprises have been capitalized by IPOs (initial public offerings). All the major healthcare corporations are publicly traded. You can learn more in a month about the real developments underway in healthcare from reading the Wall Street Journal than from attending most professional conventions or reading mainstream professional journals.

The majority of health professionals licensed for practice today in most of the major professions are engaged in private practice. What can they expect under a National Health Plan?

1. When all citizens are equally entitled to healthcare, the distinctions between public and private care will progressively evaporate.

2. Very few practitioners who continue in practice will not experience substantive change in the nature of their practice, in the case-mix they serve, in the manner in which they are reimbursed, and in the peer oversight they experience.

3. As competing health plans are organized and implemented across the country, they will begin to saturate large urban markets first. Already, in more than six centers such as Minneapolis/St. Paul, Portland, Sacramento and San Diego, managed care plans control more than 50% of the marketplace, that is, more than 50% of the residents receive their healthcare through their health plan membership. This is progressive and expanding.

4. The opportunities for salaried professional employment will expand and prove attractive to an increasing proportion of licensees, particularly younger professionals.

5. Mobility among health professionals will increase, partly in response to employment opportunities outside their area partly in response to new opportunities afforded by national licensure, partly in response to the economic pressures of professional school return-in-service training contracts, partly in response to new incentives from rural and other areas that previously did not have the funds or organization to support a practice, and partly in response to the shrinkage in their own practice.

6. There will be more continuing education but less litigation. The consuming public (patients) will be far better informed and practitioners will be more publicly accountable. A requirement of rotating relicensure will be a stimulant to advancing professional competence and thereby the quality of care available. To accomplish this continuing education will be monitored for scientific credibility and effectiveness.

7. The more that access to quality healthcare is perceived as a public right, the more there will be public, political and financial pressure to reshape healthcare delivery in the perceived public interest. A major public debate is now underway and, while the health professions will have some input, it seems very unlikely that they will make the final or fundamental decisions that will determine the future of healthcare services in this country as it will be delineated in a National Health Plan.

Acknowledgements

The original proposal has been refined in detail and expanded since its 1993 and 1994 presentations to the National Academies of Practice. Several members of an NAP Task Force on the Financing of Healthcare sent suggestions on the earlier draft which have been helpful in its reformulation: Eric Hubbard, DPM; Bettie S. Jackson, EdD, RN, MBA; Helen Rehr, DSW; and Rob Blackman, MD, via Erwin Small, DVM. In the current revision the author recognizes the input of Nicholas Cummings, Ph.D., Michael A. Cucciare, M.A., and William O'Donohue, Ph.D.

About the Author

Herbert Dörken received his PhD in clinical psychology from the University of Montreal in 1951 and was the Chief Psychologist in a 1600 bed mental hospital in the Montreal area for 8 years. His research on treatment effectiveness and on the differentiation on senile dementia and senescent decline gained visibility. In 1956 he became the Consultant in Psychology to the Canadian Department of National Health and Welfare at the time Canada's National Health Plan was being formulated and was active in a federal: provincial program to subsidize the training of professional mental health manpower under return in service contracts. As State Director of Community Mental Health Services from 1959-62 he designed, developed and directed Minnesota's network of community mental health centers bringing mental health expertise to the state's largely rural areas. In California, as Deputy Director, Chief of Psychology and Chief of Research for the Department of Mental Hygiene from 1962-73, he was active in promoting insurance coverage for mental disorder, augmenting the staffing of state facilities and redesigning and administering a multidisciplinary multi-million dollar program of applied research. From 1973-82 he was Adjunct Professor and Research Psychologist at the University of California Medical School, San Francisco, where he taught graduate courses on the Impact of Law and Regulation on Professional Practice, Cost As the Driving Force in Healthcare Reform and the Industrialization of Healthcare. He was also involved in policy research in the legislative process, drafting a number of bills which were later enacted into law. He retired in 1982 to become co-principal investigator (with Dr. N.A. Cummings, founding NAP President) of a 8 year HCFA funded research project demonstrating the positive Impact of Psychological Intervention on Total Healthcare Costs in Hawaii's Medicaid Population, including a federal employee comparison group gaining substantial cost reductions. He has since been active as a Registered Lobbyist in California, regularly writing new legislation, and also has been Scientific Director of the Foundation for Behavioral Health since 1983. Formerly the Chair of the Committee on Health Insurance (COHI), and then member of the Board of Professional Affairs, American Psychological Association, he is a fellow of its divisions of clinical psychology, public service, health psychology, and independent practice and is also, and a life fellow of the American Public Health Association. Over the past 57 years he has had an interest and involvement in various aspects of the Financing and Organization of Healthcare.

References

American Medical Association. (1989). *The impaired physician: A special report.* Chicago, IL: Author.

Cummings, N. A. (2002). The National Academies of Practice: An organization to bring the health professions together. In J. L. Thomas, J. L. Cummings, & W. T. O'Donohue (Eds.), *The entrepreneur in psychology. The collected papers of Nicholas A. Cummings, Volume 2* (pp. 95-135). Phoenix, AZ: Zeig, Tucker & Thiessen.

Dorken, H. (1994). *The financing and organization of healthcare in America: A proposal to the National Academies of Practice.* Washington, DC: National Academies of Practice.

Gingrich, N. (2004). A better way. *Forbes,* p. 36.

Institute of Medicine. (2001). *Crossing the quality chasm: A new health system for the 21st century.* Washington DC: National Academy of Sciences.

Kiesler, C. A., Cummings, N. A., & VandenBos, G. R. (Eds.) (1979). *Psychology and National Health Insurance: A sourcebook.* Washington, DC: American Psychological Association.

Chapter 4

Implementing Integrated Behavioral Health Care in TRICARE

Blake Chaffee
TriWest Healthcare Alliance

TriWest Healthcare Alliance is Phoenix-based corporation that partners with the Department of Defense (DoD) to provide access to cost-effective, high-quality health care for our nation's active and retired uniformed services members and their families. These individuals are eligible for the DoD's regionally managed health care program for the military, called TRICARE. TriWest is under contract with the DoD to manage and administer TRICARE throughout the 21-state TRICARE West Region that includes:

Alaska	Kansas	North Dakota
Arizona	Minnesota	Oregon
California	Missouri*	South Dakota
Colorado	Montana	Utah
Hawaii	Nebraska	Washington
Idaho	Nevada	Wyoming
Iowa*	New Mexico	Texas (El Paso area)

*Areas not included are certain ZIP codes in the St. Louis MO area and the Rock Island Arsenal area in Iowa.

Included in the TRICARE West Region are:

- 2,260,865 sq. mi.;
- Approximately 2.6 million TRICARE eligible beneficiaries;
- A network of approximately 80,000 providers, including 6,000 behavioral health providers;
- 7 U. S. Air Force major commands;
- 5 U. S. Army Medical Centers;
- 10 Veterans Integrated Service Networks (VISN);
- 1 Naval Medical Center;
- 5 Naval hospitals;

- 9 Naval clinics;
- 13 Coast Guard Clinics

TriWest has been a DoD contractor since 1996 and was most recently awarded its current five-year contract for the new West Region. With the West Region contract, TriWest becomes the largest DoD contractor based in the state of Arizona and holds the 10th largest DoD contract in the United States. TriWest is owned by an alliance of 15 Blue Cross Blue Shield plans and two university hospitals. TriWest currently employs more than 1,200 staff, 600 of whom are based in Arizona.

As part of its proposal to the government, TriWest outlined a program of integrated behavioral health that included in-house behavioral health staff and collaborative care programs at military treatment facilities (MTF) within the West Region. TriWest planned to develop its integrated behavioral health program in three distinct phases:

- Carving in its carve-out contract
- Developing integrated behavioral health infrastructure
- Launching integrated behavioral health pilot projects

From Carve-Out to Carve-In

Throughout its previous contract, TriWest subcontracted to Merit Behavioral Care (MBC), a subsidiary of Magellan Behavioral Health for behavioral health services. Although this traditional "carve-out" arrangement was quite successful for both companies and beneficiaries in the previous Central Region, TriWest decided to develop its own program of integrated behavioral health (IBH) for the new West Region contract. This presented more than the usual challenges because implementation of the West Region involved three separate phases, and the MBC staff was required to meet Central Region contract performance requirements until all three phases were complete.

Central Region Contract Operations

TriWest's Central Region contract behavioral health operations were located in its Phoenix headquarters which housed approximately 75 MBC staff. The MBC TRICARE operation was a classic behavioral health carve-out, including its own customer service, provider and beneficiary education, provider contracting, claims review, information services and crisis line functions. These staff implemented and operated the TRICARE behavioral health program in the 15 states of the Central Region serving approximately 1.2 million beneficiaries.

The New West Region Contract Operations

TriWest's new West Region contract behavioral health operations are located in the four functional areas of its Health Care Services (HCS) division at the Phoenix corporate headquarters and five regional hub locations:

- Tacoma
- Colorado Springs
- Phoenix
- San Diego
- Honolulu

Behavioral health staff are co-located with their medical/surgical counterparts at the corporate headquarters in utilization, quality, case management and population health improvement. The regional hub locations, designed to provide more personalized and local medical management and customer service, are staffed with both medical/surgical and behavioral health beneficiary services, utilization management and case managers, customer service representatives, and field operations personnel.

Implementation of the new West Region contract occurred in three phases with the start of health care delivery:

- June 1, 2004: Washington and Oregon
- July 1, 2004: California, Nevada and Hawaii
- October 1, 2004: the 15 states of the previous Central Region

The Transition to Integrated Behavioral Health

The current trend toward integrated behavioral health programs has developed with the recognition that large numbers of patients receiving medical/surgical care have behavioral health issues that may account for their physical symptoms or affect their medical condition. Extensive research has shown that directly addressing the psychological issues of these patients may not only relieve their distress/dysfunction but also reduce their medical utilization. As many as 70% of all health care visits have a psychosocial basis (Fries et al., 1993). Even when behavioral health involvement is observed, many of the patients presenting these symptoms will not be treated adequately (Eisenberg, 1992; Klinkman, 1997; Mumford, Schlesinger, Glass, Patrick, & Cuerdon, 1984; Saravay & Cole, 1999; Schulberg, Katon, Simon, & Rush, 1998; Simon & VonKorff, 1995; Tiemens, Ormel, & Simon, 1996; Gallo & Coyne, 2000; Williams, 1998). A primary care physician makes the initial diagnosis in 42% of patients with clinical depression and in 47% with generalized anxiety disorder. (National Mental Health Association, 2000). About 50% of all mental health care is delivered by primary care physicians. They prescribe 70% of all psychotropic medications, yet the primary care system is not prepared to deal with many of these patients. Frustrated patients often overload the primary care system because their behavioral health needs are not adequately identified and addressed. Underdiagnosis, inadequate treatment and lack of patient follow-up after treatment is initiated perpetuate medical/surgical service utilization by patients with behavioral health problems. In a carve-out system of delivery, the primary care provider's only option is referral of the patient to a mental health provider/system that is equally unprepared to deal with medical/surgical issues. Behavioral health providers frequently do not adequately address behavioral health issues in the context of disease or somatization and therefore do not provide efficient, cost-effective care. The TriWest integrated behavioral health program aims to create a clinical environment that supports early identification and more appropriate treatment of behavioral health problems associated with physical disorders and utilization of health care resources.

TriWest Model for Integrated Behavioral Care

TriWest is adopting an integrated behavioral health approach in its medical management program. TriWest's first step was to replace its previous carve-out model of behavioral care with one in which TriWest manages all health care. The expectation is that this change will improve overall care of the beneficiary population, optimize use of the military treatment facilities (MTF), improve efficiency, and raise the level of customer satisfaction.

In the TriWest model, the principals of population health improvement (PHI) will ensure a continuous focus on the entire spectrum of health. A strong emphasis on PHI will reduce the incidence of disease, promote healthy lifestyles, and improve early identification of pathologies in a system that places *equal* emphasis on physical and behavioral needs.

The transition will be completed through a graduated series of incremental changes in organizational structure and management for a seamless transition to integrated behavioral health care. Behavioral health management will be integrated with all other health care under the direction of Health Care Services. Within this framework, TriWest will focus on three populations within behavioral health care. The first will be traditional specialty behavioral care with a heavy emphasis on child and adolescent health, the "core" behavioral health business. The second will be behavioral health services for those with long-term medical illnesses, and the third will focus on high medical utilizers where behavioral intervention is likely to improve health and reduce the need for future medical services.

Concept for Transition

TriWest will introduce integrated behavioral health care in three phases. Phasing will minimize disruption and present a seamless transition to both our beneficiaries and the staff of the MTFs. During the initial conversion phase, TriWest assumed operational control of all behavioral health operations, but almost all other components of health care delivery will remained unchanged. Behavioral health staff were integrated with their medical/surgical counterparts in the hubs and corporate functional areas, including utilization management, quality management, case management and population health improvement. "Integration" of medical/surgical and behavioral health staff does *not* mean that they function interchangeably, but that their individual skill sets complement each other and are available when needed to collaborate on cases. There were no changes made at the provider/patient level. This was the "Carve-Out to Carve-In" phase.

During the next phase, we will develop the processes, technology and organization needed for full integration. Training for full integration will be initiated, still ensuring no disruption in ongoing care delivery. This is the "Infrastructure Development" phase. During this phase, integrated care management and delivery processes will be developed and refined to optimize their effectiveness within the TriWest provider network. Planning and training will also begin for the implementation of pilot projects utilizing behavioral health providers in selected MTF primary care settings. This phase will also involve identification and development of network and community resources offering behavioral health services designed for an integrated delivery model.

Phase Three is "Integrated Behavioral Health Pilot Development." This phase is the first step toward integration of traditional Primary Care with Behavioral Care done on a site-by-site basis using small, fully trained teams of providers. This phase will implement pilot projects at selected MTF primary care sites to develop the processes, technology and organization necessary for optimization of MTF primary care.

Carving-in the Carve-out

Carving-in the carve-out contract TriWest had with MBC for seven years was an essential step in developing TriWest's in-house integrated behavioral health (IBH) program and had nothing to do with MBC's contract performance. MBC had, in fact, managed the TRICARE behavioral health program extraordinarily well, as its utilization and beneficiary satisfaction measures indicated. TriWest's decision was simply based on moving with the health care industry trend toward integrated behavioral health programs. Carve-out contracts had, in fact, become the standard approach to managing TRICARE's exceptionally complex and generous behavioral health benefit.. Historically, there were several reasons for this:

- Carve-out contracts utilized managed behavioral health organizations (MBHOs) that specialized in behavioral health , bringing expertise the prime contractors, typically HMOs, lacked.
- Carving-out behavioral health gave the prime contractor predictability over its behavioral health costs.
- TRICARE carve-outs were appealing to MBHOs because TRICARE's generous benefit and high behavioral health costs presented ample management and profit opportunities.

Managed behavioral health carve-out programs in TRICARE successfully reduced behavioral health care costs without limiting access to care that was medically/psychologically necessary. Behavioral health care costs that were escalating uncontrollably in the mid-1980s are now much more in line with commercial program experience. MBHOs accomplished this with a combination of provider network discounts, utilization management of acute inpatient and RTC admissions, and increasing use of lower levels of care. In a paradoxical sense, MBHOs risk becoming victims of their own success, in the TRICARE Program and elsewhere because, by successfully managing behavioral health utilization, reducing costs and maintaining them at relatively reasonable, constant levels, the effect of their management is no longer evident to the prime contractor/payor in costs savings. This may allow the less informed and insightful payors to conclude that they no longer need the expertise of the MBHO because behavioral health costs are no longer a problem.

Consider TriWest's TRICARE contract as a case-in-point. With the generous TRICARE behavioral health benefit levels, the only reason that behavioral health care costs remain at reasonable levels is because they are well-managed. Without continued management of behavioral health utilization by behavioral health staff, utilization and costs could easily escalate. In carving-in its behavioral health carve-out contract, it will be crucial for TriWest to maintain the capacity to manage the core business of its behavioral health program, i.e., cases with exclusively behavioral health diagnoses, while developing its integrated behavioral health program. Integrated behavioral health has nothing to do with these cases because integrated behavioral health is not a substitute for behavioral health care management but an additional management program aimed at dually diagnosed cases, i.e., cases with both behavioral health and medical/surgical diagnoses. The carve-in, therefore, should seek to establish within TriWest the MBHO expertise in managing "core" behavioral health business, i.e., cases with exclusively behavioral health diagnoses. Development of an integrated behavioral health program is a separate development effort.

Continuing to operate the Central Region contract while starting up two phases of the new West Region contract presented unique problems. Many of the MBC staff employed by Magellan in the Central Region contract were interested in continued employment with TriWest for the new West Region contract; however, Magellan was under contract with TriWest to continue Central Region operations until September 30, 2004. The goals of TriWest and its subcontractor Magellan were diametrically opposite: TriWest wanted to recruit as many experienced MBC personnel as possible for its new start-up while Magellan wanted to retain as many of its staff as possible to continue to perform on the previous Central Region contract. This presented a barrier to TriWest's recruiting MBC staff in time for the start-up of two of the three phases of its West Region contract. Fortunately, TriWest and Magellan successfully negotiated a plan to accomplish both goals. TriWest agreed not to hire any MBC staff for start dates before October 1, 2004, and Magellan agreed that selected staff composing a "transition team" could work part-time on West Region start-up activities, and TriWest would reimburse Magellan for their services.

In addition to this arrangement, two other mechanisms were utilized to facilitate the transition of experienced MBC staff to positions with TriWest. First, TriWest managers recruiting several positions of the same job type for the various phases of the new contract implementation were asked to designate MBC staff for positions with October 1 start dates. Secondly, for certain positions that were critical to transition and start-up, earlier release dates were negotiated with MBC when the individual candidate's job functions could be back-filled by temporary personnel or otherwise accommodated. These two mechanisms and the leaseback arrangement turned a management conundrum into a win-win-win scenario:

- Magellan fulfilled its Central Region contract obligations
- TriWest successfully completed all 3 phases of its West Region contract implementation, and
- MBC employees were successfully transitioned to positions with TriWest

Integrated Behavioral Health Infrastructure Development

There is *some* overlap between the integrated behavioral health population and the "core" business of managed behavioral health care, i.e., patients with exclusively behavioral health diagnoses (because they also get sick), but these are essentially two distinct populations. While its approach considers each person as both a psychological and physical being, integrated behavioral health is primarily directed at those patients with psychological factors affecting their physical condition and utilization of health care resources. This approach requires specific expertise and tools to be effectively implemented. Melek (1999) offers the following list of objectives and structures that organizations include in their integration of behavioral and primary care services:

- Mental health professionals are just "one of the docs", as on-site members of the primary care medical team;
- Behavioral professionals function as on-site consultants to primary care providers (PCP);
- Smooth transitions between the medical and behavioral health portions of care (increasing the perception among users that the different providers are part of the same treatment program or team);
- Coordination of separate but related behavioral health and medical agendas and care (inter-departmental and inter-clinic planning, case management, and program development);
- Behavioral health therapy groups run in primary care settings (e.g., adolescent psychotherapy groups run in pediatric as opposed to mental health settings; newly pregnant, substance abusing women educated and treated in obstetrics clinics);
- Creation of innovative care programs to increase patient self-management and awareness (hypertension management, asthma self-management, "skills not pills", and reconditioning exercise programs);

- Multi-departmental treatment of such conditions as chronic pain or Attention Deficit Hyperactivity Disorder, allowing providers to see a more global approach to care of patients, decreasing the possibility of certain treatment elements being overlooked;
- Case-finding programs – the process by which certain cases or illnesses are sought out, with the idea that early intervention will prevent more costly care down the road (e.g., inpatient medical and surgical patients with evidence of alcohol or drug problems; emergency room patients seen for symptoms of panic disorder);
- Joint staff meetings between medical and behavioral healthcare professionals
- Increased use of technology and online medical information;
- Video conferencing teaching sessions for PCPs on behavioral healthcare topics

Most of the current literature concerns integrated behavioral health programs in health care delivery settings. Integrated behavioral health programs in health care delivery settings typically involve training behavioral health clinicians in behavioral health primary care and placing them in primary care settings where they practice in a collaborative care model with primary care physicians (Cummings, 2001). Based on research showing that a large percentage of primary care patients receive no medical diagnosis, integrated behavioral care attempts to provide behavioral health consultation, brief treatment and referral in the primary care setting. Patients are generally more receptive to behavioral health services provided in this way, and collaborative care models avoid problems with traditional referrals from primary care physicians to behavioral health specialists. Research shows that as few as 20% of patients referred for behavioral health consultation actually follow through (O'Donohue, Cummings & Ferguson, 2003). Integrated behavioral health delivery models fall into two major categories, those in which the behavioral health clinicians practices "primary behavioral health" and those in which the behavioral health clinician serves as a consultant to the PCP. In the former, the behavioral health clinician functions as an integral part of the primary care clinic team and is readily available on-site for immediate introduction to prospective patients.

In fact, the "hallway hand-off" which introduces the behavioral health clinician to the patient and initiates the behavioral health primary care intervention may actually free primary care physician time which otherwise would have been spent discussing the patient's behavioral health concerns. In the consultation model, the behavioral health clinician may maintain a more traditional group and individual psychotherapy practice in the primary care clinic. Regardless of the integrated behavioral health model employed, patients are more receptive to behavioral health intervention in a primary care clinic setting than to care in the psychiatric clinic.

Integrating behavioral health in a health care management organization presents different challenges, but the principles of integrated behavioral health still apply. Integration in this context does not mean integrating behavioral health resources into medical/surgical health care delivery operations. Instead, medical/

surgical and behavioral health staff function in a variant of the collaborative care model described above, focusing on the following subset of structure and objectives Melek (1999) provides:

- Coordination of separate but related behavioral health and medical agendas and care (inter-departmental and inter-clinic planning, case management, and program development);
- Case-finding programs – the process by which certain cases or illnesses are sought out, with the idea that early intervention will prevent more costly care down the road (e.g., inpatient medical and surgical patients with evidence of alcohol or drug problems; emergency room patients seen for symptoms of panic disorder);
- Creation of innovative care programs to increase patient self-management and awareness (hypertension management, asthma self-management, "skills not pills", and reconditioning exercise programs);
- Multi-departmental treatment of such conditions as chronic pain or Attention Deficit Hyperactivity Disorder, allowing providers to see a more global approach to care of patients, decreasing the possibility of certain treatment elements being overlooked;
- Joint staff meetings between medical and behavioral healthcare professionals
- Increased use of technology and online medical information;

Relatively little has been written or published on developing integrated behavioral health programs in managed care organizations (MCO).

TriWest considers its integrated behavioral health program an additional line of business for its behavioral health program that its staff will implement. This does not mean that all behavioral health staff are involved in both the core behavioral health business, i.e., cases with exclusively behavioral health diagnoses, and the integrated behavioral health program. There are some components of the core behavioral health business that have little or nothing to do with integrated behavioral health, e.g., residential treatment center admissions evaluation, crisis line, and peer review, and appeals processing for cases with exclusively behavioral health diagnoses. This is a major reason that integrated behavioral health programs that initially attempted "total integration" have instead developed collaborative care models. At TriWest, we have centralized and separated these "core" behavioral health functions from the utilization and case management operations in our five regional hubs. Behavioral health utilization management (UM) clinicians, case managers (CM), and behavioral health medical directors in the hubs will be involved in both the core business and the integrated behavioral health program. The medical/surgical counterparts of these staff will collaborate in implementing the integrated behavioral health program as outlined below.

Coordination of separate but related behavioral health and medical agendas: Behavioral health staff and/or program elements have been integrated into all of the functional areas within TriWest's medical management operations, including utilization management, quality management, case management, population health improvement and medical claims review. Behavioral Health managers serve on all the operational committees of Health Care Services along with their medical counterparts. This structure facilitates communication between BH and medical staff and ensures that BH issues will be addressed. This arrangement also allows BH and medical management staff to collaborate on issues that involve other TriWest departments external to Health Care Services.

In the regional hub offices, BH operational staff are co-located with their medical peers, and their actual seating arrangement facilitates their need to manage behavioral health core business and integrated behavioral health cases. Wherever possible, BH utilization management and case management staff are clustered together, surrounded by the medical peers. This facilitates communication among the BH staff on those cases with only BH diagnoses as well as communication with their medical peers on integrated behavioral health cases.

Case-finding programs: Identifying potential cases suitable for an integrated behavioral health approach requires training both behavioral health and medical/surgical staff in what to look for, but there are some types of cases that are immediately obvious. These include:

- Patients with chronic disorders including asthma, diabetes, heart disease, emphysema, chronic pain, hypertension and rheumatoid arthritis
- "Complicated" cases with multiple medical and/or psychological conditions
- Stress-related conditions
- High utilizers of health care services

In addition, there are specific case types from behavioral health's core business that frequently involve medical/surgical services. These include:

- Substance abuse detoxification
- Suicide attempts
- Eating disorders
- Medical complications of alcohol dependence

These are the obvious cases to use to start developing protocols for how behavioral health (BH) and medical/surgical staff (MS) will collaborate in an integrated behavioral health model. The protocols involve the steps MS and BH staff will take to bring their respective expertise to bear in addressing both the behavioral health and medical needs of the patient, and they form the basis of TriWest's integrated behavioral health program.

Creation of innovative care programs to increase patient self-management and awareness: TriWest's Population Health Improvement Program includes telephonic interventions aimed at increasing compliance with care regimens for patients with diabetes, asthma, coronary artery disease and depression. As an MCO, TriWest's focus includes the needs of both providers and beneficiaries in promoting positive health outcomes. Behavioral Health considers provider education an integral part of this effort, particularly on topics unique to the military population and community. Given the conflicts in Iraq and Afghanistan, post-traumatic stress disorder (PTSD) has been a concern for military medicine. TriWest has focused broadly on the psychological conditions typically associated with deployment and reunification among the family members of active duty service members and more specifically on the effects of PTSD on service members and their families. Collaborating with the University of North Texas Health Sciences Center and Pfizer Foundation, TriWest has sponsored continuing medical education seminars on PTSD for network primary care and behavioral health providers. Targeting communities with military bases that have deployed large numbers of troops, these seminars offer biographical and clinical summaries of PTSD and an overview of web-based information and local treatment resources.

Multi-departmental treatment of such conditions as chronic pain or Attention Deficit Hyperactivity Disorder, allowing providers to see a more global approach to care of patients, decreasing the possibility of certain treatment elements being overlooked: As an MCO, TriWest is not involved in direct care delivery but is involved in the business of care management. In this case, TriWest's management of cases that have both medical and behavioral health components or issues is multi-departmental, ensuring a more comprehensive approach to the management of care that accommodates both medical and behavioral issues. For example, medical directors and clinical staff consult behavioral health clinical staff on cases in which psychological and behavioral factors appear to effect the course of treatment and outcome, e.g., patient noncompliance with medication, symptoms of anxiety in patients with serious medical conditions, and symptoms of depression in patients with chronic medical conditions. Interventions consistent with TriWest's role as an MCO include offering providers and beneficiaries information on behavioral health and wellness, care coordination and case management services, and the option of mental health consultation.

Joint staff meetings: Behavioral Health staff are involved in joint staff and operational meetings within Health Care Services at TriWest. These meetings include regularly scheduled meetings with specific agenda and purpose as well as ad hoc and spontaneous opportunities to communicate and resolve unusual issues that arise. This affords BH staff opportunities to become acquainted with their medical counterparts and colleagues that are far more frequent than routine than under the previous carve-out structure. These interactions result in regular information exchange and reciprocal learning and appreciation of the issues that each department faces and for the transfer of strategies and solutions for similar management problems.

Increased use of technology and online medical information: The size of TriWest's service area and the population it serves necessitate the use of technology and online information, internally and externally. Behavioral Health utilizes TriWest's telephone and information systems capabilities to leverage the effectiveness of its staff. Behavioral Health information is integrated into TriWest's interactive voice response (IVR) system. Beneficiaries and providers can check the status of claims, get information on benefits, eligibility and TRICARE Prime enrollment, and access recorded selections in an audio health library. Providers can access several type of member-specific information including checking TRICARE eligibility for beneficiaries, the status of authorizations, and the status of claims. Providers can also access recorded information on contracting as a network provider with TriWest. In addition, both have access to recorded program information and customer service staff. The BH 24/7 crisis line outgoing message is, in fact, the first prompt that callers receive. Callers who select the option are immediately transferred to the BH crisis line staff. In addition to the IVR, Behavioral Health provides web-based information via the TriWest intranet and the company website, TriWest.com., including:

- Forms
- Newsletters
- Notices
- Referral and authorization process information
- Electronic claims submission information
- TRICARE Program information

Both MS and BH staff will require specialized training to implement an MCO integrated behavioral health program. MS staff will likely need to be educated about the behavioral health disorders they will be dealing with, their incidence among patients with particular diagnoses, and treatments. BH staff will be likely to need some training on medical terminology and the medical disorders they will encounter and the association of certain behavioral health disorders with physical conditions. Such training is particularly useful at the outset because it affirms the value of the knowledge base that respective staff members bring to the program.

Intervention changes in health care management because the MCO does not direct the beneficiary's care. The MCO's role is to review requests for authorization of health care services and to authorize care that is medically/psychologically necessary. Intervention may take several forms. The simplest approach may be to ask the requesting provider for additional information on apparent behavioral health symptomatology and issues. Such inquiries frequently result in further dialogue with the provider but, at a minimum, trigger the provider to consider the prospect that the patient has behavioral health issues that may affect his/her medical condition. Most MCOs have case management programs for complex cases requiring multiple services, and patients with both behavioral health and medical/surgical conditions may be referred to case management to develop an effective care coordination plan. Similarly, some MCOs have developed disease management programs for patients with specific chronic disorders, and disease management programs for depression have been shown to facilitate behavior change, e.g., increasing activity level and medication compliance.

Integrated Behavioral Health Care Pilots

Because integrated care is the overarching principle in TriWest's vision of health care delivery, the foundation of the system is one in which behavioral health is inextricably linked to the primary care visit. TriWest's program will be based upon the successful experience of both civilian and military health care organizations in training and placing behavioral health clinicians in primary care settings. The goal is to improve care and reduce costs in a strong medical/surgical environment complemented by the early recognition and treatment of behavioral health disorders. TriWest intends to develop pilot programs of integrated behavioral health in primary care settings at selected military treatment facilities (MTF). TriWest will collaborate with these MTFs to select and train behavioral health providers in behavioral health primary care, an approach to delivering behavioral health services in a manner similar to primary care, utilizing triage, brief assessment and focused brief interventions and referral. These pilot programs will target both MTF and community provider enrolled beneficiaries with chronic medical/surgical disorders who are high utilizers of medical services. These beneficiaries will be offered the opportunity to participate in a brief psychoeducational group program targeted at improving their capability to effectively manage their disorder. The medical/surgical utilization of these beneficiaries will be assessed before and after their participation in the program in order to evaluate any medical cost offset the program provides.

Lessons Learned

At present, the TriWest West Region contract has been fully operational for six months. During that time, Behavioral Health has completed the carve-in of the previous carve-out contract and has begun to develop the infrastructure for its integrated behavioral health program. At this point, we've had sufficient experience to recognize the importance of several issues in the successful implementation of integrated behavioral health.

1. Give both medical and behavioral health senior management a clear understanding of the organization's goals at the outset of the planning process for an integrated behavioral health implementation.
2. Utilize external subject matter experts on integrated behavioral health for ongoing consultation on strategic planning with senior management and operational planning with operations staff. Integrated behavioral health is a relatively new technology, and ongoing consultation serves to keep the new implementation on-track.

3. Clearly differentiate carving-in a carve-out contract from implementing an integrated behavioral health program.
4. Clearly define what integrated behavioral health is and what it is not and strive for consensual validation by all staff involved in the implementation.
   a. Integrated behavioral health is an additional, new line of business, separate and distinct from the "core business" of behavioral health staff (cases with exclusively behavioral health conditions).
   b. Integrated behavioral health deals with beneficiaries who have both medical/surgical and behavioral health symptoms or conditions and requires protocols that allow medical/surgical and behavioral health staff to effectively coordinate their services to improve care quality and outcomes.
   c. Integrated behavioral health does not require co-location of medical/surgical and behavioral health staff. Co-location does not equal integration.
   d. Integrated behavioral health does not involve cross-training medical/surgical and behavioral health staff to function interchangeably but rather respects the different expertise each brings to the collaboration.
5. You can never do too much education. The natural tendency for staff members is to fill in gaps in their knowledge acquisition of integrated behavioral health with erroneous assumptions from their previous behavioral health or medical/surgical training.

Opportunities

Most healthcare organizations are medical/surgical centric. In such a situation, behavioral health simply is not, and probably never will be, a priority equivalent to the medical/surgical program. Generally, this derives from the fact that behavioral health care costs are a fraction of medical/surgical costs of care. At TriWest, Behavioral Health represents approximately 6% of total health care costs. Justifying resources and expenditures in such an environment would appear to be a daunting task, but several cogent arguments can be made:

1. First, the reason behavioral health now represents only 6% of total TriWest health care costs is that behavioral health is well-managed.
2. Secondly, the core business of behavioral health is not the only arena in which significant cost-savings can be achieved through effective care management. Integrated behavioral health programs have been shown to achieve medical cost offset savings of as much as 30% among groups of high-utilizers. Potential medical cost offset savings within the primary care population of a medical/surgical organization can certainly contribute to the organization's overall business success. Behavioral health staff can contribute the technology to achieve

medical cost offset savings and improve the overall effectiveness and quality of services delivered. The potential cost savings can more than justify the necessary behavioral health resources.

3. Thirdly, a well-managed behavioral health program within a medical/surgical organization can reduce the organization's overall liability risk. In-house resources available to manage behavioral health crises are typically under-appreciated until there's a crisis.

Effective behavioral health care management is a resource- and labor-intensive effort: Current behavioral health care staffing at TriWest represents about 8% of total health care management staff and 10% of the workload. Historical levels of TRICARE behavioral health costs provide a referent within which to understand current levels of program management. In 1988 when the TRICARE Program started its first pilot program in managed behavioral health, the CHAMPUS Reform Initiative, behavioral health represented approximately 17% of total health care costs.

At this point in the transition, the carve-in of the MBC carve-out is complete. Nearly 50 MBC staff have transitioned to behavioral health positions with TriWest, and West Region contract operations are in their third week. The Behavioral Health Department now has 90 staff managing behavioral health services to 2.7 million TRICARE beneficiaries across 21 states. Behavioral health staff have been co-located with their medical/surgical counterparts within the functional areas of Health Care Services at corporate headquarters and in 5 regional hubs.

Much remains to be done to develop and implement TriWest's integrated behavioral health program. TriWest will develop integrated behavioral health approaches within the functional areas of Health Care Services, including Population Health Improvement and Case Management, to facilitate identification and early appropriate intervention with beneficiaries who have both medical/surgical and behavioral health conditions. The beneficiaries identified will be offered the opportunity to participate in disease management and case management approaches initiated by TriWest corporate and hub staff. In addition, preliminary planning for TriWest's integrated behavioral health pilot programs has begun.

Both of these programs involve working with TriWest staff and MTF and community providers to develop protocols that allow medical/surgical and behavioral health personnel to collaborate efficiently and effectively, making full use of their respective expertise. They offer behavioral health staff the opportunity to bring state-of-the-art technology to bear within a medical/surgical population with chronic disorders and concomitant behavioral health disorders to improve outcomes and achieve cost savings through medical cost offset.

TriWest will also evaluate these programs to determine their effects and to continue to improve them and the services they provide. The opportunities to develop a model integrated behavioral health program on both the care delivery and care management sides of the business are unparalleled.

References

Cummings, N. A. (2001). A new vision of healthcare for America. In N. A. Cummings, W. O'Donohue, S. C. Hayes, & V. Follette (Eds.), *Integrated behavioral healthcare* (pp.19-37). New York: Academic Press.

Eisenberg, L. (1992). Treating depression and anxiety in primary care: Closing the gap between knowledge and practice. *New England Journal of Medicine, 326* (16), 1080-1084.

Fries, J. F., Koop, C. E., Beadle, C. E., Cooper, P. P., England, M. J., Greaves, R. F., et al. (1993). Reducing health care costs by reducing the need and demand for medical services. The Health Project Consortium. *New England Journal of Medicine, 329*(5), 321-325.

Gallo, J. J., & Coyne, J. C. (2000). The challenge of depression in late life: Bridging science and service in primary care. *Journal of the American Medical Association, 284*(12), 1570-1572.

Klinkman, M. S. (1997). Competing demands in psychological care: A model for the identification and treatment of depressive disorders in primary care. *General Hospital Psychiatry, 19*(2), 98-111.

Melek, S. P. (1999). *Financial, risk and structural issues related to the integration of behavioral healthcare in primary care settings under managed care.* Denver, CO: Milliman & Robertson, Inc.

Mumford, E., Schlesinger, H., Glass, G. V., Patrick, C., & Cuerdon, T. (1984). A new look at evidence about reduced cost of medical utilization following mental health treatment. *American Journal of Psychiatry, 141*, 1145-1158.

National Mental Health Association. America's mental health survey, May 2000. Conducted by Roper Starch Worldwide, Inc. www.roper.com/Newsroom/ content/news 189.htm.

O'Donohue, W., Cummings, N.A., & Ferguson, K. E. (2003). Clinical integration: The promise and the path. In N.A. Cummings, W. T. O'Donohue, & K. E. Ferguson (Eds.), *Behavioral health as primary care: Beyond efficacy to effectiveness* (pp.15-30). Reno, NV: Context Press.

Saravay, S. M., & Cole, S. A. (1999). Mental disorders in the primary care sector: A potential role for managed care. *American Journal of Managed Care, 4*(9), 1319-1322.

Schulberg, H. C., Katon, W., Simon, G. E., & Rush, A. J. (1998). Treating major depression in primary care practice: An update of the Agency for Health Care Policy and Research Practice Guidelines. *Archives of General Psychiatry, 55*(12), 1121-1127.

Simon, G. E., & VonKorff, M. (1995). Recognition, management, and outcomes of depression in primary care. *Archives of Family Medicine, 4*(2), 99-105.

Tiemens, B. G., Ormel, J., Simon, G. E. (1996). Occurrence, recognition, and outcome of psychological disorders in primary care. *American Journal of Psychiatry, 153*(5), 636-644.

Williams, J. W., Jr. (1998). Competing demands: Does care for depression fit in primary care? *Journal of General Internal Medicine, 13*(2), 137-139.

Chapter 5

Rural Mental Health: Challenges and Opportunities Caring for the Country

Dennis F. Mohatt, Mimi M. Bradley, and Scott J. Adams
WICHE Mental Health Program, Boulder, Colorado

In announcing his *New Freedom Commission* (NFC) *on Mental Health* in Albuquerque, New Mexico, President George W. Bush (2002) stated: "our country must make a commitment: Americans with mental illness deserve our understanding, and they deserve excellent care." He also observed that the "fragmented" mental health delivery system is often an obstacle to obtaining needed care, as too many people fall through the cracks in the current mental health system.[1] The challenges to closing the gaps and transforming mental health care are especially significant for rural and frontier America. The *New Freedom Commission* made a specific effort to examine mental health care in rural and frontier America and to make note of its special needs in its final report and recommendations to the President.

The Subcommittee on Rural Issues (SRI), appointed by the *New Freedom Commission*, found a convergence of unique issues pertaining to mental health services in rural areas. Specifically, the SRI (2004) reported that the vast majority of barriers to mental health care for rural Americans regard limited availability, accessibility, and acceptability. This chapter will explore ways to improve mental health systems in rural and frontier communities from the aspect of availability, accessibility, and acceptability of mental health treatment. Each section will include recommendations to address identified barriers. However, prior to addressing the barriers noted above, it is necessary to provide a brief contextual look at mental health in rural and frontier America, including a presentation of urban myths versus rural reality, a discussion of the definition of *rural*, rural demographics, and the prevalence of mental health disorders in rural America.

Rural America in Context

The *New Freedom Commission Subcommittee on Rural Issues* presented a table (reproduced below) that contrasted a number of urban myths about rural areas with the reality of rural life. While this chapter will not discuss all these issues, this table is useful in providing an overview of the kinds of problems rural Americans face with regard to mental health care.

	URBAN ASSUMPTION	RURAL REALITY
Specialized Mental Health Services	There is duplication and lack of coordination and integration of services.	There is a lack of availability of services but effective (informal) coordination and integration of existing services.
Resources	Resources would be adequate if they were managed effectively or if resources were available. It is just a matter of competing for them.	Resources are scarce and inadequate.
Specialized Mental Health Professionals and Providers	There is an oversupply of specialized mental health professionals and providers.	There are severe shortages of specialized mental health professionals and providers.
Access to Specialized Mental Health Services	Access to services is fundamentally a problem of removing barriers related to ability to pay, racial or ethnic discrimination, and convenience of location or hours.	Access to services is fundamentally a problem of the lack of availability of services, and solving other access problems will do little until this fundamental problem is addressed.
Mental Health Service Utilization	Specialized mental health services are overused.	Specialized mental health services are underused.
Stigma	Stigma is simply an attitudinal barrier to the appropriate use of mental health services that can be overcome with education.	It is very difficult for a person seeking mental health services not to publicize that fact throughout their entire social network and for that knowledge to be taken into account in all their personal and professional relationships, with very real consequences.
Specialization	Certain kinds of specialization are cost-effective and considered best practices.	Specialization is not practical.
Meeting Client Needs	The obligation is to meet the client's need for specialized mental health services and refer them to other supportive services to meet other needs.	The obligation is to meet the full range of mental health and supportive needs of clients because no other supportive services are available.

Table 1. Mental Health Practice: Urban Assumptions and Rural Realities

	Urban assumption	Rural reality
Organizational Capacity of Mental Health Providers	Mental health providers have the staff (e.g., office managers, grant writers, evaluators) and the information systems (e.g., Internet access, electronic billing) that will allow them to participate effectively in state-of-the-art programs and opportunities.	Many rural mental health providers do not have the administrative staff to perform specialized functions (e.g., grant writing, insurance billing); or the telecommunications connections to operate effectively in the modern world of electronic commerce and communication; or the information technology capacity to conduct outcome measurement, sophisticated cost accounting, and so forth.
Professional Ethics	Ethical mental health practice demands clear and distinct boundaries between one's professional and personal life and requires one to avoid entering into a treatment relationship with people with whom you have a previous personal or professional relationship.	Practical realities make it impossible for one to totally separate one's professional and personal life and make it not feasible to totally avoid dual relationships.
Service Delivery Issues and National Public Policy	National public policy issues, such as homelessness, AIDS, intravenous drug use, and so forth, are critical issues for major segments of the population needing specialized mental health services, and specialized programs are needed.	National public policy issues are critical issues for only special segments of the population needing specialized mental health services, and developing specialized programs should be secondary to developing sound, basic mental health services.
Policies on Cost Control	With an excess supply of mental health professionals and providers, costs can be managed or controlled by organizing providers into competing networks.	An inadequate supply of mental health professionals and providers, scarcity of resources, relatively low costs, and providers and informal caregivers distributed across large geographic areas make competition counterproductive and requires cooperation and sharing resources.
The Role of Primary Care	Primary care providers manage a significant number of patients with mild to moderate mental disorders, but refer most patients with serious mental disorder to psychiatrists.	Primary care providers manage patients representing the full range of mental disorder and often provide the only medical oversight for people with serious mental illnesses.
Indigenous Healers and Informal Caregivers	Indigenous healers and informal caregivers are parts of clients' lives that must be dealt with but are not an integral part of service delivery.	Indigenous healers and informal caregivers are essential ingredients in delivering services and meeting the needs of local populations.

The Definition of Rural

The Department of Health and Human Services (HHS) reported that there is no consistent definition of *rural* used across agencies or programs (HHS, 2002). This lack of consensus can lead to confusion and difficulty targeting grants, evaluating services, developing policy, and calculating HHS investment in rural communities (HHS, 2002; NFC-SRI, 2004).

For instance, consider definitions used by the United States Census Bureau and the Office of Management and Budget (OMB). The Census Bureau (1990) distinguishes between "urban" and "rural," and bases its definition on population density. The former is defined as: 1) central places with a population of 50,000 or more, together with contiguous territory having population density of 1000 or more per square mile, *and* other areas outside these central places with a population of 2,500 or more. All other areas (i.e., areas with less than 2,500 residents and open territory) are classified as "rural" (NFC-SRI, 2004). Furthermore, the term "frontier" is defined by having low population density, generally fewer than 6 or 7 people per square mile (Ciarlo & Zelarney, 2002; NFC-SRI, 2004).[2]

The Office of Management and Budget (OMB), however, bases its operational definition of "rural" on county types in terms of the degree of social and economic interaction between "core" and "adjacent" communities (Hewitt, 1989; OMB, 1990; NFC-SRI, 2004). That is, adjacent communities with a high degree of social and economic integration with core communities (population $\geq$ 50,000) are classified as "metropolitan," whereas those with low integration are identified as "non-metropolitan." Thus, one can see that the OMB definition also uses different terminology than the Census Bureau, for example, using "nonmetropolitan" in place of "rural."

A system developed by Goldsmith, Holzer, Ciarlo, and Woodbury (1999) uses a "Grade of Membership" (GOM) analysis of numerous socio-economic variables. The data from such methodology would yield richer information that could be used to plan and mobilize rural initiatives (NFC-SRI, 2004). The socio-economic variables used by the GOM system include:

- Social rank (i.e., economic, occupational, and educational status),
- Household/family composition,
- Housing,
- Mobility,
- Travel-to-work characteristics,
- Ethnicity,
- Local economic activities,
- Tax structure, and
- Expenditures for police and fire services (NFC-SRI, 2004).

While the uniqueness and diversity of rural communities from one another should be respected, a formalized definition would be valuable in creating a baseline from which to begin discussions regarding rural issues.

Rural Demographics

Many Americans equate rural areas with farming and agriculture. However, only approximately 6.3% of rural Americans live on farms and 50% of those families have

Nonmetropolitan and metropolitan counties, 2003

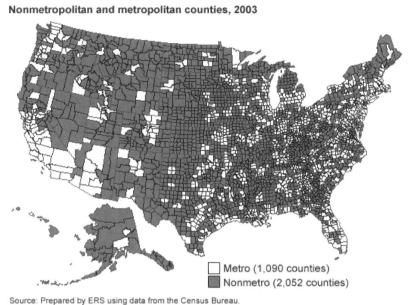

Metro (1,090 counties)
Nonmetro (2,052 counties)

Source: Prepared by ERS using data from the Census Bureau.

Figure 1. Nonmetropolitan and metropolitan counties, 2003

income from off-farm activities (United States Congress, 2002). Even in areas of the U.S. with the greatest percentage of farm employment, non-farm employment still accounts for nearly 80% of jobs. In other words, the majority of rural farmers supplement their farm-based income with non-farm employment (NFC-SRI, 2004). (Source: Figure 1 from NFC-SRI, 2004)

In contrast to Americans in urban areas, rural individuals have low paying jobs and lower incomes, are more likely to be unemployed, and less likely to be promoted out of lower wage positions (NFC-SRI, 2004). In 1996, 23% of rural workers were employed in the service sector and were almost twice as likely as their urban counterparts to earn a minimum wage (U.S. Congress, 2002).

Poverty continues to be a fact of rural life, with over 25% of rural workers earning less than the federal poverty rate. Child poverty is also higher in rural areas, with more than half of all rural children (3.2 million) in female-head-of-households living in poverty. Children of color are of particular risk, with 46.2% of rural African American, 43% of rural Native American, and 41.2% of rural Hispanic children living in poverty (NFC-SRI, 2004; U.S. Congress, 2002). People of color constituted approximately 17% of the rural population in 1997, compared with about 25% of the overall U.S. population.

During the 1990's, several million more people moved from the city to the country, representing a new trend of rural migration that contrasts with the out-migration trends of the early 20th Century. In the early 1990's, 70% of rural counties

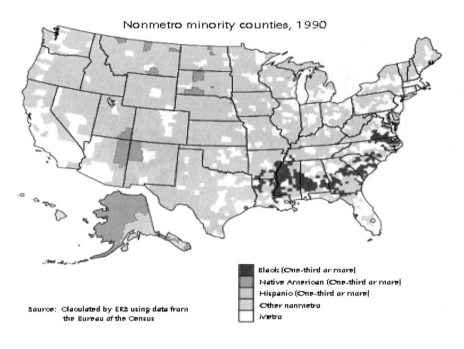

Figure 2. Nonmetro minority counties, 1990

grew in population, but the pace of growth decreased by the end of that decade (U.S. Congress, 2002; NFC-SRI, 2004). Although immigrants generally settle in urban areas, those who do move to rural areas (2% of total rural population) tend to be concentrated in only a few locations (Effland & Butler, 1997; NFC-SRI, 2004). For instance, 17% of the total rural immigrant population of the United States lives in Texas. The largest group of rural immigrants, individuals of Mexican descent, continue to be the largest group of rural immigrants, increasing from 48% in the 1980s to 57% in the 1990s (NFC-SRI, 2004).

Rural educational levels are often lower than those in urban environments. Fewer rural adults have a college education compared to urban adults (15% versus 28%), and the number of rural adults without a high school diploma is greater than in urban areas (20% versus 15%). Rural high school graduation rates match or surpass urban rates, however, it appears that rural graduates tend to leave their rural communities more frequently than rural students who do not graduate (NFC-SRI, 2004; U.S. Congress, 2002). Thus, the out-migration phenomenon has implications regarding rural health workforce shortages and workforce development. Many capable individuals leave their rural community resulting in itinerant service provision by persons living and trained in urban areas (NFC-SRI, 2004).

Prevalence of Mental Disorders in Rural Areas

Demographic, socio-economic, and cultural factors influence mental health and mental health care in any given community (Mohatt, Bradley, Adams, & Morris, pre-press). However, the most comprehensive and recent data indicate that the prevalence and incidence of mental health problems are similar between rural and urban populations (Kessler et al., 1994; Wells, Sturm, & Burnam, 2001). Current prevalence rates show that approximately 20% of the United States population is affected by mental health issues each year (Kessler et al., 1994).

The overall prevalence of substance abuse disorders among adults has also been shown to be comparable between rural and urban areas. According to the Epidemiological Catchment Area (ECA) Study, which compared rural and urban prevalence rates for a large variety of psychiatric disorders, the rural lifetime prevalence rate of co-occurring (i.e., psychiatric and substance abuse disorders) disorders was 32%, only slightly lower than the 34% rate in urban areas (Robins & Reiger, 1991).

In a review of studies investigating the prevalence of psychiatric disorders in rural primary care settings, Sears and colleagues (2003) found that 34 to 41% of patients had a mental health disorder. Additionally, results of studies of seriously mentally ill individuals indicate that rural residents have poorer outcomes (e.g., reliance on inpatient services, increased symptom severity) when compared to urban residents, especially if there are co-occurring substance abuse issues (Fischer, Owen, & Cuffel, 1996; Rost, Owen, Smith, & Smith, 1998).

One striking difference between rural and urban populations is the higher rate of suicide in rural communities, which has been a consistent trend for more than a decade (Institute of Medicine, 2002; NFC-SRI, 2004; Stack, 1982; Wagenfeld, Murray, Mohatt, & DeBruyn, 1994). Specifically, the suicide rate for older adult (elderly) males and Native American youth in rural populations is significantly higher than in urban populations (Eberhardt, Ingram, & Makuc, 2001). Adults suffering from depression, who live in rural areas, tend to make more suicide attempts then their urban counterparts (Rost et al., 1998). However, Rost, Fortney, Fischer, and Smith (2002) suggest that it is difficult to attribute these elevated suicide rates to rurality per se because suicide comparisons have not been adjusted for other variables such as income and education.

Barriers to Mental Health in Rural America

"SAMSHA [Substance Abuse and Mental Health Services Administration], in collaboration with the National Institute of Mental Health (NIMH), is urged to ensure research is supported that seeks to improve the depth of knowledge available on the prevalence, incidence, and etiology of behavioral disorders across a wide array of rural environments, to better support the ability to precisely focus limited resources on specific areas of need (NFC-SRI, 2004)."

While the prevalence of mental and substance use disorders is not significantly different in rural compared to urban areas, the Subcommittee on Rural Issues articulated that the difference lies in the *experience* of individuals with such problems, including their families, caretakers, and communities (NFC-SRI, 2004). The lack of available mental health services, access to these services, and acceptability of these services all contribute to rural residents' differential experience and outcomes. Problems with availability, accessibility, and acceptability will be discussed in detail in this section.

Availability

Rural America has been underserved for over 40 years. The availability of mental health services and the number of mental health providers in rural areas continues to be severely inadequate. Over 85% of the 1,669 federally designated mental health professional shortage areas are rural (Bird, Dempsey, & Hartley, 2001). According to the National Advisory Committee on Rural Health (1993), of the 3,075 rural counties in the United States, 55% had no practicing psychologists, psychiatrists, or social workers, and all of these counties identified were rural (NFC-SRI, 2004). There are approximately 605 rural counties in the United States without a medical health care provider and approximately 1600 rural counties that do not have accredited mental health care providers (Rosman & Van Hook, 1998). It is estimated that approximately two-thirds of individuals with symptoms of mental illness receive no care at all. Of those who do receive treatment in rural areas, approximately 40% receive care from a mental health specialist and 45% from a general medical practitioner (Regier et al., 1993).

Primary care physicians and other general medical practitioners are often the first-line providers for rural residents. Primary care physicians, however, often have limited training in identifying and treating mental illness and behavioral disorders (Ivey, Scheffler, & Zazzali, 1998; Little, Hammond, Kollisch, Stern, & Dietrich, 1998; Susman, Crabtree, & Essink, 1995). In addition to training concerns, primary care physicians may also lack the time and resources to adequately diagnose mental health disorders.

The public mental health system is commonly the only provider in rural areas that serves individuals with serious mental health issues. In the absence of a formal system of providers (e.g., public hospital systems, Federal, State, and locally supported Community Health Centers, and local public health departments), the "informal" system (e.g., private professionals and organizations that provide free or low-cost care) is forced to bear the responsibility of treating the majority of mental health issues in rural communities (Hartley & Gale, 2003; Taylor et al., 2003). Additionally, informal system providers utilize lay community health workers (also known as indigenous paraprofessionals) as providers of mental health care in rural communities (Hollister, Edgerton, & Hunter, 1985; Wagenfeld, Murray, Mohatt, & DeBruyn, 1994). In fact, providers with Bachelor's level education (i.e., paraprofessionals) often have the most contact with individuals in need of mental health care. However, they often are not adequately trained to triage and make appropriate treatment decisions. Additionally, the families and caregivers of mentally ill rural residents also lack resources and support to aid in caring for their loved ones. In addition, Medicare reimbursement rates are often lower in rural areas, which affect the earning potential for rural mental health professionals (Meyer, 1990).

The availability of specialty mental health services (e.g., neuropsychology, geriatric) is even lower than that of general mental health services. Most specialty mental health services are available through larger trade centers or locally by periodic visits made by providers (Wagenfeld et al., 1994). Rural areas also contain fewer hospital-based inpatient and outpatient services for both psychiatric and substance abuse (Hartley & Gale, 2003). Often when individuals are released from inpatient care to the community, there are few social services and rehabilitation agencies to provide follow-up care.

In the past ten years, many rural hospitals have closed or been converted to Critical Access Hospitals that provide a more limited array of services. As a result, rural residents with immediate mental health needs (i.e., psychosis, suicidality) often have law enforcement as their emergency responder (Larson, Beeson, & Mohatt, 1993). These individuals are frequently transported out of their community to the nearest facility with staff who can direct triage and stabilization (NFC-SRI, 2004).

There are significant differences in the distribution of rural Community Health Centers (CHCs). Many Eastern and Southern states have approximately 30 to 40 rural CHC sites, but many Midwestern and Mountain states (Iowa, Minnesota, Nebraska, Kansas) have few or none (e.g., North Dakota) (Hartley & Gale, 2003; National Advisory Committee on Rural Health, 1993). The Farm Bill of 1987 included the Rural Crisis Recovery Act, which helped support direct funding of rural mental health services. However, community efforts are often limited by the lack of long-term funding to ensure sustainability.

There is recent support for the expansion of mental health services within the Community and Migrant Health Centers programs. These Federally Qualified Health Centers (FQHCs) could potentially improve and expand the availability of and access to mental health treatment. However, there is not yet a mandate for the FQHCs to collaborate and coordinate with already existing community mental health centers, which has the potential to duplicate services and render the system less efficient (NFC-SRI, 2004).

The recruitment and retention of certified mental health professionals is of major concern in rural communities (Kimmel, 1992). There has been a steady decline in the number of training programs specifically created for rural mental health professionals (NFC-SRI, 2004; Wagenfeld et al., 1994). The shortage of mental health professionals prompted the National Health Service Corps (NHSC) to offer loan repayment in exchange for service in mental health professional shortage areas. From 1995 to 1999, the NHSC placed 244 mental health professionals in rural areas (Bird et al., 2001). Additionally, two national organizations, the American College of Mental Health Administration and the Academic Behavioral Health Consortium, hosted a national meeting in 2001 regarding workforce issues (NFC-SRI, 2004). The conference gave birth to the Annapolis Coalition on Behavioral Health Workforce Development whose mission is "to build a national consensus on the nature of the workforce crisis and to promote improvements in the quality and relevance of education and training by identifying and implementing change strategies." Because of the unique nature of rural environments, mental health training programs need to establish core competencies for individuals working in rural areas.

Recommendations

After a review of the current literature and research on the availability of mental health services in rural America, recommendations seem to be best organized in three categories: policy, training, and services:

Policy

1. Convene an expert panel to develop a single definition of rural. After this definition has been applied consistently, the definition should be further measured for accuracy.
2. The Subcommittee on Rural Issues (2004) made the following recommendations related to rural mental health workforce development, 1) establish a cross-agency work group to examine existing workforce enhancement programs, 2) articulate a rural mental health workforce strategy that supports mid-level and non-traditional mental health providers, and 3) ensure the financial support of training programs that prepare rural mental health professionals.
3. Support flexible use of providers through "any-willing provider" laws and expand state practice laws that allow rural professionals to maximize the use of their established competencies (Ivey, Scheffler, & Zazzali, 1998).
4. The Subcommittee on Rural Issues (2004) encouraged the National Health Services Corps (NHSC) to allow mid-level mental health professionals (e.g., Master's level psychologists, social workers, and counselors) to qualify for the loan repayment and scholarship programs. The Subcommittee pointed out that mid-level professionals are more likely to be found and remain in rural underserved areas.
5. Continue to educate state legislators about the mental health workforce needs in rural communities.
6. Encourage legislators to enact legislation to increase Medicare reimbursement for rural providers.

Training

1. Existing funding streams and training programs should mandate a set of skills that lead to rural competency (National Advisory Committee on Rural Health, 1993).

2. Encourage rural educational institutions to partner in order to maximize and expand availability of training options.

3. Encourage training institutions to institute a clearly articulated pathway for mental health professions in rural communities.

4. Increase the number of available programs with a specific focus on rural mental health.

5. Explore distance delivery strategies to meet needs of trainees.

6. Evaluate the current training programs for rural mental health professionals at all levels (e.g., relevance of training to "real-world" rural living, cultural competence).

7. Increase training for mid-level providers (primary care providers and mental health professionals).

Services

1. The Subcommittee on Rural Issues (2004) proposed that SAMSHA in partnership with NIMH, "initiate and support research to identify, verify, and disseminate evidence-based practices suitable for rural practice environments. Resources could be made available to support transferring this knowledge to rural providers and systems of care."

2. Federal agencies and other funding agencies should require the collaboration of new rural mental health services with already existing services.

3. The Subcommittee on Rural Issues (2004) encouraged the Department of Health and Human Services "to explore the creation of a limited program – similar to the former Community Mental Health Centers Act – to provide a basic safety net continuum of rural mental health care for underserved areas. The Subcommittee advises that this program ensure integration with the Community and Migrant Health Centers."

4. Fold in the use of evidence-based practices into grant award contracts.

5. Evaluate the effectiveness of treatment by non-mental health care specialists in rural areas.

Accessibility

Although research has shown that rural and urban residents have comparable prevalence rates for mental disorders, rural residents are much less likely to have access to services or providers (Lambert & Agger, 1995). The Subcommittee on Rural Issues (2004) identified three significant components of access to mental health services which are particularly limiting for rural residents: knowledge, transportation, and financing.

Mohatt and Kirwan (1995) found that rural residents lacked an awareness of the need for mental health care, which often leads to seeking care later during the course of their illness. Acute symptoms, especially if they are novel to the person, may not immediately be recognized as mental health related or requiring treatment (Rost et al., 2002). In addition to knowing that one needs care, individuals need to know what treatment options exist in their communities or where the nearest care is located (NFC-SRI, 2004). According to Lambert and Agger (1995), studies have shown that reduced access to mental health services is directly related to limited availability of mental health centers and providers.

Recent research indicates that the knowledge that one needs mental health care is so low in rural areas that the smallest obstacles may discourage that individual from seeking treatment (NFC-SRI, 2004; Rost et al., 2002). Many outreach interventions in rural areas have failed to convince mentally ill individuals that they need to seek care (Fox, Blank, Berman, & Rovnyak 1999). While we know from experience that these outreach strategies have not been successful, there is still a need to clearly understand the reasons for their ineffectiveness.

Rural Americans are hindered by their inability to travel to or pay for mental health services (NFC-SRI, 2004). Transportation barriers for people living in rural communities include the lack of personal transportation to travel to service providers; limited, inefficient, or inconvenient public transportation (Schauer, & Weaver, 1993; U.S. Senate, 1992); and long distances to the nearest provider of mental health services. In addition, the use of catchment areas can complicate access to services for rural residents. The catchment area system may require individuals to seek services in an area that they do not usually frequent due to the allocation of funding streams (Mulder et al., 2000). In other words, funded services are not available everywhere and the nearest catchment area may be in an unfamiliar location or community.

Socio-economic factors (e.g., low paying jobs, limited insurance) also have an impact on the accessibility of services for rural Americans (NFC-SRI, 2004). For instance, inability to pay limits accessibility to mental health services, either because of insufficient insurance coverage or high co-payments for appointments (Buckwalter, Smith, Zevenbergen, & Russell, 1991). Of the people living in rural areas who do have health insurance, many do not have comprehensive benefits and do not have coverage for psychotherapy (NIMH, 2000). Many rural residents are self-employed or are employed by a small business and, thus, may not have employer-based health insurance. In response to increased insurance premiums (by an average of 16.4% in 2001), many small businesses are either discontinuing insurance coverage for their employees, dropping coverage for dependents, increasing the employee's contribution to the premium and deductibles, or not providing health insurance at all (Hartley & Gale, 2003; Levitt, Holve, & Wang, 2001). Employers with 50 or fewer employees, which is often the case with rural businesses, are exempt from the Mental Health Parity Act of 1996 (NFC-SRI, 2004). As a result, more rural residents are paying out-of-pocket for basic primary care services (Hartley & Gale, 2003).

Two-thirds of the uninsured living in rural areas are poor or near-poor, meaning their family income is less than 200% of the poverty level (Kaiser Commission, 2003). Generally, small group or individual comprehensive health insurance policies (i.e., with adequate prescription drug benefits) include high deductibles with limited or no behavioral health care coverage (McDonnell & Fronstin, 1999). As a result of being unable to pay for services, rural residents are more likely not to seek services due to pride and the lack of free or reduced fee treatment (Mueller, Patil, & Ullrich, 1997). For families with children with Serious Emotional Disturbance (SED), having no insurance can be particularly distressing. Many families who cannot pay for treatment for their children are confronted with the choice of giving up custody in order for their child with SED to receive appropriate treatment (NFC-SRI, 2004).

The cost of health services that are only partially reimbursed by Medicare and Medicaid may be too expensive for some rural residents. Low-income adults, who comprise almost half of the rural uninsured, only qualify for Medicaid if they are disabled, pregnant, elderly, or have dependent children (Kaiser Commission, 2003). Approximately one-fourth of the rural poor qualify for Medicaid, compared to 43% of low-income urban residents. The lack of prescription privileges for older adults is also concerning, with only 16% of rural elderly, compared to 79% of urban elderly, having access to Medicare+Choice plan with drug coverage (MedPAC, 2000). According the Health Care Financing Administration (1998), over 9 million Medicare beneficiaries (nearly one in four) live in rural America and nearly 1 million (one in 10) rural beneficiaries are age 85 or older.

The use of new technology and telehealth strategies have increased access to services for rural residents. Telehealth technology has been instrumental in increasing the availability of health services, consultation, and training (NFC-SRI, 2004). Although most grantees under the Federal Office for the Advancement of Telehealth indicated that mental health was an area of service delivery, the actual prevalence of telehealth mental health care projects was quite minimal. In addition, these projects were often not connected with formal systems of care for adults or children, especially those with serious mental illness (LaMendola, Mohatt, & McGee, 2002; NFC-SRI, 2004). The data support the fact that telehealth mental health care has increased access for rural residents in general. However, there is a lack of data on the effectiveness of telehealth mental health interventions (NFC-SRI, 2004). Research in this area is significantly lacking and will be important in order to demonstrate its value and to inform future telehealth treatment interventions.

Finally, it is difficult for mental health agencies, especially those that serve persons with serious mental illness or children with SED, to operate without financial assistance from the government. In addition, rural programs often operate in areas with limited sources of financial resources to leverage as matching funds for other grant support (NFC-SRI, 2004). Finally, although the actual numbers of individuals with serious mental illness may be relatively small (Gale & Deprez, 2003), the geographic limitations, fragmented delivery of mental health services, and limited insurance coverage make it difficult for this population to access services.

Recommendations

Similar to the issue of availability, a review of the current literature and research on the accessibility of mental health services in rural America indicates that recommendations can be organized in three categories: policy, training, and services:

Policy

1. Premium costs and deductibles need to be structured in a way that allows rural residents to have equitable access to affordable health care insurance (Rural Policy Research Institute, 2000).
2. Improve access to prescription drugs for rural Medicare beneficiaries (Rural Policy Research Institute, 2000).
3. The Subcommittee on Rural Issues (2004) encouraged HHS to "develop Federal policies that will enable rural individuals and small businesses to enter insurance-purchasing pools as a means to enhance access to more affordable health insurance options."
4. The Subcommittee on Rural Issues (2004), encouraged SAMHSA to "ensure that non-Federal matching fund requirements are not places at levels unrealistic for rural entities competing for Federal funding opportunities."

Training

1. The Subcommittee on Rural Issues (2004) encouraged SAMSHA to collaborate with HHS and the Surgeon General, to create a public information campaign to increase rural residents' understanding of mental illnesses and best practices for treatment. They also noted that this initiative might be coordinated with local systems of care.

Services

1. The Subcommittee on Rural Issues (2004) suggested that SAMSHA and the HRSA Office for the Advancement of Telehealth and NIMH, fund rural demonstrations of, and performance measurement of, Telehealth Mental Health Care for adults with SMI and children with SED. Federal agencies should encourage the coordination of telehealth systems and public mental health systems.
2. The Subcommittee on Rural Issues (2004), suggested that SAMHSA and the HHS "implement a study and tracking mechanism to monitor the relinquishment of child custody to obtain mental health treatment for children."
3. Increase operational funding for rural mental health providers to provide transportation services for consumers.
4. Research the effectiveness of in-home mental health visits for individuals in remote areas.
5. Encourage legislation on parity of funding for mental and physical health.

Acceptability

Many factors limit the acceptability of mental health services in rural areas, including cultural beliefs, values unique to rural culture, and the stigma surrounding mental health (Intermill & Rathbone-McCuan, 1991); incompatibility of urban training with rural reality; limited cultural competence regarding rural ethnic minority groups; and disparities in research and policies between urban and rural areas. Each of these issues will be described.

Rural residents tend to value self-reliance and view help-seeking behavior in a more negative light than urban residents (Rost et al., 2002). Other cultural attitudes often observed in rural communities include the concern that fellow rural community members will discover they are in treatment for emotional issues (Berkowitz & Hedlund, 1979; Bushy, 1993; Wagenfeld et al., 1994). Many rural individuals may be fearful of being labeled "insane," of being shunned by friends and other community members, or of being institutionalized (Buckwalter, Smith, & Caston, 1994). These fears are not completely unfounded, as rural or frontier communities, by definition, have small populations in which most residents know one another either directly or through shared acquaintances. While this closeness among rural residents is often valued and contributes to a strong sense of community, it brings with it the very real likelihood that one's private life will become public. According to Rost, Smith, and Taylor (1993), the more negative the labeling of a rural individual struggling with depression, the less likely they are to seek treatment.

Strategies to reduce the stigma around mental disorders and encourage individuals to seek treatment when needed may be accomplished by increasing educational campaigns and enhancing social and professional network referrals (Kenkel, 2003). Outreach efforts will be challenged to generate innovative strategies to reach rural residents, especially the elderly and those in extremely remote locations. Understanding and utilizing the work of indigenous healers or other natural supports could be particularly helpful in this regard (Buckwalter, 1992; Neese, Abraham, & Buckwalter; 1999).

It is common for public mental health programs and services to be based on urban models and experiences, and are merely applied to fit rural communities (Beeson, Britain, Howell, Kirwan, & Sawyer, 1998; Bergland, 1988; Gamm, Tai-Seale, & Stone, 2002; Larson et al., 1993; Mohatt, 2000; NFC-SRI, 2004). Mental health professionals are generally trained with urban-centered standards that often do not directly apply to rural communities (Wagenfeld & Buffum, 1983). For instance, although there has been increased national attention and support for evidence-based practices, there have been only minor efforts with rural mental health providers and systems to increase the utilization of such practices. While parts of the established urban models may be applicable to rural society, parts that do not fit will be, at best, ineffective and, at worst, will alienate rural residents through insensitivity to the uniqueness of rural culture, people, and daily realities.

Thus, when programmatic goals and treatment approaches are misaligned with rural reality, one cannot expect residents to seek treatment or treatment to be effective.

Mental health providers in rural areas need an understanding of and appreciation for cultural similarities and differences within, among, and between groups (NRHA, Issue Paper, 1999). Many ethnic minority individuals are unable to access providers who are of similar ethnic or cultural background, speak their native language, or are knowledgeable about their particular culture (Martin, 1997; NFC-SRI, 2004; U.S. Public Health Services Office of the Surgeon General, 2001). Because of this barrier, ethnic minority individuals may be more hesitant to enter treatment based on fear that the provider may not understand their culture and traditions. Although this phenomenon is similar in urban settings, rural culture and values may further compound the fear of seeking treatment for ethnic minorities and other minority groups. Additionally, a survey of rural mental health outreach programs by the National Association for Rural Mental Health (NARMH) found that even the best programs felt unprepared to meet the cultural and clinical needs of recent immigrants to rural areas (Lambert, Donahue, Mitchell, & Strauss, 2001; NFC-SRI, 2004).

The American Psychological Association (1995) identified five important goals of cultural competence: 1) identifying social, economic, political and religious influences affecting rural communities, 2) understanding the importance of ethnic and cultural influences in rural communities and the importance of the oral tradition, 3) understanding the impact of the interaction between social institutions and ethnicity on the delivery of mental health services, 4) recognizing the impact of the provider's own culture, sensitivity and awareness as it affects his or her ability to deliver mental health care, and 5) understanding alternative treatment sources in the ethnic minority culture. The National Center for Cultural Competence (NCCC) website includes checklists and other self-assessment measures and information on obtaining training and technical assistance by NCCC faculty. However, it should be noted that cultural competence is a dynamic process that, in addition to reading and training, requires interaction and experience with the population. That is, enhancing understanding about ethnic and other minority groups requires an experiential component that is less tangible than traditional training programs.

In addition to increasing the acceptability of rural residents, efforts need to be directed at increasing attention to and acceptability of the needs of rural communities. Some advancements have been made in this area including the creation of both the Federal Office of Rural Health Policy and a National Advisory Committee on Rural Health within the Health Resources and Services Administration. However, attention to rural mental health remains eclipsed by the larger mental health field with its adherence to urban models and culture. The invisibility of rural America has been documented in several publications (Bergland, 1988; HHS Rural Task Force, 2002; NFC-SRI, 2004; Pion, Keller, & McCombs, 1997), as evidenced by the following five examples:

1. The lack of research and presentation of evidence-based practices specific to rural communities.
2. Rural programs already stretched thin due to personnel shortages are often at a disadvantage when Grant Funding Applications and Requests for Proposals insist on short turnaround times.
3. Matching fund requirements often do not account for the available resource pool in rural communities. For example, programs on Native American reservations are mandated to provide the same non-Federal match as other programs, however, most health resources on reservations are Federally funded.
4. Research on rural health provision has supported a generalist model, however, there is continued focus on specialty-driven practice and legislation (Pion, Keller, & McCombs, 1997).
5. Rural needs are often seen as fitting into urban-tested and urban-based policies and practices.

Recommendations

Recommendations regarding acceptability of mental health issues and services generally fall under the policy category, and at least one recommendation from a previous section applies here:

1. The Subcommittee on Rural Issues (2004) suggested that the "HHS require a 'rural impact statement' of all behavioral health rules, policies, and initiatives within the department retrospectively and prospectively to ensure rural equality of access."
2. The Subcommittee on Rural Issues (2004) encouraged SAMSHA to "establish an Office of Rural Mental Health and a National Advisory Committee on Rural Mental Health, specifically staffed and tasked to exclusively coordinate SAMSHA activities relating to rural areas and ensure coordination with other HHS offices relating to those rural areas."
3. The Subcommittee on Rural Issues (2004) suggested that HHS "require the creation of a SAMHSA Rural Mental Health Plan, with specific targets (similar to Healthy People 2010), as a means to establish a rural mental health benchmark and method for gauging progress."
4. Pass legislation to support innovative outreach efforts (e.g. using rural community members to provide outreach; train the trainer model).
5. The Subcommittee on Rural Issues (2004) encouraged SAMSHA to collaborate with HHS and the Surgeon General, to create a public information campaign to increase rural residents' understanding of mental illnesses and best practices for treatment. They also noted that this initiative might be coordinated with local systems of care.

Summary

This chapter sought to clarify issues related to mental health care in rural and frontier America. Among the most salient contextual factors to understanding these issues are that 1) rural has no single definition, 2) rural economics have switched from a predominantly agriculture-centered basis to non-farm employment (although wages are still much lower in rural than urban areas), 3) outmigration of rural residents (especially those with higher education levels) to more populated areas continues, and 4) despite comparable prevalence rates for mental health and substance use disorders to urban peers, rural America has a woefully lacking supply of mental health professionals.

The identified contextual issues help to frame three primary barriers to pursuing and/or receiving mental health care in rural and frontier America: availability, accessibility, and acceptability. As indicated, the significant lack of mental health professionals in rural areas limits the availability of treatment and places a heavy burden on primary care providers and, in emergency situations, law enforcement to help individuals with mental health or substance abuse problems. As a result, rural residents often enter care later in the course of their disorders, with more severe symptoms. Limited knowledge of symptoms of mental health problems, available treatment, and where to receive treatment, as well as limited transportation or vast geographic areas, and restricted financial resources negatively impact the accessibility of mental health services. Finally, mental health care is often not considered acceptable due to stigma associated with such problems, limits on privacy due to living in small communities, the misapplication of urban-based treatment models to rural areas, and limited cultural understanding of rural and ethnic minority populations.

On the positive side, rural mental health has been elevated to a higher priority status within the mental health community. In particular, federal interest in rural mental health initiatives has helped to increase attention to the needs of rural communities. At the federal level, the New Freedom Commission on Mental Health, Subcommittee on Rural Issues was one of only four subcommittee reports (out of 16) to be released, and overall goals of the Commission directly target rural issues. Additionally, the Office of Mental Health Research at the National Institute of Mental Health (NIMH) and the Office of Rural Health Policy in the Health Resources and Services Administration (HRSA) have been responsible for creating research and service delivery opportunities. However, there is a lot of work to be done at multiple levels to create and sustain viable mental health systems in rural areas.

Previous sections listed recommendations for improving mental health care in rural and frontier America. In brief, four areas of future focus to develop rural mental health are education and training, clinical programs and services, administration, as well as research and evaluation. Education and training for clinicians and consumers in rural areas should regard evidence-based practices (EBPs), collaborative care, and knowing when and how to access services. EBPs are continuing to be a focus of service delivery across mental health systems in the U.S., but the applicability of these treatments to rural still needs to be determined. The emergence of telehealth has made progress in linking rural mental health consumers with providers in urban areas, especially psychiatrists. The Internet is also becoming a vehicle for increased communication in rural areas. New developments in health care financing (e.g., managed care and for-profit health care corporations) are restructuring delivery systems. Specifically, the semi-privatization of public health insurance programs (e.g., Medicaid and Medicare) has created more incentives for corporate health care providers and insurance companies to enter rural markets.

A consistent theme emphasized in the literature is the importance of involving consumers in research and the planning of services. While this makes intuitive sense, it is common that consumers are left out of the planning processes for transforming mental health delivery systems. Rural communities and consumers should be allowed to speak authentically about their perspectives of their own needs. In order to advocate for the needs of rural communities to policy-makers, it is critical that solid research identifying the most effective services for rural residents is available. Outcome data based on current model programs will also be helpful in marketing the needs of rural communities.

Rural communities comprise much of the American landscape, and while the populations may be small, the issues they face are real, under-addressed, and sometimes ignored. Mental health and other professionals who understand the pulse of rural America will be instrumental in educating other professionals, legislators, and Americans to advance positive change for rural communities.

References

American Psychological Association. (1995). *Caring for the rural community: An interdisciplinary curriculum.* Washington, DC: Office of Rural Health.

Beeson, P. G., Britain, C., Howell, M.L., Kirwan, D., & Sawyer, D. A. (1998). Rural mental health at the millennium. In R.W. Manderscheid & M.J. Henderson (Eds.), *Mental Health United States 1998* (pp. 82-97). Rockville, MD: Center for Mental Health Services, SAMHSA, U.S. Department of Health and Human Services.

Bergland, B. (1988). Rural mental health : Report of the National Action Commission on the Mental Health of Rural America. *Journal of Rural Community Psychology, 9*(2), 29.

Berkowitz, A., & Hedlund, D. (1979). Psychological stress and role congruence in farm families. *Cornell Journal of Social Relations, 14,* 47-58.

Bird, D. C., Dempsey, P., & Hartley, D. (2001). *Addressing mental health workforce needs in underserved rural area: Accomplishments and challenges.* Portland, ME: Maine Rural Health Research Center, Muskie Institute, University of Southern Maine.

Buckwalter, K. (1992). *Mental and social health of the rural elderly.* Paper presented at the Health and Aging in Rural America: A National Symposium, San Diego, CA.

Buckwalter, K., Smith, M., & Caston, C. (1994). Mental and social health of the rural elderly. In R. Coward, N. Bull, G. Kulkulka, & J. Gallager (Eds.), *Health services for rural elders* (pp. 203-232). New York: Springer Publishing Co.

Buckwalter, K. C., Smith, M. Zevenbergen, P., & Russell, D. (1991). Mental health services of the rural elderly outreach program. *The Gerontologist, 31*(3), 408-412.

Bush, G. W. (2002, April). Remarks by President Bush in announcing the New Freedom Commission on Mental Health at the University of New Mexico, Albuquerque. Available online: http://www.mentalhealthcommission.gov/address.html

Bushy, A. (1993). Rural women: Lifestyles and health status. *Nursing clinics of North America, 28*(1), 187-197.

Ciarlo, J. A., & Zelarney, P. T. (2002). Focusing on the frontier: Isolated rural America. *Journal of the Washington Academy of Sciences, 86*(3), 1-24.

Coburn, A. F., Ziller, E. C., (2000). *Improving prescription drug coverage for rural Medicare beneficiaries: Key rural considerations and objectives for legislative proposals.* A joint policy paper of the Maine Rural Health Research Center and the RUPRI Rural Health Panel, P2000-8.

Eberhardt, M. S., Ingram, D. D., & Makuc, D. M. (2001). *Urban and rural health chartbook: Health United States 2001.* Hyattsville, MD: National Center for Health Statistics.

Effland, A. B. W., & Butler, M. A. (1997). Fewer immigrants settle in nonmetro areas and most fare less well than metro immigrants. *Rural Conditions and Trends, 8*(2), 60-65.

Fischer, E.P., Owen, Jr., R.R., & Cuffel, B.J. (1996). Substance abuse, community services use, and symptoms severity of urban and rural residents with schizophrenia. *Psychiatric Services, 47*(9), 980-984.

Fox, J., Blank, M., Berman, J., & Rovnyak, V. G. (1999). Mental disorders and help seeking in a rural impoverished population. *International Journal of Psychiatry in Medicine, 29*(2), 181-195.

Gale, J. A., & Deprez, R. D. (2003) A public health approach to the challenges of rural mental health service integration. In B. H. Stamm (Ed.), *Rural behavioral health care: An interdisciplinary guide* (pp. 95-108). Washington, DC: American Psychological Association.

Gamm, L., Tai-Seale, M., & Stone, S. (2002). *Meeting the mental health needs of people living in rural areas.* Rockville, MD: Center for Mental Health Services, SAMHSA, U.S. Department of Health and Human Services.

Goldsmith, H. F., Holzer, C. E., Ciarlo, J. A., & Woodbury, M. A. (1999). Low density counties with different types of sociodemographic, economic and health/mental health characteristics. In *Letter to the Field, 18* (Frontier Mental Health Services Resource Network). Boulder, CO: WICHE Mental Health Program.

Hartley, D., & Gale, J. (2003). Rural Health Care Safety Nets. In R. M. Weinick, M. Robin, & J. Billings (Eds.), *Monitoring the health care safety net. Book III: Tools for monitoring the health care safety net* (AHRQ Pub. No. 03-0027). Rockville, MD: Agency for Healthcare Research and Quality.

Health Care Financing Administration Office of Strategic Planning. (1998). *Data from Medicare current beneficiary survey.*

Hewitt, M. (1989). *Defining rural areas: Impact on health care policy and research* (Office of Technology Assessment). Washington, DC: U.S. Congress.

Hollister, W., Edgerton, J., & Hunter, R. (1985). Alternative services in community mental health: programs and processes. Chapel Hill, North Carolina. University of North Carolina.

Institute of Medicine (2002). *Reducing suicide: A national imperative.* Washington, DC: National Academies Press.

Intermill, N. L., & Rathobone-McCuan, E. (1991). *Mental health services for elders in rural America.* Kansas City, MO: National Resource Center for Rural Elderly.

Ivey, S. L., Scheffler, R., & Zazzali, J. L. (1998). Supply dynamics of the mental health workforce: Implications for health policy. *Milbank Quarterly, 76,* 25-58.

Kaiser Commission on Medicaid and the Uninsured. (2003). The uninsured in rural America. Publication Number: 225202. Available online: http://www.kff.org/uninsured/kcmu225202factsheet.cfm

Kenkel, M. B. (2003). Rural women: Strategies and resources for meting their behavioral health needs. In B. H. Stamm (Ed). *Rural behavioral health care: An interdisciplinary guide,* (pp. 181-192). Washington, DC: American Psychological Association.

Kessler, R. C., McGonagle, K. A., Zhao, S., Nelson, C. B., Hughes, M., Eschleman, S., et al. (1994). Lifetime and 12-month prevalence of DSM-III-R psychiatric disorders in the United States: Results from the national comorbidity survey. *Archives Of General Psychiatry, 51,* 8-19.

Kimmel, W. A. (1992). Rural mental health policy issues for research: A pilot exploration. Rockville, MD: National Institute of Mental Health, Office of Rural Mental Health Research.

Lambert, D., & Agger, M. (1995). Access of rural Medicaid beneficiaries to mental health services. *Health Care Financing Review, 17*(1), 133-145.

Lambert, D., Donahue, A., Mitchell, M., & Strauss, R. (2001). *Mental health outreach in rural area: Promising practices in rural areas.* Rockville, MD: Center for Mental Health Services, Substance Abuse and Mental Health Services Administration.

LaMendola, W. F., Mohatt, D. F., & McGee, C. (2002). *Telemental health: Delivery models and performance measurement.* Boulder, CO: WICHE Mental Health Program.

Larson, M. L., Beeson, P. G., & Mohatt, D. F. (1993). *Taking rural into account: A report of the National Public Hearing on Rural Mental Health.* St. Cloud, MN: National Association for Rural Mental Health and the Federal Center for Mental Health Services.

Levitt, L., Holve, E., & Wang, J. (2001). *Employer health benefits 2001 annual survey.* Menlo Park: Henry J. Kaiser Family Foundation.

Little, D. N., Hammond, C., Kollisch, D., Stern, B., & Dietrich, A. J. (1998). Referrals for depression by primary care physicians. A pilot study. *Journal of Family Practice, 47,* 375-377.

Martin, P. (1997). Immigration and the changing face of rural America. In *Increasing understanding of public problems and policies* (pp. 201-212). Oak Brook, IL: Farm Foundation.

McDonnell, K., & Fronstin, P. (1999). *EBRI health benefits data book* (1st ed.). Washington, DC: Employee Benefit Research Institute.

MedPAC. (2000). Report to the Congress: Selected Medicare Issues, June 2000. Washington, DC: Medicare Payment Advisory Commission (MedPAC).

Meyer, H. (1990). Rural American: Surmounting the obstacles to mental health care. *Minnesota Medicine, 73,* 24-31.

Mohatt, D. F. (2000). Access to mental health services in frontier areas. *Journal of the Washington Academy of Sciences, 86*(3), 35-45.

Mohatt, D. F., Bradley, M. M., Adams, S. J., & Morris, C. D. (pre-press). *Mental health and rural America: 1994-2004.* Publication of the United States Department of Health & Human Services, Office of Rural Health Policy.

Mohatt, D. F., & Kirwan, D. (1995). *Meeting the challenge: Model programs in rural mental health.* Rockville, MD: Office of Rural Health Policy.

Mueller, K., Patil, K., & Ullrich, F. (1997). Lengthening spells of uninsurance and their consequences. *The Journal of Rural Health, 13*(1), 29-37.

Mulder, P., Kenkel, M. B., Shellenberger, S., Constantine, M. G., Streiegel, R., Sears, S. J., et al. (2000). *The behavioral health care needs of rural women.* Washington, DC: American Psychological Association, Committee on Rural Health. Available online: http://www.apa.org/rural/ruralwomen.pdf

National Advisory Committee on Rural Health. (1993). *Sixth annual report on rural health.* Rockville, MD: Office of Rural Health Policy, Health Resources and Services Administration, HHS.

National Institute of Mental Health. (2000). *Rural mental health research at the National Institute of Mental Health.* Available online: http://www.nimh.nih.gov/publicat/ruralresfact.cfm

National Rural Health Association. (1999). Mental health in rural America: An issue paper prepared by the national rural health association. Available online: http//www.nrharural.org/dc/issuepapers/ipaper14.html

Neese, J. B., Abraham, I. L., & Buckwalter, K. C. (1999). Utilization of mental health services among rural elderly. *Archives of Psychiatric Nursing, 13*(1), 30-40.

New Freedom Commission on Mental Health. *Subcommittee of Rural Issues: Background Paper.* DHHS Pub. No. SMA-04-3890. Rockville, MD: 2004.

Office of Management and Budget (1990). OMB Circular A-11. Preparation and Submission of Budget Estimates.

Pion, G. M., Keller, P., & McCombs, H. (1997). *Mental health providers in rural and isolated areas: Final report of the ad hoc rural mental health provider work group.* Rockville, MD: Center for Mental Health Services.

Regier, D. A., Narrow, W. E., Rae, D. S., Manderscheid, R. W., Locke, B. Z., & Goodwin, F. K. (1993). The de facto United States mental and addictive disorders services system. *Archives of General Psychiatry, 50,* 85-94.

Robins, L. N., & Reiger, D. A. (Eds.). (1991). *Psychiatric disorders in America: The Epidemiologic Catchment Area Study.* New York: The Free Press.

Rosman, M., & Van Hook, M. P. (1998). *Changes in rural communities in the past twenty-five years: Policy implications for rural mental health.* Available online: http://www.narmh.org/pages/refone.html

Rost, K., Fortney, J., Fischer, E., & Smith, J. (2002). Use, quality and outcomes of care for mental health: The rural perspective. *Medical Care Research and Review, 59*(3), 231-265.

Rost, K., Smith, R., & Taylor, J. (1993). Rural-urban differences in stigma and the use of care for depressive disorders. *Journal of Rural Health, 9,* 57-62.

Rost, K. M., Owen, R. R., Smith, J., & Smith, Jr., G. R. (1998). Rural-urban differences in service use and course of illness in bipolar disorder. *Journal of Rural Health, 14*(1), 36-43.

Schauer, P. M., & Weaver, P. (1993). Rural elder transportation. In J.A. Krout (Ed.), *Providing Community-Based Services to the Rural Elderly* (pp. 42-64). Thousand Oaks, CA: Sage.

Sears, S. F., Jr., Evans, G. D., & Kuper, B. D. (2003). Rural social services systems as behavioral health delivery systems. In B. H. Stamm (Ed.), *Rural behavioral health care: An interdisciplinary guide* (pp. 109-120). Washington, DC, American Psychological Association.

Susman, J. L., Crabtree, B. F., & Essink, G. (1995). Depression in rural family practice. Easy to recognize, difficult to diagnose. *Archives of Family Medicine, 4,* 427-431.

Stack, S. (1982). Suicide: A decade of review of the sociological literature. *Deviant Behavior: An Interdisciplinary Journal, 4,* 41-66.

Taylor, P., Blewett, L., Brasure, M., Call, K. T., Larson, E., Gale, J., et al. (2003). Small town health care safety nets: Report on a pilot study. *Journal of Rural Health, 9*(2), 125-34.

United States Census Bureau. (1990). *Selected Historical Decennial Census Urban and Rural Definitions and Data.* Available online: http://www.census.gov/population/www/censusdata/ur-def.html

United States Congress. (2002). Why rural matters. In *Fast Facts* [Electronic version]. Washington, DC: Congressional Rural Caucus, U.S. House of Representatives.

United States Health and Human Services Rural Task Force. (2002). *One department serving rural America* (Report to the Secretary). Washington, DC: U.S. Department of Health and Human Services.

United States Public Health Service Office of the Surgeon General. (2001). *Mental health: Culture, race, and ethnicity.* Rockville, MD: Department of Health and Human Services.

United States Senate, Special Committee on Aging. (1992). *Common beliefs about the rural elderly: Myth or fact?* Serial No. 102-N. Washington, DC: U.S. Government Printing Office.

Wagenfeld, M. O., & Buffum, W. E. (1983). Problems in, and prospects for, rural mental health services in the United States. *International Journal of Mental Health, 12*(1-2), 89-107.

Wagenfeld, M. O., Murray, J. D., Mohatt, D. F., & DeBruyn, J. C. (Eds.). (1994). *Mental health and rural America: 1980 – 1993* (NIH Publication No. 94-3500). Washington, DC: US Government Printing Office.

Wells, K. B., Sturm, R., & Burnam, A. (2001). *National survey of alcohol, drug, and mental health problems* [Healthcare for Communities], 2000-2001 [Computer file]. ICPSR version. Los Angeles, CA: University of California, Los Angeles, Health Services Research Center. Available online: http://webapp.icpsr.umich.edu/cocoon/HMCA-STUDY/04165.xm

Footnotes

1. For more information, go to http://www.mentalhealthcommission.gov/address.html
2. United States Census Information is available online: http://www.census.gov/population/www/censusdata/ur-def.html

Chapter 6

Behavioral Health Policy and Eliminating Disparities through Cultural Competency

Melanie P. Duckworth
Department of Psychology, University of Nevada, Reno

It is commonly recognized and lamented that culturally diverse individuals are likely to suffer greater physical and mental disability consequent to receiving less health care and poorer quality health care (New Freedom Commission on Mental Health, 2003). Whether captured by age, ethnicity, gender, race, or socioeconomic status, cultural diversity has traditionally translated to a greater rate of errors in identification of mental health risks, diagnosis of mental disorders, and application of psychological treatments (United States Public Health Service Office of the Surgeon General, 1999). For example, African-Americans and Hispanic-Americans experiencing affective disorders are disproportionately misdiagnosed as having schizophrenia (Mukherjee, Shukla, Woodle, Rosen, & Olarte, 1983; Trierweiler et al. 2000). Thus, in trying to improve the provision of mental health care to individuals who are disproportionately underserved by the current mental health care system, Paul's (1986) fundamental clinical question may be better conceptualized as "for what person, presenting with what symptoms, to what facility, with what expectation for care, under what care provider, with what clinical expertise, is behavior change and health improvement likely to take place?"

The current state of mental health care can be characterized in terms of the burden borne by Americans who experience mental health problems and in terms of the adequacy of access to mental health services. Mental health problems are common, impacting persons of all backgrounds and occurring across the developmental lifespan. Epidemiological studies suggest that between 5% and 7% of adults experience serious mental disorders (Kessler et al., 2001; United States Public Health Service Office of the Surgeon General, 2001). Mental health problems have been identified as the leading cause of disability in the United States (World Health Organization, 2001), with treatment costs estimated at 71 billion dollars (Coffey et al., 2000). Although substantial, these treatment costs do not capture the full cost of mental health service delivery due to the number of undiagnosed and untreated suffers of mental disorders.

Persons of culturally diverse backgrounds are disproportionately represented among individuals for whom access to health care is limited. They are less likely to have access to mental health services, less likely to receive needed mental health care, and more likely to receive health care that is of poorer quality (United States Public Health Office of the Surgeon General, 2001). Additional barriers preventing culturally diverse persons from seeking mental health care include stigma and fear of treatment, different cultural ideas about mental illness and racism and discrimination by individuals and institutions (United States Public health Office of the Surgeon General, 2001). Clearly, the mental health care system has not attended well to understanding the relevant histories, languages, and values of diverse cultural groups.

Rural living residents have also been disenfranchised in the mental health care system. Rural Americans make up 25% of the United States population (New Freedom Commission on Mental Health, 2003). Rural residents with mental health care needs tend to enter mental health care later in the course of mental illness, enter care with more serious and disabling symptoms, and require more expensive and intensive treatment (Wagenfeld, Murray, Mohatt, & DeBruyn, 1994). Moreover, rural dwellers have lower income and are less likely to have private health insurance benefits for mental health care (McDonnell & Fronstin, 1999).

At the President's charge, the New Freedom Commission on Mental Health undertook the study of problems and gaps in mental health care with the aim of developing recommendations for transforming mental health care (New Freedom Commission on Mental Health, 2003). The Commission identified six goals as key to a transformed mental health system. Numbered among these six goals is the goal of eliminating disparities in mental health services by improving access to culturally competent mental health care and by improving access to quality care in rural and geographically remote areas across the nation. Although not targeted directly in this chapter, some of the major barriers to access (e.g., socioeconomic status and education) experienced by Americans dwelling in rural and geographically remote areas are similar to those experienced by culturally diverse populations and can be reduced using similar improvement strategies. The current chapter will outline strategies for reducing disparities in mental health care delivery and mental health outcomes for persons who are representatives of cultural diversity. Specifically, the chapter will address the following questions:

1. What are the factors that impede access to culturally competent mental health services among culturally diverse backgrounds?
2. What are the factors that would improve perceptions regarding the acceptability and benefit of mental health services among persons of culturally diverse backgrounds?
3. How is culturally competent mental health care to be defined and measured?
4. What will ensure the increase of culturally competent mental health care providers?

Before addressing these questions, definitions of key terms are provided to increase clarity in the use of these terms for the current chapter. Draguns (1997) defines *culture* as "the shared social experiences of a group defined on the basis of its origin and/or morphological or 'racial' characteristics" (p. 214). Examples of grouping that arise out of this definition of culture include African Americans, Italian Australians, and Finnish Canadians. Culture has also been equated with *ethnic identity*, ethnic identity referring to the historical and cultural patterns and collective identities shared by groups of people from a specific geographical region of the world (Betancourt & Lopez, 1993). Ethnic identity is considered to provide more insight into an individual's heritage and value system than would be provided by knowledge of race (Atkinson, Morten, & Sue, 1993). Hays (1996) defines culture as referring to "all the learned behaviors, beliefs, norms, and values that are held by a group of people passed on from older members to newer members, at least, in part to preserve the group" (p. 333), this definition of culture emphasizing the interpersonal and social aspects of culture rather than mere geographic or physical similarities. *Human diversity* refers to group-specific factors salient for the individual (Roysircar, 2004). These include gender, socioeconomic status, age, religion, race, ethnicity, regional/national origin, sexual orientation, and ability status. *Cultural competence* would imply knowledge of those factors which render a particular group distinct from other groups, knowledge of the shared interpersonal and social experiences that characterize a particular cultural group, knowledge of the salience of between and within-group experiences for a given group member, and knowledge of the relevance of salient group experiences to the therapeutic process.

What are the factors that impede access to culturally competent mental health services among persons of culturally diverse backgrounds?

The higher order goal of providing culturally competent mental health care to persons of culturally diverse backgrounds presupposes unimpeded access to mental health care and an unquestioning acceptance of Western health care practices on the part of such persons. However, for many persons of culturally diverse backgrounds, access to mental health care is not unimpeded. Utilization of mental health care services by culturally diverse populations is documented in the Surgeon General's Mental Health: Culture, Race, and Ethnicity Supplement (2001). This report suggests that only 9% of Hispanic Americans with a diagnosed mental disorder access mental health care providers. The mental health care utilization rate among Asian Americans and Pacific Islanders was described as extremely low, with utilization rate among Asian Americans and Pacific Islanders estimated at 17%. African Americans are said to access mental health services at a rate less than half of that for all Americans combined (33%). There is a dearth of representative community studies addressing mental health care utilization among persons who self-identify as being of American Indian or Alaska Native heritage; however, data from small scale studies suggest a mental health care utilization rate for American Indians and Alaskan Natives of 32%.

Primary among factors that impede access to mental health care are socioeconomic status and educational attainment. Lower socioeconomic status and lower educational attainment translate to decreased access to health care, in general and mental health care, in particular (New Freedom Commission on Mental Health, 2003). Persons from culturally diverse backgrounds comprise a disproportionately large percentage of persons living in poverty. Persons from culturally diverse and rural backgrounds also suffer higher rates of unemployment and number predominantly among the nations uninsured. Economic and educational factors that impinge upon mental health care access and delivery require national economic policies emphasizing job development and a livable wage and national educational policies emphasizing a match between educational curricula and the needs of the 21st century job force.

Other factors important to the issue of mental health care access and utilization may be addressed at the national public health level as well as at the level of the individual service provider or health care agency. These factors include:

- provider diversity
- language
- cultural beliefs regarding mental disorder and disease
- cultural influences on the evaluation and labeling of mental health concerns
- cultural prescriptions for management of mental health concerns
- cultural beliefs regarding the absolute and relative effectiveness of Western approaches to managing mental health concerns

Provider diversity. According to data compiled by the United States Census Bureau (2001), Caucasian Americans comprise the largest proportion of the U.S. population (69%), followed by African Americans (12.7%) and Hispanic Americans (12.6%). By the year 2050, the U.S. Census Bureau projects that the population of Caucasian Americans will decrease by approximately 19% and that Hispanic American and Asian American populations will at least double in size. A slight increase of several percentage points for the African American population is expected. Currently, the number of culturally diverse mental health professionals available to culturally diverse populations is less than optimal. There are 101 American Indian and Alaskan Native mental health professionals available per 100,000 American Indians and Alaskan Natives; 70 Asian American and Pacific Islander mental health professionals available per 100,000 Asian Americans and Pacific Islanders; and 29 Hispanic Americans mental health professionals available per 100,000 Hispanic Americans (United States Public Health Service Office of the Surgeon General, 2001). African Americans are reported to account for only 2% of psychiatrists, 2% of psychologists, and 4% of social workers.

Although the numbers reported reflect the current availability of culturally diverse mental health professionals, any legitimate hope for an increase in culturally diverse representativeness among mental health professionals would rest upon the rates of recruitment and retention of culturally diverse persons into mental health training programs. The percentage of people of color numbered among Bachelor's of Arts degree recipients, enrolled graduates, new doctorates, and currently employed doctoral degree recipients has more than doubled over the past 25 years (Wicherski & Kohout, 1997). Although demographic shifts in the field of psychology are in the desired direction, these shifts do not portend a sufficient increase in cultural representativeness among mental health care professionals.

Language. Accurate diagnosis of mental health concerns and provision of appropriate and effective mental health care depend upon the clarity and precision of the informational exchange between the mental health care provider and the consumer of such care. For persons from culturally diverse backgrounds, language can pose a significant barrier to obtaining mental health services. American Indians and Alaskan Natives speak over 200 indigenous languages; Asian Americans and Pacific Islanders speak over 100 languages and dialects; and approximately 40 percent of Hispanic Americans surveyed deny speaking English or do not speak English well (United States Public Health Service Office of the Surgeon General, 1999).

The restrictions on mental health care access imposed by language barriers are even greater than what would be expected by virtue of the level of cultural diversity that characterizes mental health care professionals. It must be remembered that cultural identification does not imply language capabilities among mental health professionals. As important as any effort to increase cultural diversity among mental health care providers are efforts to increase the capacity of mental health care professionals to provide services to non-English speaking mental health consumers. These efforts might include providing economic incentives to English-speaking mental health care providers who are or become proficient in languages other than English. Mental health care agencies may also wish to determine the economic feasibility and practical workability (e.g., scheduling) of having translators available when the percentage of non-English speaking health care consumers presenting to the agency exceeds some critical number.

Cultural beliefs about mental disorders. As important as any of the system level factors (i.e., socioeconomic and educational factors) already discussed is the impact of cultural beliefs on an individual's tendency to seek care for mental health concerns. Asian Americans and African Americans often forego seeking mental health services for management of mental health concerns because of the stigma associated with mental illness (Sue & Sue, 1999; Sussman, Robins, & Earl, 1987). These cultural beliefs tend to lessen the likelihood that a given individual will seek assistance from the mental health care system. Mental health care providers are again reminded of the need to acknowledge and be knowledgeable of the cultural context in which mental health problems occur and in which mental health problems will be managed (Duckworth & Iezzi, in press). Such cultural beliefs require tactful but direct questioning and address by mental health care providers.

If not addressed, these unspoken cultural beliefs may influence mental health care assessment and treatment.

Cultural influences on the evaluation and labeling of mental health concerns. Cultural factors may influence the degree to which any mental health care professional is considered "the authority" when it comes to recognizing, diagnosing and managing health concerns. Persons of culturally diverse backgrounds may view disease diagnosis and treatment as a communal process. A health care professional may be consulted only after "local authorities" have been consulted and have provided input and guidance regarding the import of a particular health concern. Local authorities may include family members and/or friends, community leaders, and spiritual representatives who are perceived as having special knowledge regarding mental health concerns and management strategies. Efforts to increase access to mental health services among persons of culturally diverse backgrounds would necessarily include educational initiatives aimed at "local authorities" within the cultural community of the identified mental health consumer. Such efforts would ensure more timely and efficient access to mental health services, increase compliance with recommendations made by mental health care providers, and improve mental health outcomes.

Cultural prescriptions for management of mental health concerns. Alternative therapies are employed by persons of culturally diverse backgrounds for the management of mental health concerns and these strategies are employed at a rate generally equal to that of Caucasian Americans. African Americans and Hispanic Americans are more likely to present to emergency departments and/or to primary care providers for management of mental health concerns than to mental health professionals (United States Public Health Service Office of the Surgeon General, 1999). Mental health care approaches that respect and, where appropriate, incorporate culturally sanctioned alternative therapies would improve consumer perceptions regarding the mental health care experience.

Cultural beliefs regarding the effectiveness of mental health care. Cultural beliefs regarding the effectiveness of mental health services are often predicated upon direct experiences with mental health care providers and agencies. Negative opinions of mental health care services among persons of culturally diverse backgrounds arise from experiences of symptom negation, misdiagnosis, inappropriate treatment, culturally insensitive treatment, and worse, failure to treat. The Surgeon General's report on mental health (1999) documents the following inequalities in diagnosis and treatment between Caucasian Americans and persons of culturally diverse backgrounds. These inequalities call into question the appropriateness of mental health services currently provided to culturally diverse populations:

- When compared to Caucasian Americans who exhibit the same symptoms, African Americans tend to be diagnosed more frequently with schizophrenia and less frequently with affective disorders (Trierweiler et al., 2000).

- Fewer African Americans receive antidepressant medications than Caucasian Americans, and when antidepressant medications are prescribed, the newer SSRI medications that have fewer side effects are prescribed less often to African Americans than to Caucasian Americans (Melfi, Croghan, Hanna, & Robinson, 2000).
- Only 24% of Hispanics with depression and anxiety receive appropriate care, compared to 34% of Caucasian Americans (Young, Klap, Sherbourne, & Wells, 2001).

Although culturally competent mental health care might serve to improve diagnostic accuracy and treatment effectiveness, the above examples suggest a breakdown in care provision that challenges basic professional practices. The primacy of cultural factors in explaining inequalities in care between Caucasian Americans and culturally diverse populations need to be evaluated systematically. The contribution of provider bias and stereotyping to the observed inequalities in care between Caucasian Americans and culturally diverse populations can not be ignored or minimized. A part of the work of becoming a culturally competent mental health care provider is acknowledging that differences in power and privilege exist and often impact everyday interactions between providers and consumers of mental health services. The provider's self-awareness is viewed as essential in establishing a therapeutic alliance with consumers of health care. Daniel, Roysircar, Abeles, and Boyd (2004) suggest that health care providers residing in the United States are likely to be exposed to cultural stereotypes that could lead to unwarranted assumptions about culturally diverse health care consumers. To prevent premature conclusions, Hays (2001) recommends examining the functional value of assumptions, asking how the therapist has come to a given understanding about the client, asking whether other alternative explanations are possible for the client's experience, and trying to generate a more positive interpretation of culturally-influenced behaviors, beliefs, or feelings.

What are the factors that would improve perceptions regarding the acceptability and benefit of mental health services among persons of ethnically diverse backgrounds?

Concerted efforts to improve the accuracy of diagnosis and the appropriateness and effectiveness of mental health care delivery will serve to improve perceptions of mental health care among culturally diverse populations. There are process variables that influence consumer willingness to contact mental health services and actively participate in treatment. Mental health care providers can better ensure successful interactions with and beneficial outcomes for culturally diverse mental health consumers by attending to all relevant cultural factors (Duckworth & Iezzi, in press). Mental health care providers are encouraged to attend to the entire spectrum of cultural factors present in any individual health care consumer, to enlist the consumer's help in prioritizing those cultural factors, and to attend to the entire spectrum of culture factors that characterize their own experiential histories. Providers are also encouraged to seek feedback from clients, peers, supervisees, and relevant others as a means of increasing self-awareness (Daniel et al., 2004).

Placing mental health concerns in cultural context is also considered important. Mental health care providers need to balance the emic and etic approaches in assessing and managing culturally diverse populations (Draguns, 1997). The emic approach views culture as permeating all aspects of psychological distress. Culture and psychopathology are intertwined and are part of a holistic experience. Alternatively, the etic approach denies the role of culture in defining psychological experiences, and instead, focuses on examining psychological experiences that are common across cultures. The emic approach provides the mental health care professional with information about abnormal behavior and experiences that is unique in terms of the historical and sociocultural background of the individual while the etic approach provides the mental health care professional with a nomothetic framework for conceptualizing and managing mental health concerns.

How is culturally competent mental health care to be operationalized and measured?

The context of federally funded studies of mental health disorders and their treatments presents a unique opportunity to formalize the practice of culturally competent mental health assessment and intervention and to measure the benefit of such practices to mental health care consumers. Empirical research into the multiple aspects of the mental health care experience is required. Use of a component analysis approach to measuring mental health care consumer, provider, and system variables and their interaction is recommended. Variables of import include consumer-specific cultural factors that influence the initiation and maintenance of mental health concerns; provider-specific cultural factors that influence mental health care provision; and mental health care system influences, including accessibility of services and flexibility in meeting the needs of mental health care consumers and providers.

What will ensure the increase of culturally competent mental health care providers?

Any increase in cultural competence across mental health care providers will be consequent to a formal embrace and measurable integration of diversity knowledge requirements into of clinical training program curricula, professional licensing procedures, discipline practice guidelines, and continuing education requirements. Diversity knowledge requirements within training programs should be mandated and evaluated as satisfactory or not as part of the routine training program accreditation process, with diversity training requirements explicated clearly and at a sufficiently detailed level. While respecting the independence and autonomy of clinical training programs, the accrediting agency should provide course minimums and minimum standards of subject expertise for instructors that are designed to ensure culturally competent practice. Accrediting agencies may wish to forward the following clinical training program curriculum recommendations:

- incorporation of the American Psychological Association-sponsored reports on culture, ethnicity, age, gender, and sexual orientation as required readings for Ethics and Diversity courses
- incorporation self-awareness exercises (that require clinical trainees to examine those aspects of culture by which they might be characterized) into formal Assessment and Intervention courses
- routine overt discussion of cultural factors during conduct of comprehensive assessments and throughout intervention as the relevance of such factors are highlighted by therapeutic processes and outcomes
- routine overt discussion of cultural factors during supervisory meetings, with address of the impact of cultural factors of the trainees' interactions with and expectations of mental health consumers and address of cultural factors impacting the trainees' interaction with clinical supervisors.

Accrediting agencies may wish to forward the following Diversity course instruction recommendations: 1) that Diversity course instructors be selected, not based on ease of course coverage or course scheduling priorities, but based upon the instructor's active involvement in research that either addresses directly matters of culture and diversity or directly targets persons of diverse cultural backgrounds as research participants; and 2) that Diversity course instructors acknowledge the limits of their world-view and routinely include other professionals who represent aspects of cultural diversity to participate in course instruction. In weighing these formal program mechanisms for promoting diversity against the less formal measures of commitment to diversity (e.g., representatives of diversity present as faculty members and as graduate students), training programs should ensure that evidence of both formal and informal commitment to diversity is present.

Licensing boards and agencies monitoring the practice of mental health care providers can do much to ensure the cultural competence of mental health practitioners. Licensing boards can structure written and oral examination items so that knowledge of cultural factors is tested and cultural competence in applied circumstances measured. Requirements can be put into effect stipulating that a percentage of continuing education credits be earned through participation in approved cultural diversity courses, presentations, and workshops.

Mental health research is another arena ripe for the formalization of diversity knowledge and practice requirements. Currently, federally funded research grants and contracts are awarded based on the investigators committing to 1) structure recruitments efforts to better ensure the inclusion of members of underserved populations among research participants; and 2) include individuals with cultural diversity expertise among research staff. While diversity requirements should not be so stringent that federally funded mental health research is crippled, diversity requirements should have some teeth. Grantees should not be allowed to avoid the duty of including underserved populations in mental health research by pointing to the burden associated with including such populations. Funding priority should be given to research groups and agencies with an established record of conducting research and/or providing services to underserved populations.

Persons serving as diversity consultants on federally funded grants and contracts should demonstrate expertise in conceptualizing and measuring the impact of cultural factors identified as relevant to the research question under study. This should not be taken to an absurd extreme. Research protocols that target members of ethnically diversity populations for study participation need not include diversity consultants who represent different ethnic groups. Instead, cultural diversity consultants should be selected based on the following: 1) the breadth of their knowledge of cultural factors; 2) their contributions to literature on cultural factors; 3) their professional experience in providing services to culturally diverse mental health consumers; 4) their comfort in identifying and addressing cultural factors that may be relevant to the research protocol; and 5) their commitment to addressing cultural factors present in the research group that may be relevant to the research protocol.

Conclusions

The current state of the mental health care system falls short in being able to meet the mental health care needs of many Americans. This is particularly true for culturally diverse Americans. The New Freedom Commission on Mental Health (2003) represents a significant policy plan directed towards transforming mental health care. As part of that plan, it is crucial that disparities in health care access and delivery across the many aspects of culture be eliminated. A number of suggestions for eliminating disparities in mental health care delivery and mental health care outcomes for persons of culturally diverse backgrounds were forwarded in the current chapter. A concerted effort by all agents of health care to fulfill the promise of transforming mental health care in America will result in policies and practices that will markedly reduce the mental health burden borne by the individual, the community, and ultimately, the nation.

References

Atkinson, D. R., Morten, G., & Sue, D. W. (1993). *Counseling American minorities: A cross-cultural perspective*. Dubuque, IA: William C. Brown.

Betancourt, H., & Lopez, S. R. (1993). The study of culture, ethnicity, and race in American psychology. *American Psychologist, 48*, 629-637.

Coffey, R. M., Mark, T., King, E., Harwood, H., McKusick, D., Genuardi, J., et al. (2000). *National Estimates of Expenditures for Mental Health and Substance Abuse Treatment, 1997* (Rep. No. SAMHSA Publication SMA-00-3499). Rockville, MD: Substance Abuse and Mental Health Services Administration.

Daniel, J. H., Roysircar, G., Abeles, N., & Boyd, C. (2004). Individual and cultural diversity competency: Focus on the therapist. *Journal of Clinical Psychology, 60,* 755-770.

Draguns, G. (1997). Abnormal behavior patterns across cultures: Implications for counseling and psychotherapy. *International Journal of Intercultural Relations, 21,* 213-248.

Duckworth, M. P., & Iezzi, T. (in press). Recognizing and dealing with cultural influences in psychotherapy. In N. Cummings, W. O'Donohue, & J. Cummings (Eds.), *Clinical strategies for becoming a master psychotherapist.* New York: Elsevier.

Hays, P. A. (1996). Addressing the complexities of culture and gender in counseling. *General Counseling and Development, 74,* 332-338.

Hays, P. A. (2001). *Addressing cultural complexities in practice: A framework for clinicians and counselors.* Washington, DC: American Psychological Association.

Kessler, R. C., Berglund, P. A., Bruce, M. L., Koch, J. R., Laska, E. M., Leaf, P. J. et al. (2001). The prevalence and correlates of untreated serious mental illness. *Health Services Research, 36,* 987-1007.

McDonnell, K., & Fronstin, P. (1999). *EBRI Health Benefits Databook.* Washington, DC: Employee Benefit Research Institute.

Melfi, C., Croghan, T., Hanna, M., & Robinson, R. (2000). Racial variation in antidepressant treatment in a Medicaid population. *Journal of Clinical Psychiatry, 61,* 16-21.

Mukherjee, S., Shukla, S., Woodle, J., Rosen, A. M., & Olarte, S. (1983). Misdiagnosis of schizophrenia in bipolar patients: A multiethnic comparison. *American Journal of Psychiatry, 140,* 1571-1574.

New Freedom Commission on Mental Health. (2003). *Achieving the promise: Transforming mental health care in America, Final report.* Rockville, MD: Department of Health and Human Services.

Paul, G. L. (1986). Can pregnancy be a placebo effect? Terminology, designs, and conclusions in the study of psychosocial and pharmacological treatments of behavior disorders. *Journal of Behavior Therapy & Experimental Psychiatry, 17,* 61-81.

Roysircar, G. (2004). Cultural self-awareness assessment: Practice examples from psychology training. *Professional Psychology: Research and Practice, 35,* 658-666.

Sue, D. W., & Sue, D. (1999). *Counseling the culturally different: Theory and practice,* (3rd ed.). New York, NY: John Wiley & Sons, Inc.

Sussman, L. K., Robins, L. N., & Earls, F. (1987). Treatment-seeking for depression by black and White Americans. *Social Science and Medicine, 24,* 187-196.

Trierweiler, S. J., Neighbors, H. W., Munday, C., Thompson, S. E., Binion, V. J., & Gomez, J. P. (2000). Clinician attributions associated with diagnosis of schizophrenia in African American and non-African American patients. *Journal of Consulting and Clinical Psychology, 68,* 171-175.

United States Census Bureau. (2001). *Profiles of general demographic characteristics 2000: 2000 Census of Population and Housing: United States.* Washington, DC: Author. Retrieved from http://www.census.gov/ipc/www/usinterimproj/>.

United States Public Health Service Office of the Surgeon General (1999). *Mental Health: A Report of the Surgeon General.* Rockville, MD: Department of Health and Human Services, U. S. Public Health Service.

United States Public Health Service Office of the Surgeon General (2001). *Mental Health: Culture, Race, and Ethnicity: A Supplement to Mental Health: A Report of the Surgeon General.* Rockville, MD: Department of Health and Human Services, U.S. Public Health Service.

Wagenfeld, M. O., Murray, J. B., Mohatt, D. F., & DeBruyn, J. C. (1994). *Mental health in rural American, 1980-1993: An overview and annotated bibliography.* Washington, DC: Department of health and Human Services, U.S. Public Health Service.

Wicherski, M., & Kohout, J. (1997). *1995 Doctorate Employment Survey.* Washington, DC: American Psychological Association.

World Health Organization. (2001). *The World Health Report 2001 - Mental Health: New Understanding, New Hope.* Geneva: World Health Organization.

Young, A. S., Klap, R., Sherbourne, C. D., & Wells, K. B. (2001). The quality of care for depressive and anxiety disorders in the United States. *Archives of General Psychiatry, 58*, 55–61.

Chapter 7

Evidence-Based Practices and Behavioral Healthcare Policy

Anil Godbole

Advocate-Illinois Masonic Medical Center, Advocate-Bethany Hospital, and the University of Illinois at Chicago

Introduction

Evidence-based practices are a subject of debate and discussion throughout the entire behavioral health field. The promise and relevance of this initiative are balanced against its barriers and limitations. The very phrase "evidence-based practices" has different meanings to diverse segments and stakeholders depending on their viewpoints and expectations. This chapter examines the complexities, tensions, and solutions inherent in the roles played by science, the practitioner workforce, consumers and payers. Challenges and opportunities are explored in order to develop a coherent set of achievable goals. Policy recommendations are presented that will involve public/private partnership, a consumer/clinician collaboration and funding/technology support.

Context

Evidence-based medicine is more than an isolated movement, trend or fad. It is a statement regarding the culture and practice of medicine that is now receiving particular attention as the healthcare system undergoes continual transformation. Advances in science and technology, fiscal constraints, demographic changes and consumer expectations drive this transformation, as the healthcare field undergoes a sea change in the post World War II era. The European countries, along with Australia and Canada, elected to organize healthcare as a social good, to be supported by taxpayers and to be organized and led by a unified national effort. The United States adopted a hybrid of public and private enterprise and each of those components has undergone substantial change in its size, structure and mechanisms affecting delivery of care. The benefits and limitations of the divergent pathways taken by these nations are often a subject of public debate, with no clear conclusion to be drawn by examining either of these systems.

Relman (1988) has described three periods of this modern revolution in U.S. healthcare, defining them as expansion (1940-60's), cost containment (early

1980's), and assessment and accountability (late 1980's). The last phase, in his words, denotes 'our efforts to achieve an equitable healthcare system of satisfactory quality at a price we can afford.' In the United States, the healthcare system accounts for approximately 15% of the GDP. Although a significant portion is publicly financed, the delivery of healthcare is predominantly based on free market system subject to principles of supply and demand, competition, varying degree of consumer choice and limited government controls. The result has been termed a two-edged sword. On the one hand, it has produced an advanced, superb state-of-the-art medical system. On the other, it has led to growing disparities that have made the field vulnerable to pressure brought forth by a market-based system. The conventional rules of product or service-oriented business are being brought into play in healthcare, despite its poor fit with true market principles. Because healthcare is seen as another large scale business enterprise, it has been expected to undergo similar changes as other manufacturing or service industries moving from a cottage industry stage to a modern, complex, technologically advanced and efficiency-based model of industry. The variances in amount and quality of care available to citizens are substantial and are not consistent with the efficiency model. As part of this profound change in healthcare, Deming (1986) emphasized the role of 'Total Quality Control' in bringing about efficiency, improvement in quality and responsiveness to consumer choice. Donabedian (1966) described the importance of the entire medical care bureaucracy that influences and defines healthcare, and issues of access, early and acute diagnosis, ancillary and support services, etc. He refers to quality as reflection of a triad of forces: structure, process and outcome. Uwe Reinhardt (1991) has described the varying relationship between cost and quality from an analytic perspective that influences the emerging debate on health policy. Ellwood (1988) and Berwick (1989) have described the 'outcomes management model' as an important paradigm espoused for organizing and conducting continuous quality assessment activity. In adopting these principles of management efficiency, quality control and enhancement, and consumer choice and centeredness, the healthcare field as a whole has made great progress, but closer scrutiny reveals substantial challenges yet to be addressed and overcome.

In spite of rapid progress in science, technology and consumer sophistication, it has become apparent that there is an ever present lag between our scientific knowledge and actual day-to-day practice. The Surgeon General's report (1999) was a landmark document that concluded that a range of treatments of documented efficacy exist for most mental disorders. The report encouraged people with mental disorders to actively seek treatment. It emphasized the importance of a range of available treatments supported by evidence, and the patients' right to choose the treatment of their preference. It looked at the mental health system through the lens of life-span and public health perspective and pointed to the glaring problems of fragmentation, inequity and the wide gap between what we know works well and what is available or actually practiced. The report identified courses of action that included the need to build the science base and the research agenda that includes neuroscience as well as science-to-service aspects. It emphasized special areas of mental health promotion, illness prevention, risk reduction and strengthening of protective factors and resiliency. The Institute of Medicine, in its published report 'Crossing the Quality Chasm' (2001), challenged the field to embrace patient-centered care with an agenda that included redesign of care processes, effective use of information technology, knowledge and skills management, development of effective treatment teams, coordination of care and the use of performance/outcomes for continuous quality improvement and accountability. The development, dissemination and practice of evidence-based medicine is embedded in this vision of a transformed system.

President Bush's 'New Freedom Commission on Mental Health' (2003) published its final report calling for transformation of the behavioral health system. The report identified fragmentation, stigma, barriers to access, disparity, mismatched and uncoordinated funding, lack of comprehensive planning at Federal, State and local levels, as well as the obvious delays and deficiencies in moving evidence-based practices to the community level as essential barriers to a responsive and efficient behavioral healthcare system. The Commission appointed a special subcommittee on the topic of 'Evidence-based Practices'. The full report of that committee is soon to be published but Howard Goldman (2003) who was consultant to the committee, published a paper that had served as a background to the committee's work. The Committee's findings and recommendations are embedded in Goal 5 of the Commission, namely 'Excellent Mental Health Care is Delivered and Research is Accelerated' which focuses on the need to expand science, service delivery research, dissemination and implementation of evidence-based practices, demonstration projects, workforce training and development and financial incentives in support of effective treatments. It is evident that across the various stakeholders including academic centers, professional organizations, consumers and advocacy groups, the research and science community, policy makers and payers, accreditation and licensing bodies, there is a growing awareness of the importance of promulgation and practice of evidence-based treatments, which is reflected by the inclusion of this topic in their respective responsibilities and agendas.

Factors Influencing Evidence-based Practices (see Figure 1)

In reviewing factors influencing the spread of the evidence-based practice movement within the behavioral health field, it becomes apparent that external pressures from the environment representing the priorities of relevant interest groups, as well as internally driven strivings for improving care, are at work. Payers are asking for cost effective care that produces demonstrable effects and benefits; treatments that are safe and thus reduce exposure to risk; and accountability by individual professional and organized systems to be accountable for what they do and the decisions they make in rendering or withholding treatment. Consumers are pushing for a voice and choice in decisions regarding treatment. Consumer expectations also include issues of affordability and some promise of hope in the effectiveness of the treatment. These trends among payers and consumers are not

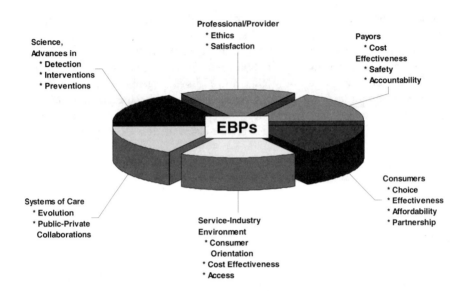

Figure 1. Factors Influencing EBPs.

limited to healthcare but are also being expressed in their purchase of airline tickets, choice of rental cars, hotels and the service they receive at their neighborhood bank and grocery store. Internal forces within the field itself are a reflection of expanding science, early detection, introduction of safer and more effective medications, advances in psychosocial rehabilitation and development of more effective therapies. The technological revolution that makes it possible to obtain current research information, communicate electronically with other members of the team involved in the care of the patient, and obtain longitudinal clinical information with a click of the mouse, along with an increasing awareness of the importance of outcomes and consumer satisfaction, equip the practitioners to adopt and adapt to evidence-based practices. The systems of care within institutional or community based programs are improving their infrastructure and the new technology and management competencies make it possible for managers and administrators to strive for a performance based clinical system. Finally, it must be acknowledged that all practitioners enter the field of behavioral health because of a genuine desire to help the mentally ill. Thus an ethical, moral and professional desire to provide the best possible care motivates the practitioners to work toward the provision of effective evidence-based practices whenever circumstances allow and support it.

Definition

There is not as yet a universally accepted definition of 'evidence-based practice', but the key elements of any such definition must include *science, clinician* and *consumer*. The Institute of Medicine (IOM) states that 'Evidence-based practice is the integration of best research evidence with clinical expertise and patient values.' This definition was adopted by the 'New Freedom Commission'. Drake (2001) and his colleagues have described 'the purpose of evidence-based medicine is to enable patients – through the process of collaboration with their healthcare providers – to take advantage of the best available scientific evidence when they are making healthcare decisions.' Sackett, Rosenberg, Gray, Haynes, and Richardson (1996) have noted that 'evidence-based medicine calls for physicians to combine judicious use of scientific evidence and patient's preferences for interventions and outcomes in making decision about healthcare'. Dawes (1999) has described it as "Partly a philosophy, partly a skill and partly….a set of tools." We will consider the *three key elements* identified in these definitions in more detail.

1. Development of Science/Best Practice Research

How much of the clinical practice of behavioral health is a scientific pursuit and how much is art and intuition, is an ongoing debate. In fact, this discussion has historical roots going back over two thousand years to Galen's description of two schools of practitioners, the empiricists and the subjectivists. Although the field of psychiatry is increasingly moving towards an empirical and phenomenological base for the diagnosis and treatment of mental disorders, the field still lags behind other medical specialties in establishing a more robust scientific base. Non-psychiatric medicine relies on anatomical pathology, chemical histology, volumetric studies, imaging data and such to yield a cellular, tissue, organ or system level diagnosis, and treatments are designed to bring about observable and quantifiable normalcy. In the field of mental health the DSM-IV, which provides the underlying language for the entire clinical practice, research, reimbursement and public policy, is premised on a descriptive nosology with diagnosis related to specific clusters of symptoms (subjective). Although DSM-IV represents a significant advance over earlier models of diagnosis and treatments, which were based on theoretically and ideologically driven schools of psychiatric thought – Freudian, Adlerian, Jungian, interpersonal, Gestalt, biological, etc,– it still lacks precision, specificity, quantitative dimensions and conclusive evidence.

Thus, it is important to recognize that the entire discussion of evidence-based practices is set on a foundation of science that is not robust and always replicable. Also, it is important to recognize other limitations of evidence-based practices, in that no intervention is applicable to all populations, all settings and to all outcomes. In spite of these limitations, progress in science and research has led to break-throughs in pharmacological agents (e.g., Lithium, neuroleptics, anti-depressants, mood stabilizers); advances in effective interventions such as cognitive behavioral and dialectical therapies; and milieu-related treatment systems, , such as assertive community treatment, therapeutic foster care, integrated treatment for dual diagnosis, and supported employment. All of these promise stable psychosocial rehabilitation and recovery. The development of these agents and interventions is based on varying degrees of scientific evaluation and evidence. Drake (2003) has provided an excellent survey of the robustness of evidence underlying specific interventions. He categorizes various levels of evidence, with the highest standard set by randomized clinical trials, and compares each practice to alternative practices or to no interventions. The evidence begins to soften as we move further downwards to clinical trials with standardized approaches and some comparison groups; meta-analysis; consensus expert panels; practice guidelines; algorithms, etc.

In addition, there is a whole range of practices that are emerging and innovative in nature which lack widespread, replicable scientific evidence and are less thoroughly documented, but which show promise and have shown some effectiveness on outcome measures in specific and special circumstances (jail diversion, re-entry programs and consumer operated services, school mental health services, wraparound services, multifamily group therapy, trauma specific interventions, peer support services, etc.).

Although we have greatly increased our ability to effectively treat schizophrenia, bipolar disorder, major depression, anxiety disorder, attention deficit disorder, etc., we still do not have evidence-based interventions for several mental disorders such as borderline personality disorder, post traumatic stress disorder, obsessive compulsive disorder and a number of disorders of childhood. Even the so-called evidence-based practices have not been thoroughly tested in complex clinical situation such as co-morbidities, culturally diverse populations, urban/rural locales, as well as along the lifespan. Research on prevention is also woefully lacking. The emerging science of Genomes, neuro-imaging and identification of biological markers may provide aid in developing preventative strategies.

Tom Insell (2003) sounded an optimistic note in offering the possibility of cure, as science begins to take advantage of emerging knowledge regarding the full sequence of human genome, in-vivo brain studies for functional imaging and neurochemistry. He expresses an opinion that major breakthroughs in our field for prevention and cure will come out of basic science development. Research is just beginning on protective factors as well as factors fostering resiliency. The heterogeneity of mental disorder, its vicissitudes of manifestations, relapses and reoccurrences over a span of several years, and its devastating effects on family, social, and occupational aspects of life pose a unique challenge to the scientific and research community. The research community must include experts in biology, psychology, social and community sciences; and often the work needs to be done across these fields in a multi-disciplinary team approach with consensus on objectives, methodology and outcomes. The relevance of science depends on who is asking the question, what it is, why it is being asked, how the answer is being arrived at, the number of possible answers, who benefits from each answer, and at what cost and to whom. Our field is just beginning to grapple with these questions and we are far from articulating the persuasive answers required to convince policymakers to assign a high priority for resource allocation to the mental health field. This is in spite of the fact that the World Health Organization (2001) reports that mental illness, along with substance abuse, constitutes almost 25% of disabilities in the industrialized world; and as such poses a major public health hazard.

There is clear recognition that mental health care is no longer delivered only in the traditional mental health system. Several parallel, at times overlapping, but essentially uncoordinated, delivery systems are in play. A closer look points to mental illness as a major challenge in juvenile justice, child welfare, schools, nursing homes, jails and prisons, on the streets and in disability programs. Primary healthcare acts as the front door for a range of mental health problems including severe mental illness, and this is particularly true for children and the elderly. Ron Kessler (2003) has pointed to the epidemiological data showing that most serious mental disorders begin in childhood or adolescence, but that research on the impact of early intervention, its cost effectiveness, identification of risk and protective factors is clearly lacking. His data also show that the earlier the disorder starts the longer it takes to get into treatment. This is very disturbing, because early–onset disorders often are more severe and persistent than later-onset disorders. It is obvious that research regarding effective treatments needs to consider this epidemiological evidence and also address how to educate practitioners outside the mental health area about the effective identification and treatment of mental disorders. 'The Psychiatric Clinics of North America' recently devoted an entire issue to the subject of evidence-based practices in mental healthcare. In it, Burns (2003) presented an update on the status of current knowledge in the area of children mental health, described some of the evidence-based practice initiatives; outlined a vision for the future in bringing together research and practice sites; and suggested roles for various stakeholders. Similarly, Bartels et al. (2003) have described the emerging evidence base in geriatric care, stressing collaboration with primary care and long term care. They also identified existing barriers and potential strategies for overcoming them. There are similar updates on substance abuse, by McGovern and Carroll (2003), and schizophrenia, by Lehman, Buchanan, Dickerson, Dixon, Goldberg, Green-Paden, et al (2003). The service delivery research will have to include areas outside of specialty mental health that are intimately, if sometimes secondarily, involved in providing mental healthcare.

There is much to be learned from our international colleagues. A centralized healthcare system has afforded them an opportunity for emphasizing prevention and adopting a public health approach, particularly in areas of resource allocation and data collection. Goldner and Blisker (1995) from Canada made one of the first contributions to the literature of evidence-based practices. There is considerable international effort in development and implementation of evidence-based medicine. Geddes and Carney (2001) have established a center for evidence-based mental health that has 181 members in 32 countries across five continents; all members are actively involved in teaching or promoting evidence-based mental health. There is also considerable additional work on this subject in Canada, Australia, New Zealand and South Africa.

2. Clinical Expertise

This key element comprises three essential components: dissemination of knowledge, acquisition of clinical skills and implementation in the field.

• Dissemination of knowledge

The report of the New Freedom Commission confirmed the previous findings of the Surgeon General's report and IOM report that there is generally a lag of almost 15 - 20 years between what we know works and what is actually practiced. This problem of dissemination and implementation of evidence-based practices delays the journey from science to service. It has been noted that most of the community practice settings do not offer evidence-based practices: even if one or two of the effective treatments are available, fidelity to the practice model is often compromised. Efforts at wide publication of practice guidelines by the American Psychiatric Association, American Psychology Association, Publication of PORT study by Lehman and Steinwachs (1998), TMAP initiative by Rush et al. (1999), have led to minimal observable change in practitioner behaviors.

It is recognized that disseminating and operationalizing evidence-based practices in behavioral health significantly differ from disseminating a product or procedure. New technologies or procedures in medicine, such as the Swan-Ganz catheter, modified flexible gastroscope or laparoscopic procedure, gain wide acceptance and application in a relatively short time. There is a straightforward explanation for this: A technology company with its marketing and sales force is actively promoting the equipment; both public and private payers are quick to include these procedures in their benefit packages for physicians and facility reimbursement; and the practitioners' desire for a 'competitive edge' incentivizes the acquisition of these skills, making possible the widespread rapid adoption of the product and the intervention. In Psychiatry, only pharmaceutical agents seem to follow this course of widespread and rapid use, but even there, adherence to recommended protocols and algorithms that are supported by research is poor. In the field of mental health, evidence-based practices face some unique challenges. The practices often tend to include more than one practitioner; may be enacted over a period of several months or years the treatment may involve more than one setting, and thus essentially depend on a given practitioner's skills and collaboration. Quite often the entire intervention or components of intervention are not reimbursed by either private or public payers. There is no profit incentive or margin for researcher or provider to encourage the dissemination of the new practice or for a clinician to acquire the skills to provide the intervention. The end result is often maintenance of the status quo, with practitioners continuing to provide treatment that may be ineffective or at times even harmful. There is very limited research in the science of dissemination. We seem to know more about what doesn't work than what is successful. Everett Rogers (1995) has described the many determinants of how new innovations are widely adapted in the society. He suggests that regardless of the characteristics of the innovation, the nature of potential adopters and the broader system into which they are being introduced will determine how the innovation is dispersed or reinvented.

There is growing evidence that simple publication of guidelines and lectures and seminars on evidence- based practices are not successful in bringing about change in practitioner behavior. Green and Kruefer (1991) have described a model in which three elements are prescribed: predisposing or disseminating strategies, such as educational events and/or written materials; enabling methods, such as practice guidelines and decision support; and reinforcing strategies such as practice feedback mechanisms. There is growing knowledge regarding various strategies for the adoption of evidence-based practices at the practitioner level as well as within systems of care. Corrigan, Steiner, McCraken, Blaser, and Barr (2001) have summarized the successes and limitations of dissemination research at the staff level and have considered dissemination from the varying perspectives of staff therapist, supervisor, administrator and policy maker. They have outlined method-ologies of training, supervision, tool kits and manuals, work incentives, culture change, organization support, role of innovators and champions, outcome and feedback, consumer involvement and satisfaction, resource allocation, etc. as all important elements in successfully embedding an evidence-based practice in the culture of an organization. Torrey, Finnerty, Evan, and Wyzik (2003) have described strategies for leading the implementation of evidence-based practices within organizations. They outline a three phase process starting with the motivational phase – Why Do It? – through the enacting phase – How To Do It? – to the sustaining phase – How to Maintain and Extend Gains over time? In each phase they describe a series of activities both at system level and program level. Robert Rosenheck (2001) has suggested constructing decision-making coalitions, linking new initiatives to goals and values, qualitatively monitoring implementation and performance, and organizing self-sustaining communities of practice and learning in order to facilitate and sustain transfer of research-based interventions to actual practice.

In recent years, consumers are asserting an important voice in favor of adoption of evidence-based practices. The role of consumer advocacy groups in transfer of science to service initiatives can be a valuable asset. NAMI has been a major supporter of such efforts and has been a coalition partner with federal agencies, academic centers and private foundations in supporting the 'Evidence-Based Practices Project'. It has also run a national technical support center and, with the help of state and local chapters, aided in promoting assertive community treatment. It performs a valuable function of providing education to family members and has developed family-to-family education programs. NAMI also has conducted nation-wide surveys to monitor implementation of evidence-based practices at state level and obtain feedback on consumer and family satisfaction with access and quality aspects of evidence-based practices. Many of these functions are organized through the 'Treatment/Recovery Information and Advocacy database' (TRIAD).

- Acquisition of clinical skills

This component of evidence-based practices refers to the acquisition and practice of evidence-based intervention at the level of the practitioner as well as at an organizational level. It also notes the disconnect between researchers and practitioners. The practitioner may be situated in a solo or group practice or may be working within a small or large healthcare system, and thus be variably influenced and affected by the setting in which he works. During the last decade as the concept of evidence-based practices began to permeate the field, it has met with varying degrees of enthusiasm and skepticism; and sometimes with outright ridicule. Researchers look at evidence in terms of level of its truth or validity, while the rest of the world looks at evidence primarily for its usefulness (Druss, 2003). Druss also points out that the research process is slow, methodical and conservative, while policy makers overwhelmingly identify timeliness and relevance as the most important qualities that would lead them to use information in their decisions. Policymakers also have difficulty in reconciling ambiguity and qualifications attached to the evidence.

Drake (2003) has raised issues of differing value systems and how they form the basis of resistance and skepticism. He points out that existing practice often is based on tradition, convenience, clinical preference, political correctness, marketing and/ or clinical wisdom. The objective and systematic evaluation of outcomes is generally not incorporated in current practice, whereas evidence-based practices are based on interventions that are standardized, replicable, and outcome- based, with demonstrated effectiveness. Practitioners are faced with the monumental task of reviewing the research literature, discriminating between claims made by proponents of various treatments; identifying a specific intervention that applies to a specific patient with a unique set of problems and resources; and then being in a position to follow the patient consistently over a period of time to evaluate the outcome. This is a demanding task for a practitioner, particularly if he or she was not grounded in theory and practice skills related to any or all evidence-based practices, and has not learned to objectively review the nature and robustness of scientific evidence as part of his or her professional training. This knowledge and skill are rarely acquired while on the job, as the cost, time and available resources pose a formidable challenge. If a practitioner is working within a small or a large institution or a community-based program, then the program sets the overarching mission, priorities, clinical care system, decision making authority, available supervision, infrastructure, reimbursement, etc. The organizations also decide what patient populations are to be served the level of necessary staffing and their skills; and what interventions and programs are supported. The individual practitioner is then expected to conform to the system's needs and decisions. Quite often evidence-based interventions require more than one practitioner's skills, and may need a team of multidisciplinary professionals to work collaboratively for a single patient, thus requiring system support or coordination across several systems (e.g., housing, vocational, justice, etc.). In spite of these barriers, there is reason for optimism: Professional organizations, GME accreditation bodies and academic centers are increasingly promoting inclusion of evidence-based practices in the core curriculum, and larger healthcare systems and managed care organizations are emphasizing or requiring the demonstration of specific outcomes through application of evidence-based practices, disease state managements or following of practice guidelines and protocols. It will be critical how the incentives, both professional and financial, are designed to promote practice of evidence-based interventions.

• Implementation in the field

The major thrust for systematically moving evidence-based practices to the field has come from Federal leadership and its support of State initiatives. Each state functions as a distinct laboratory. The state mental health agency may be either stand-alone or combined with one or more other agencies such as substance abuse, child welfare, family services, developmental disabilities, rehabilitation, public health or health and human services. This affords an advantage for wide experimentation but also acts as an impediment to developing uniformity, predictability and national standards based on data from the States, and thus poses a great challenge in operationalizing evidence-based practices. In spite of these challenges, there are a number of national initiatives underway dedicated to promoting evidence-based practices.

The state authorities across the country, through their national organization (NASMHPD) have embarked on adopting evidence-based practices within their States. There is significant variance in the number of practices selected, whether they are limited demonstration projects or applied statewide, the degree of fidelity to the practice model, etc. But this effort has had significant impact in bringing evidence-based practices to the field and the community level. An outgrowth of this national effort is the 'Evidence-Based Services Project' which is a collaborative effort involving the New Hampshire Dartmouth Psychiatric Research Center, Robert Wood Johnson Foundation, the Federal Center for Mental Health Services and other funders. National organizations such NASMHPD and NAMI are working closely with this project. This project is being implemented in three phases. Phase 1 involved identifying six specific evidence-based practices that have significant research support, and then developing implementation materials that are referred to as 'tool kits' for each of the six practices. Specific tool kits were prepared for varying constituencies such as consumers, family and other supporters, mental health practitioners and supervisors, mental health program directors and public mental health authorities. The purpose of these toolkits was the training and ongoing support of each stakeholder, and helping to develop overall consensus amongst them. Phase 2, currently underway, is a study of the feasibility and effectiveness of these teaching and support materials, as well as the effectiveness of these procedures and interventions. The evaluation will also include measurement of outcomes. Phase 3 will be a national demonstration effort with the goal of embedding all six evidence-based practices across all participating states after having received feedback on barriers to implementation, effectiveness of the toolkit methodology, etc.

3. Consumer Choice/Participation

The Surgeon General's report, IOM report and the report of the New Freedom Commission on Mental Health were unanimous in emphasizing that the entire healthcare system needs to be designed to achieve 'Patient Centeredness'. This can be understood to mean that one looks thru the lens of the primary or potential user of healthcare and his or her family. The needs, preferences and expectations of patients become the bedrock for research, delivery system design, offerings of interventions and desired goals and outcomes. One can develop all kinds of drugs in a laboratory, and a plethora of specific interventions for specific disease states in academic and research venues, but without engagement, acceptance, and adherence on the part of patients, none of these will achieve the projected effectiveness. There is ample evidence as to the drop-out rates in therapy and discontinuation rates for medications to suggest widespread disconnect between researchers and providers on one side, and consumers on the other. The fact that almost 50% of patients with severe mental illness do not receive any care during a year points not only to problems of insurance availability and access to providers, but also to major distrust between the consumer and provider communities.

Historically, the providers of mental health have been skeptical about including consumers in treatment decisions, because of a perception that the patient is unable to make an informed decision, or is seen as deficient in sound judgment. Providers have also questioned a patient's cognitive and affective stability to make rational choices. The consumer and family movement led by advocacy organizations has appropriately challenged this paternalistic point of view. The healthcare field as a whole now promotes consumer participation and collaboration between provider and consumer. Consumers need to be involved at every level of the healthcare system. They should have meaningful input in setting research agendas, participating in research design, defining desired outcome, etc. They also need to be similarly involved in the design and setting of priorities of delivery systems.

The Recovery movement has challenged the field to go beyond settling for symptomatic improvements or reduction of relapses and reoccurrences or reduction of side effects and morbidities, and push the system to help patients on their journey to achievable recovery. The New Freedom Commission defined recovery as 'the process in which people are able to live, work, learn and participate fully in their communities. For some individuals, recovery is the ability to live a fulfilling and productive life despite a disability. For others, recovery implies the reduction or complete remission of symptoms. Science has shown that having hope plays an integral role in individual's recovery.' The Commission emphasized 'recovery' as fundamental in formulating its six goals and for achieving transformation of the behavioral health system. William Anthony (1993), a pioneer in the recovery model, describes recovery as "a deeply personal, unique process of changing one's attitude, values, feelings, goals, skills and/or roles. It is a way of living a satisfying, hopeful and contributing life, even with limitations caused by the illness. Recovery involves the development of new meaning and purpose in one's life as one grows beyond the catastrophic effects of mental illness."

The consumer or advocacy movement does not represent a homogenous group or a single point of view. It represents a wide variety of perspectives on consumer roles, level of participation, control over decision-making, family role and partici- pation, the role of professionals, and priorities and methods for advocacy. This variance includes a wide spectrum from purposeful collaboration with the provider community to overt militancy and threat of legal recourse. Munetz and Frese (2001) have described the "two apparently very different approaches to treatment of mentally ill persons that are emerging. The scientific, objective evidence-based approach emphasizes external scientific reality, whereas the recovery model stresses the importance of the phenomenological, subjective experiences and autonomous rights of persons who are in recovery." There is a natural tension and at times obvious conflict between the two models, and the two authors have suggested a model for reconciling these differing perspectives into a phased approach with increasing level of decision-making moving in the direction of consumer as progress is made on the journey toward recovery. The suggested compromise would be for researchers and providers to be able to identify and offer a menu of possible alternative treatment options and an outcome probability distribution of efficacy and adverse effects of each option. Then it would be the consumer's preference based on his values and resources that should determine the choice of treatment. Although the evidence in this area of consumer-operated services, value of consumer participation, peer group support etc. is so far quite limited and not quite robust, collaborative partnership with consumers is still a moral and political imperative, and should have a priority in advancing research.

We have already stressed the important role consumers and their families play in dissemination and implementation of evidence-based practices at the state and local levels. It can be argued that the best way to ensure the use of evidence-based practice is for the consumer to be well-informed, resourceful and thus demand the practitioner and the system to provide the state-of-the-art care. The consumer thus empowered can also be a major voice in persuading policy makers and payers to ensure that best-evidence treatments and supports are available to all who are in need. In summarizing critical success factors in achieving science-to-service transformation, the following conditions need to exist:

Science-to-Service Critical Success Factors

1. Any Door

Regardless of when, where and how a patient seeks help for an emotional problem or mental illness, he or she should be assured of receiving predictable and responsive care. Patients may surface at primary healthcare sites, social service agencies, emergency rooms, correction or justice systems, child welfare, nursing homes, etc. Regardless, the evaluation, triage, and treatment plan needs to be based on uniform standards of care.

2. Individualized Treatment Plan

The treatment and recovery plan should be specific to the needs and resources of the patient and the patient has to have a choice in decision about treatment intervention, provider and site of care. The consumer should own his treatment plan and should be able to transport it as necessary. The plan should be periodically updated.

3. Relevant Scientific Development

The research agenda both for basic science and service delivery should emphasize the entire 'science to service' cycle and 'field to science' cycle and continually expand its agenda to include real-life practice conditions, co-morbidities, and conditions not yet amenable to known treatments. Research should also inform us about best ways to disseminate related knowledge and skills and about proven teaching methods.

4. Menu of Options

Providers should be able to offer a range of treatment options and alternatives with their relative efficacy, safety and limitations described to the patients and family, and then engage the patient in the decision about the choice of treatment.

5. Attention to Diversity

The research community needs to include cultural, gender, age and geographic aspects into consideration in determining the effectiveness of drugs, therapies and other interventions. The studies should be longitudinal, to more accurately reflect the predicted course of illness and recovery.

6. Best Practices

There should be a mechanism for identifying evidence-based practices and denoting their level of evidence. This process needs to be dynamic and self-renewing as science expands and as new data is received from the field. For the psychotropic drugs, agencies like the FDA perform part of that function. There needs to be a similar entity, whether governmental or private, based on consensus of the entire field, that provides unbiased, current information on state-of-the-art treatments to providers, consumers and payers.

7. Aligned Incentives

Incentives for work enhancement, skill acquisition, system organization, reimbursement, licensing and accreditation must be aligned to promote practice of evidence-based treatments.

8. Trained Workforce

A motivated, skilled workforce trained in evidence-based practices is a cornerstone for successful implementation of effective treatments. There is need for this process to be team-based with periodic updates to absorb new knowledge and skills.

9. Consumer Education and Participation

A well-informed consumer and family, given a seat at the table at every level of decision-making, is needed to help ensure that the system will maintain patient-centeredness.

10. Designed Reimbursements

Public and private payers need to re-examine their inventory of eligibility criteria, covered benefits, reimbursed interventions, rates of payments, etc. to bring them in line with current scientific knowledge and consumer preference. There should also be careful attention to coordination and alignment of expenditures within the diverse sources of funding and reimbursement.

Special Areas for Consideration

Certain areas have especially significant impact on the emergence and future of evidence-based practices – specifically *Information Technology, Financing Issues, Workforce Development and Psychotropic Medications.*

Information Technology

It is obvious that the use of modern technology should lay the groundwork for conduct of day-to-day clinical practice, provider and consumer education, and for collection of the data on efficiency and outcomes, necessary for payers and policymakers to make decisions about appropriate and timely allocation of resources. Despite this, behavioral health practitioners have lagged behind in embracing new technological advances. In the field of behavioral health, the clinical practice depends more on subjective or descriptive evidence, and successful longitudinal treatment depends in large part on communication and transfer of information between various providers. Freedman (2003) has provided an update on development of a common language, structured interviews or assessments, automated sub-reports, a core set of severity rating scales and outcome measures, static or active electronic medical records with automated clinical decision supports, prompts for risk factors, laboratory and pharmacology data, drug interactions, follow-up schedules and other reminders. He also points to the inherent resistance within the behavioral health community in adopting current capabilities offered by information technology. Additionally, there are significant cost barriers in transforming the current 'paper-and-person' system to automated information platforms. Federal and state agencies have not supported such transfers at the community level of care, and are themselves slow in adopting current technology in measuring their own performance and promoting support for evidence-based practice. Private payers and behavioral health carve-outs have concentrated on fiscal and administrative efficiency data and are just beginning to support clinical protocols, decision support system and disease management programs. There are only a few stand-alone information platforms for behavioral health which require continuous updating as the field evolves and customization needs proliferate, making it difficult for a single provider or agency to make an informed choice and invest in a reliable and predictable information system. A few large-scale initiatives are underway, particularly within the VA system and at some academic centers, which signals a promising trend. Eventually it will be necessary to develop an integrated information system through which behavioral health data is well coordinated or integrated within the general health system.

The New Freedom Commission report has called for development of person-centered, integrated, comprehensive electronic health records that would aid providers and researchers, and it also stresses the need for consumers to have the choice and capability to obtain, store and share personal health information. Consumers should be able to use Internet assessment services and other health information sources to enable them to

- Evaluate the quality of care provided
- Participate in on-line support groups
- Evaluate best practices
- Learn about the most recent treatment breakthroughs and emerging best practices

Financing Issues

The issues of financing this entire enterprise of evidence-based practices will require priority and proportionate funding support for research in areas of scientific development and refining of interventions that include multi center replication of evidence. Historically, NIMH has been the lead agency for supporting research. It has supported service research for Community Mental Health Centers (CMHC's) in the 1970's and expanded its role in service delivery research through its extramural branch through the 1980's and onwards. SAMHSA has generally taken the lead in implementation of evidence-based practice through its funding of various dissemination and implementation projects. Now these two federal agencies are going forward in the 'Science to Service' initiative to promote evidence-based practices. At the state level, several factors contribute to inadequate and uneven investment and support: reluctance to use Federal block grant monies, constraints on use of general revenue funds because of state priorities, provider vested interests, a lack of long range goals, leadership turnover, and state funding dispensed through multiple agencies such as criminal justice, Medicaid, housing, education, child welfare, etc. With each agency defining its own eligibility criteria, reimbursed benefits and priorities for funding, significant barriers are created to the development of a state-wide, long range, comprehensive and coordinated plan for implementing and sustaining evidence-based practice. The individual provider and community agencies are struggling with survival issues and, at best, planning on a year-to-year budget. Medicaid, which has become the largest payer of services for the severely mentally ill, does not cover many of the evidence-based practices or covers only some components of care. Additionally the rates for such services may be below the cost of providing the care, and thus providers are reluctant to institute a long range plan involving infrastructure development, workforce training and supervision and measurement of outcomes, particularly as there is no mechanism in place to pay for the transition cost, and no guarantees of enhancing revenues by implementing evidence-based practices. Most of the current evidence-based practices have been developed for management of the severely mentally ill and involves the public sector; and thus leadership will need to be at the federal, state, county and other governmental agencies' level. The private sector in behavioral health is largely managed through the for-profit behavioral health carve-outs, who are contracted by states, large insurance companies or health plans that determine the eligibility and benefit structures. These contracts are short term, with fluctuating enrollment, and have no incentives built in for implementing evidence-based practice.

Medicaid is becoming the largest single payer for services delivered to seriously mentally ill children and adults. Although it is a federal program, it grants considerable autonomy to the States in how it is designed and implemented, resulting in 50+ different Medicaid programs. It functions as an insurance benefit and concentrates on eligibility determinations and claims payment for defined benefits. It has had no role in advancing research, in supporting systems of care, in ensuring appropriateness, effectiveness or quality of care. It is only recently that it has started looking into sponsoring demonstration projects, running pilots for innovative case management and community residential care as an alternative to institutional care. Within its own structure, Medicaid has several different funding streams that pay for hospitals, pharmacy, nursing homes, outpatient clinics, rehabilitation and physician services, etc. without any coordination of these benefits or designation of accountability to any single entity. In states where Medicaid is contracted out to a behavioral health carve-out, there are some state formulated parameters for performance and outcome. This environment as a whole is not conducive to the practice of evidence-based interventions.

Medicare shares a smaller responsibility for paying for mental health services. The lack of parity and other limitations and co-payment requirements act as additional barriers to development of a comprehensive evaluation of outcomes. Medicare also serves as an insurance program for the elderly and the disabled and although administered centrally through a federal agency it also lacks in ensuring connectivity between the defined benefits, claims payment and evidence-based interventions. Steve Bartels (2003) points to evidence that, although collaborative care has been found to be effective in the treatment of depression in the elderly who present themselves predominantly in the primary care health system, its common-place application is prevented by lack of payment support for some critical elements of the intervention.

As long as we have a system of healthcare where the public and private payers function as insurance and claims payment entities, important public health issues such as parity, universal coverage, and adoption of evidence-based practices do not assume priority and support.

Workforce Development

The New Freedom Commission underscored the fact that without an adequate trained workforce, realization of any of the Commission's goals would be very difficult. There is considerable information on workforce shortages particularly in the treatment of children and the elderly, as well as in rural communities. The disciplines of child psychiatry, geriatric psychiatry and nursing face formidable challenges as the demographic changes and increased demand for services impact the field. In addition to the issues of sheer numbers, other complex issues include cultural competence, diversity of workforce, and skills training. The recruitment and retention of workforce is affected by the appeal of the field, work environment, quality of life, comparative compensation and opportunities for personal and professional growth. The stigma associated with mental illness and misconceptions regarding its incurability add to the discouragement of young people who might otherwise be interested in entering the field or remaining in it. The training programs are based on their "guild" identity, tradition and history. Often the curricula are not rapidly updated to include the most current knowledge, and the experiences are not designed to impact skill for practicing evidence-based interventions. The rigidly drawn boundaries among various disciplines do not expose the trainees to the kinds of collaborative, team-based approaches and inter-disciplinary work often necessary in the treatment of mental disorders.

Hoge, Tondora, and Staurt (2003) have reported that routinely employed teaching methods may impact knowledge but do not successfully change practitioner behaviors and have very little effect on patient outcomes. They have recommended strategies for teaching that are derived from learning theory and research that demonstrates positive effects in changing provider behaviors. Methods such as interactive sessions, academic detailing, reminders, audit and feedback, use of opinion leaders, patient-mediated interventions and social marketing are listed as effective. They also emphasize that using any one of these methods is usually not sufficient and they suggest that combining several of these methods, particularly practiced over a period of time with several repetitions and feedback can have a cumulative positive effect on learning and behavior. It needs to be stressed that in addition to embedding a culture of excellence in the curricula and training methods, appropriate supervision and incentives need to be built into the system that emphasize recovery outcomes and consumer participation. Adequate workforce training will be a key to acquisition of skills at the practitioner level – an essential element of evidence-based practices, as discussed earlier.

The Annapolis Coalition on Behavioral Health Workforce Education (2002) has published a detailed analysis of problems encountered in workforce development and they have made a comprehensive set of recommendations for reform. They have called for a voluntary assessment conducted by all training programs across the country to address a standard list of desired domains and each program's adherence to them. These include:

- Evidence based practices are taught.
- Teaching methods are of demonstrated effectiveness in building skills.
- Competencies to be acquired are identified and assessed for individual's training.
- The training curriculum covers skill development related to recovery, consumer centeredness, patient safety, co-occurring disorders, interface with primary care/ managed care and cultural competence.
- Training is interdisciplinary and training sites and student composition is reflective of the community to be served.
- Consumers and families have a role as educators in training program.

Any discussion of workforce development for practicing evidence-based behavioral healthcare will be incomplete unless we take a broader view of the workforce. The personnel within schools, correctional facilities, primary care settings, nursing homes, etc. need to be included as adjuncts and collaborators in providing first-line interventions and often in continued care. The licensing and accrediting organizations have begun to address these issues but we are far from a coordinated, well-planned comprehensive agenda for meeting the workforce challenges.

Psychotropic Medications

The pace of innovation in psychotropic drugs has been remarkable during the last 15 years. An array of new drugs in the atypical antipsychotic, antidepressants, mood stabilizer categories have established widespread use. None of these drugs have a curative effect and at best are partially effective in achieving varying degrees of symptomatic relief. They all have similar side effect profiles, with some unique features; but no drug in any of these categories has established a clear superiority. The unprecedented rise in their use is driven by scientific advances, expanding insurance coverage, growth of managed care, greater willingness of physicians to make pharmacotherapies a central component of treatment of mental disorders. As much as this practice has contributed to facilitating rehabilitation and recovery, it has also posed problems as the rapid rise of related expenditures leads to payers adopting strategies that may impact access and choice. There are several problems and limitations associated with drug treatment. These drugs do not work for all who have a mental disorder and even when they do work, they often achieve only partial remission and do not always prevent relapse. This problem is heightened by the fact that physician adherence to established practice guidelines, algorithms and protocols is quite unsatisfactory. This disparity has been particularly noted in rural areas and in the care of minorities. Research for FDA approval is limited to short-term trials and is conducted under tightly-controlled conditions for specific disease and age cohorts and thus the results are not often comparable to practice conditions. This problem is experienced particularly for co-morbid conditions and in the treatment of children and elderly. The course of mental illness and its recovery may span several years and there is very limited research on the effectiveness and complications associated with continuation and maintenance treatment with medications. The psychotropic drugs are widely used in the primary healthcare system and there is some evidence that inappropriate dosages and inadequate duration of treatment are quite common. There are other problems such as polypharmacy, as well as wide geographic variations in prescription utilization not explained by clinical rationale.

The American Psychiatric Association has published practice guidelines for several disease-specific states but these are lengthy and detailed, and although the APA has made efforts to develop briefer, more focused and user friendly guidelines, their use is far from commonplace in actual practice. Mellman et al. (2001) have reviewed the nature and limitation of evidence in medication treatment, current status of protocols/guidelines, algorithm development, barriers to implementation and problems in access and patient adherence. They conclude that for improving care there would be a need for administrative support, participation of non-physician members in the treatment team, an active role for consumers and families in discussing therapeutic options, and improved access and affordability. This requires a joint effort by administrators, clinicians, policy makers, consumers and families to ensure the appropriate use of psychotropic medications as a key component in the overall treatment for recovery.

Goals: Courses of Action

The President's 'New Freedom Commission on Mental Health' adopted the eight courses of action recommended in the Surgeon General's report. These actions, taken together, will aid in overcoming systemic barriers and promote the mental health of the nation. These actions involve all stakeholders, and call for the entire field to mobilize its energy for a planned, coordinated and sustained effort to achieve the following goals:

- Continue to build the science base
- Overcome stigma
- Improve public awareness of effective treatments
- Ensure the supply of evidence-based services and providers trained in evidence-based practices
- Ensure delivery of state-of-the-art treatments
- Tailor treatment to age, sex, race and culture
- Facilitate entry into treatment
- Reduce financial barriers to treatment

It is obvious that in order to achieve these goals we will need more than just goodwill on the part of all stakeholders. Specific policies will need to be adopted and enacted by federal agencies, state authorities, professional and provider organizations, academia, regulatory and licensing bodies, and accrediting organizations. Consumers and elected officials will have to insist on these policy changes and provide oversight in their successful implementation. The 'evidence-based subcommittee' of the 'New Freedom Commission' formulated eight specific policy recommendations to achieve the above goals.

Policy Recommendations

In enacting the following policy changes, a range of options exists. The Governmental agencies (federal, state, licensure, etc.) can assume a more hands-on prescriptive role in initiating the changes and moving them forward. Alternatively, they can perform a facilitating function in providing appropriate forums, technical assistance and funding support to bring about gradual transformation. These agencies can also adopt a relatively passive role, relying more on the effort and momentum generated by the stakeholders. These decisions will be shaped by the political environment, leadership qualities within the governmental agencies and the degree of consensus and collaboration developed within the stakeholder community.

1. Partnership for National Leadership

The relevant federal agencies – particularly at the National Institutes of Health (NIH) and Substance Abuse and Mental Health Services Administration (SAMHSA) but also at the Agency for Healthcare Research and Quality (AHRQ) and the National Institute on Disability and Rehabilitation Research (NIDRR) – should establish a working relationship specifically related to developing and implementing evidence-based practices throughout the life cycle. They should work with diverse elements within the Federal Government and within other organizations in the public and private sectors to advance knowledge, disseminate findings, and implement evidence-based practices.

Topics to be encompassed by this process should include the following:

- Expanding mental health outreach partnerships and mental health awareness activities;
- Developing and strengthening quality improvement programs linked to evidence-based practices in the public and private sectors, including licensure, credentialing, accreditation, and treatment guidelines and algorithms;
- Creating a national infrastructure for leadership in evidence-based practices, such as through a renewed staff college operated jointly by the partnership involving NIH and SAMHSA;
- Building infrastructure for a national multidisciplinary mental health professional training program to focus on disseminating and implementing evidence-based practices; and
- Advancing knowledge, including rigorously evaluated service demonstration programs.

2. Expand Mental Health Outreach Partnerships and Mental Health Awareness Activities

A number of organizations and initiatives have been and can continue to be useful for improving public awareness of effective treatments such as evidence-based practices. Some are actually sponsored directly and exclusively by Federal agencies, such as the National Institute of Mental Health (NIMH) Outreach Partners Program and several SAMHSA communications contracts. Others are in the private sector, funded by a mix of public and private resources, such as the National Mental Health Association and National Alliance for the Mentally Ill (NAMI) anti-stigma campaign and the National Mental Health Awareness Campaign. The NIMH Outreach Partners form a network of outlets in each state for NIMH and its science-based messages and information about evidence-based practices. The outlets often are state and local affiliates of NAMI, the Mental Health Association or the National Depressive and Manic Depressive Association. The Mental Health Awareness Campaign was launched at the first White House Conference on Mental Health in 1999 and is funded privately and by Federal contracts. It develops public service announcements and places them in a range of media outlets directing individuals to its website and links to others that encourage individuals to seek evidence-based practices. These activities are critical for increasing the demand for evidence-based practices. An informed consumer and family make a powerful source of pressure for implementing new practices, especially those with such clearly delineated benefits. Variety and involvement of multiple organizations is probably beneficial for reaching many audiences with solid messages about different evidence-based practices. More such programs can be encouraged. What is missing, however, is a point of coordination to reduce fragmentation and promote collaboration and efficiency in the use of scarce resources. In particular, mass media awareness activities are expensive to develop and to field. Duplication of effort should and can be avoided.

3. Develop and Strengthen Quality Improvement Programs Linked to Evidence-based Practices in the Public and Private Sectors

One important vehicle for implementing evidence-based practices widely is through quality improvement strategies. These strategies take many forms and involve numerous organizations. Mechanisms include licensure, credentialing, and accreditation offered by a range of organizations in both the public sector (governmental licensure) and the private and quasi-public sector (formal training program credentials and their links to accreditation bodies). Professional associations also develop standards for empirically supported treatments (the American Psychological Association) and practice guidelines (American Psychiatric Association), which include best practices as well as evidence-based practices. Some degree of diversity is welcomed to encourage multiple perspectives on what constitutes "evidence" and who should decide. There are differences of opinion on these matters. Perhaps there will never be a consensus, but currently there is no national leadership on these issues—again to encourage discourse and collaboration and to work to efficiently develop quality assurance mechanisms for everyone to use. The proposed national partnership for leadership on evidence-based practices should develop and strengthen quality improvement strategies using evidence-based practices. The goal is not to preclude individual initiative but to promote sharing and learning among the partners and to avoid inefficient and unnecessary fragmentation and duplication of effort.

4. Create a National Infrastructure for Leadership in Evidence-based Practices, such as through a Renewed Staff College

There is need for an infrastructure at many levels of organization in the public and private sectors to promote the dissemination and implementation of evidence-based practices. Nationally, the proposed partnership could sponsor and support a center or collaborative network to review practices and the evidence supporting their effectiveness, to develop quality improvement tools, as well as to conduct training. In addition, such a center could develop training materials, present conferences, and provide ongoing consultation and support to organizations wishing to promote and implement evidence-based practices. As described earlier, various organizations already have developed centers on implementing evidence-based practices: NAMI, NASMHPD, and several of the individual states have provided examples. The partnership could form an umbrella organization for them and help establish new centers. In addition, some activities, such as review of the evidence for various practices, might best be done in a single collaborative consortium of interested parties.

Up until the early 1980s the NIMH operated a Staff College, a national training and implementation support center for mental health programs. Frequently in these days of discussion of evidence-based practices individuals long-experienced in the mental health field have lamented the passing of this highly valued organization and its functions.

5. Revive Infrastructure for a National Multidisciplinary Mental Health Professional Training Program focused on Disseminating and Implementing Evidence-based Practices

With the creation of the NIMH after World War II, the Federal Government encouraged the development of national workforce of mental health providers through its staff development and professional training programs. These programs have been slowly phased out since the 1980s, leaving this major responsibility to the various elements of the field itself – professional and post-professional training sponsored by public and private universities, professional associations, and other private entities. Successful in creating a professional and para-professional workforce, the field has fallen down in its efforts to train these providers in newer practices, particularly evidence-based practices. This failure is not a matter of unwillingness or lack of interest, but the many structural barriers to learning and implementing evidence-based practices in everyday services. Everyone agrees that there is a need for new leadership and support for the training of a workforce skilled in evidence-based practices. However the desirable goal of offering updated knowledge and skills through quality improvement and continuing education Is hampered by the usual barriers: the need for multidisciplinary training in a world that emphasizes disciplinary training; financial considerations; and resistance to new practices within the organizations that provide services.

6. Advance Knowledge, Including Rigorously Evaluated Service Demonstration Programs

Historically various Federal agencies and private foundations – sometimes in partnership with each other and often in partnership with local providers and mental health authorities – have sponsored mental health service demonstration programs. It is common to evaluate these demonstration programs to add to the knowledge base about the feasibility and effectiveness of innovative service models and to derive lessons from the experience to pass on to others. After several decades of service demonstration programs, there is now a lull in activity in mental health services. The one exception has been in the area of evidence-based practices – to learn how to better implement these practices in real world settings.

Although there have been some initial efforts at service demonstrations, they have just begun, and there are many more areas for advancing knowledge that have yet to be planned or developed. For example, although Phase 2 of the project in the public sector for adults with severe mental illness (described above as the "Evidence-Based Services Project" in eight states) has begun, there are several dozen states ready to move forward with the demonstration. It will be difficult, however, for them to organize and fund their efforts. Phase 3 has yet to be planned and funded. Projects for children and adolescents with severe emotional disturbance are just being conceptualized – based on some groundbreaking work with multi-systemic treatment out of South Carolina. Work is also just beginning on the study of implementing evidence-based practices for individuals with late life disorders, such as depression. Foundations have sponsored private sector projects, mostly focused on treating depression, particularly in primary care settings. None of these projects, however, is specifically focused on learning about the *process* of dissemination of innovation and the implementation of evidence-based practices throughout the life cycle.

The Federal Government, particularly NIMH and later the Center for Mental Health Services (CMHS), has taken the lead in planning, fielding, and evaluating mental health service demonstrations. As noted in Recommendation No. 1, above, a national partnership for leadership in evidence-based practices must be identified to take responsibility for coordinating these knowledge development activities. This involves more than designing service demonstrations. It also includes involving all stakeholders in advising research funding agencies about sponsoring research that is more likely to result in services that will move from scientific study into practice.

This specific recommendation however focuses principally on service demonstrations, moving both from science to services and from services to science.

7. Assure that Existing Funding Mechanisms Will Encourage the Use of Evidence-based Practice

As noted in the earlier discussion of the course of action devoted to reducing financial barriers, it is essential to find a range of strategies and tactics to finance evidence-based practices. The failure of most mental health service financing to pay adequately for these practices is one of the most important reasons for problems with implementation. Depending upon the source of funding for mental health services, the barriers differ. For an individual with private insurance it is uncommon for services more complex than an office visit, such as multi-systemic therapy or assertive community treatment, to be included in the benefit package. Some services, such as supported employment, fall outside the scope of traditional health insurance. Occasionally, a managed care company can 'flex the benefit' to cover such services, but that is the exception rather than the rule. Uninsured individuals may have the greatest access to some of these services in the public mental health system, although resources are scarce and Medicaid match requirements are eroding categorical dollars for these services. Tragically, on occasion parents must relinquish custody of a child in order to access such services. Medicare views many of these services as outside their rigid coverage rules. Even disease management strategies, such as collaborative care, which have been demonstrated effective with a range of chronic illnesses including depression, have not been approved for coverage by Medicare or other payers. There are other broader and more basic deficiencies in some financing for evidence-based practices, such as lack of medication coverage for specific agents (e.g. novel anti-psychotic drugs) or for any drugs at all (e.g. in Medicare). Recommendations for these eliminating these barriers are not discussed here – nor are barriers in receipt of services from other human services agencies that fund mental health services for individuals under their jurisdiction, such as rehabilitation services and the criminal justice system.

- As discussed above, there is a need to cover evidence-based practices in Medicaid benefits. It is also critical that the rates paid to providers create an incentive for them to deliver evidence-based practices. The Center for Medicaid and Medicare Services (CMS) is the largest single payer for mental health services and Medicaid is its largest component. CMS needs to partner with SAMHSA in providing guidance and technical assistance related to existing opportunities, waivers and demonstration projects. Priority should be given to the six evidence-based practices identified through the SAMHSA/Dartmouth project, to collaborative care in primary health settings and to children's mental health (treatment foster care, multi-systemic therapy).
- As discussed above, it is essential to cover evidence-based practices in Medicare benefits, particularly the disease management interventions that cannot be paid

for in their "bundled" form. These practices should be brought to the attention of the Medicare National Coverage Process to add them to the list of covered services. In the case of collaborative care for chronic disease management this probably requires special attention to how to "bundle" or "un-bundle" the services.

8. Using the Mental Health Services Block Grant to Initiate Evidence-based Practices

In an era of scarce resources one of the most important existing funding streams available for initiating service innovations is the Federal Mental Health Services block grant. Without increasing the level of funding in the block grant the resources could be used to shift services from existing practices to evidence-based practices. Although the FY 2002 funding is only $433 million (representing at most a few percent of any state's mental health budget), the block grant is a source of flexible financing that would permit funding for evidence-based practices that might not otherwise be part of a state's Medicaid plan. It also could serve as an extra source of funding to go beyond what is expected by service providers from state and local governmental sources. Several of the states already involved in projects for implementing evidence-based practices are using block grant resources to do so.

As noted earlier, it is critical to develop an infrastructure for implementing evidence-based practices within each state. A first step in the Federal-state partnership should be the creation of a state center (or centers) for implementing evidence-based practices. Both centralized and decentralized models exist in several states, often funded with Federal block grant resources. These centers are involved in training, consultation and support, as well as in providing leadership and monitoring programs for fidelity to the intended model of evidence-based practices.

The Federal CMHS within SAMHSA administers the block grant. Originally created in 1981 by the first Omnibus Budget Reconciliation Act during the Reagan Administration, the block grant was designed to bring all Federal funding for general mental health services into a single stream of resources. This legislation repealed the Mental Health Systems Act and the block grant replaced a number of previous programs, including the Community Mental Health Centers Program. The block grant represents a centerpiece of new Federalism and gave the state mental health authority broad latitude in the use of these Federal funds to pay for community based mental health services. The block grant spending was subject to state mental health plans and a system of Federal monitoring. States use the block grant for a wide range of mental health services – some of them are evidence-based and others represent best practices where no evidence-based practices exist. Still others are innovations waiting to be tested. Recent efforts to expand the block grant have been only modestly successful. Legislators are asking for evidence that the appropriations are for effective services and that states can be accountable for the services funded through the block grant. These two characteristics – effectiveness and accountability – are hallmarks of evidence-based practices with their track record of positive research findings and fidelity measures for assessing adherence to proven models of care and treatment.

Some changes in the use of the block grant can be accomplished through guidelines or regulations while others may require legislation.

Future: A Promising Project

Following the publication of the President's 'New Freedom Commission on Mental Health' report, SAMHSA has begun a vigorous and far-reaching effort in achieving the transformation. The activities include (Hennessy, 2005):

- Establishment of a special office of 'Science to Service' project and an intradepartmental work group comprised of SAMHSA, NIH, and AHRQ senior staff to facilitate and oversee the project.
- National Institutes of Mental Health (NIMH)/CMHS partnership funding for state planning grants for implementation of evidence-based practices.
- Plan for a rollout meeting for major stakeholders.
- Targeted meetings on implementation of evidence-based practices, outreach and engagement with CMS and HRSA.
- Technical assistance and a national website under 'mental health system transformation'.
- One promising effort, consistent with the goals outlined in the President's 'New Freedom Commission on Mental Health' report, is the expansion and evolution of SAMHSA's National Registry of Evidence-based Programs and Practices (or NREPP). NREPP is a system to determine the quality of scientific evidence and the effectiveness of interventions to prevent and/or treat mental and addictive disorders. The system was initiated in 1998 in the area of substance abuse prevention with support from SAMHSA's Center for Substance Abuse Prevention (CSAP), but the system is currently being revised and expanded to include all interventions to prevent and/or treat mental and addictive disorders. SAMHSA's Center for Mental Health Services (CMHS) and Center for Substance Abuse Treatment (CSAT) are participating in this expansion.

NREPP will provide timely and accurate information about the scientific, evidence-based support for substance abuse and mental health treatment and prevention interventions. In addition, NREPP will provide a variety of audiences, including the general public, with information about the adaptability of these programs and practices to real-world prevention and treatment settings. In short, SAMHSA is committed to making the NREPP a leading national resource of practical, contemporary and reliable information for stakeholders interested in identifying and implementing evidence-based interventions to prevent and/or treat mental and addictive disorders.

By Fall 2005, the NREPP website will be substantially redesigned, and will include information – searchable by outcome – on effective prevention and treatment interventions in both mental health and substance abuse. The website address is www.nationalregistry.samhsa.gov.

- Planned creation of 'national implementation research network' (NIRN) through Florida Mental Health Institute.
- Influence SAMHSA discretionary and block grant incentives.
- Act as a resource to states and communities.
- Provide an important tool for both public and private purchasers in selection of effective services.

This project ensures the centrality of patient choice described by Hope (2002) with all the essential four elements: patient choice; high-quality evidence; patient-accessible unbiased information; and information which can be used by a patient within and outside of treatment settings.

Conclusion

Let us visualize concentric circles with evidence-based practices at the center, as a component of the behavioral health system, which in turn is a component of the general healthcare system. This system is being encircled by a host of other human services such as welfare, disability, housing, corrections, education, labor, etc. The outermost circle includes all other important national priorities such as defense, agriculture, environment, social security, etc. It becomes obvious that with all these powerful complex forces and systems in play, it will be nearly impossible to chart a predictable course for evidence-based practices. It may gain momentum but would it be sustained? Would it get widespread acceptance and support? Would technology and science facilitate this or make it more complex and expensive? What is the extent of consumer and policymaker demand for it? How will over-arching policies evolve in the areas of parity, universal healthcare, and a single payer system, and what would be their impact? As Don Berwick has aptly said 'Some is not a number, soon is not a time'. These and many other questions and their answers will guide the course of evidence-based practices. In this chapter, we have examined the strengths and limitations of evidence-based practices, identified key partners in this enterprise, and suggested specific policies that will facilitate transformation of a mental health system into one which will embrace evidence-based practices at its core. Regardless of all the uncertainties mentioned, the value of evidence-based practices as central to good healthcare is compelling.

Acknowledgments

The entire section on 'Recommendations' is based on a background paper prepared for the 'Evidence-based Practices Subcommittee' of the President's 'New Freedom Commission on Mental Health' by Howard Goldman, M.D.

References

Annapolis Coalition on Behavioral Health Workforce Education. (2002). Behavioral health workforce education and training. *Administration and Policy on Mental Health, 29,* 4-5.

Anthony, W. (1993). Recovery from mental illness: The guiding vision of the mental health service system in the 1990's. *Psychosocial Rehabilitation Journal, 16*(4), 11-23.

Bartels, S. J., Dums, A. R., Oxman, T. E., Schneider, L. S., Arean, P. A., Alexopoulos, G. S., et al. (2003). Evidence-based practices in geriatric mental health care: An overview of systematic reviews and meta-analyses. *Psychiatric Clinics of North America, 26*(4), 971-990.

Berwick, D. M. (1989). Continuous improvement as an ideal in healthcare. *New England Journal of Medicine, 320,* 53-56.

Burns, B. (2003). Children and evidence-based practice. *Psychiatric Clinics of North America, 26,* 955-970.

Corrigan, P., Steiner, L., McCraken, S. G., Blaser, B., & Barr, M. (2001). Strategies for disseminating evidence-based practices to staff who treat people with serious mental illness. *Psychiatric Services, 52*(12), 1598-1606.

Dawes, M. (1999). Preface. In M. Dawes (Ed.), *Evidence-based practice: A primer for health professionals.* New York, Churchill Livingstone.

Deming, W. E. (1986). *Out of crisis.* Cambridge, MA: MIT.

Donabedian, A. (1966). Evaluating the quality of medical care. Milbank Memorial Fund Q: *Health Society, 44*(3), 166-203.

Drake, R. E. (2001). Implementing evidence-based practices in routine mental service setting. *Psychiatric Services, 52,* 179-182.

Drake, R. E. (2003). Fundamental principles of evidence-based medicine: Applied to mental health care. *Psychiatric Clinics of North America, 26,* 811-820.

Druss, B. (2003, November). Evidence and transformation. Paper presented at the Nineteenth Annual Rosalynn Carter Symposium on Mental Health Policy.

Ellwood, P. M. (1988). Outcomes management: A technology of patient experience. *New England Journal of Medicine, 318,* 1549-1556.

Freedman, J. (2003). The role of information technology in evidence-based practice. *Psychiatry Clinics of North America, 26,* 833-850.

Geddes, J., & Carney, S. (2001). Recent advances in evidence-based psychiatry. *Canada Journal of Psychiatry, 46*(5), 403-406.

Goldman, H., & Azrin, S. (2003). Public policy and evidence-based practice. *Psychiatric Clinics of North America, 26,* 899-917.

Goldner, E. M., & Bilsker, D. (1995). Evidence-based psychiatry. *Canada Journal of Psychiatry, 40,* 97-101.

Green, L., & Kruefer, M. (1991). *Application of precede/proceed in community settings: Health promotion planning: An educational & environmental approach.* Mountainview, CA: Mayfield.

Hennessy, K. (2005, January). *Delivering excellent mental health care and accelerating research: A SAMHSA update.* Paper presented at the Kansas Freedom Commission Initiative Goal 5 Summit.

Hoge, M., Tondora, J., & Staurt, G. W. (2003). Training in evidence-based practice. *Psychiatric Clinics of North America, 26,* 851-865.

Hope, T. (2002). Evidence-based patient choice and psychiatry. *Evidence-based Mental Health, 5,* 100-101.

Insel, T. (2003, November). *Research for recovery: The National Institute of Mental Health perspective.* Paper Presented at The Nineteenth Annual Rosalynn Carter symposium on Mental Health Policy.

Institute of Medicine Committee on Quality Healthcare in America. (2001). *Crossing the quality chasm: A new health system for the 21ˢᵗ century,* Washington, DC: National Academic Press.

Kessler, R. (2003). *The importance of new epidemiological findings for policy.* Paper presented at the Nineteenth Annual Rosalynn Carter Symposium on Mental Health Policy.

Lehman, A., Buchanan, R. W., Dickerson, F. B., Dixon, L. B., Goldberg, R., Green-Paden, L., et al. (2003). Evidence-based treatment for schizophrenia. *Psychiatric Clinics Of North America, 26,* 939-954.

Lehman, A. F., & Steinwachs, D. M. (1998). Translating research into practice: The schizophrenia patient outcome research team (PORT) treatment recommendations. *Schizophrenia Bulletin 24,* 1-10.

McGovern, M. P., & Carroll, K.M. (2003). Evidence-based practices for substance abuse disorders. *Psychiatric Clinics of North America, 26,* 991-1010.

Mellman, T. A., Miller, A. L., Weissman, E. M., Crismon, M. L., Essock, S. M., & Marder, S. R. (2001). Evidence-based pharmacological treatment for people with severe mental illness: A focus on guidelines and algorithms. *Psychiatric Services, 52*(5), 619-625.

Munetz, M. R., & Frese, F. J. 3ʳᵈ. (2001). Getting ready for recovery: Reconciling mandatory treatment with recovery vision. *Psychiatric Rehabilitation Journal, 25*(1), 35-42.

President's New Freedom Commission on Mental Health. (2003). *Achieving the promise: Transforming mental health care in America.* Washington, DC: Department of Health & Human Services.

Reinhardt, U. E. (1991). *The importance of quality in the debate on national health policy healthcare Quality management for 21ˢᵗ Century.* American College of Physician's Executives.

Relman, A. S. (1988). Assessment of accountability: The third revolution in medical care. *New England Journal of Medicine, 319,* 1220-1222.

Rogers, E. M. (1995). The challenge: Lessons for guidelines from the diffusion of innovations. *Journal on Quality Improvement, 21,* 324-328

Rosenheck, R. (2001). Organization process: Missing link between research and practice. *Psychiatric Services, 52*(12), 1607-1612.

Rush, A. J., Rago, W. V., Crismon, M. L., Toprac, M. G., Shon, S. P., Suppes, T., et al. (1999). Medication treatment for the severely and persistently mentally ill: The Texas Medication Algorithm Project. *Journal of Clinical Psychiatry, 60*(5), 284-91.

Sackett, D. L., Rosenberg, W. M., Gray, J. A., Haynes, R. B., & Richardson, W. S. (1996). Evidence-based medicine: What it is and what it isn't. *British Medical Journal, 312,* 71-72.

Torrey, W. C., Finnerty, M., Evan, A., & Wyzik, P. (2003). Strategies for leading the implementation of evidence-based practices. *Psychiatric Clinics of North America, 26,* 883-897.

U.S. Public Health Service Office of the Surgeon General. (1999). *Mental health: A report of the Surgeon General.* Rockville, MD: Department of Health & Human Services, U. S. Public Health Services.

World Health Organization World Health Report. (2001). *Mental health: New understanding, new hope.* Geneva: World Health Organization.

Chapter 8

Improving Care for the Chronic Mentally Ill Patient: A Policy Perspective

John A. Talbott
Professor of Psychiatry, University of Maryland School of Medicine

Abstract

In this chapter I will give some of the history of the prior two national mental health commissions, then after a word on some definitions of terms I will use, I will review the historical background of various reform movements that our country's mental health services have undergone since colonial times, especially as they apply to the chronic mentally ill. I will then summarize the state of the chronic mentally ill in America today as others, the commissioners of the President's New Freedom Commission, and I see it. To facilitate discussion of the existing situation regarding the six areas or issues the Commission has identified for attention, I have reworded their "goals" as "issues" and will give the data or arguments used by the commissioners to justify their concerns, what their ultimate goal is regarding each issue, what they concretely propose that the federal and local governments do, and then add my own comments about the issue and solutions. I will then try to explain how the newest Presidential Commission puts this all together, give a general critique of the Report and relate what some experts have already said about the report. To specify what further steps need to be undertaken to fulfill the Commission's worthy goals, I will discuss four areas: good intentions, leadership, funding and administrative flexibility and change. Finally, I will add a personal appreciation of the Commission's work.

Introduction

In 1955, the first national Commission on Mental Illness and Mental Health was appointed, largely as a result of the published reports of inhumane conditions in the nation's state (Musto, 1977) and Veteran's Administration mental hospitals. In 1961, their report on the mentally ill – "Action for Mental Health"– was published, calling for an end of large state hospitals and the building of smaller facilities in the community. In 1964, President John F. Kennedy's administration adapted this report into a call for treatment in the community through community mental health centers (Public Law, 1963). President Jimmy Carter appointed the second Presidential Commission in 1977, at a time when the disasters of badly implemented and unplanned community care, later known as deinstitutionalization, became overwhelming, and their report (President's Commission, 1978) called for a comprehensive approach to addressing these problems. In 2002, President George W. Bush appointed the third such commission and it has recently published its report (New Freedom, 2003).

What is the state of the chronic mentally ill in America today, how does the newest Presidential Commission address it, and what further needs to be done to fulfill its worthy goals? This chapter will review these three questions, beginning with some historical background to set 21st Century developments in context (Talbott, 1994). But first, some discussion of terms.

Definitions

I will employ the contentious word "chronic mentally ill" in its most widely used and understood definition, i.e., that proposed by Leona Bachrach, a sociologist, in 1976, designating specifically, "those individuals, who are, have been, or might have been, but for the deinstitutionalization movement, on the rolls of long-term mental institutions, especially state hospitals." To counter the usual objections, the term includes those persons who are seriously, persistently or episodically ill as well as occasionally, continually or never hospitalized and has no implication of not improving, never recovering or deteriorating. The Commission uses the term "serious" for DSM-III-R illnesses that result in "functional impairment" (New Freedom, 2003, p. 2). I believe the word "serious" implies that there are illnesses that are not serious, i.e., that are frivolous, which I do not believe we mean to imply. Therefore, in quoting the Commission report, I will preserve their "serious" wording, but in my writing, I will use the word "severe."

Historical Background

At our beginnings as a nation, in colonial times, there was no health or mental health care. The mentally ill were either cared for at home by their families, in out-dwellings on their family's grounds or later in public, largely city or county-run, "houses". While much is made of the difference in intent of the three types of places mentally ill persons were sent to; that is, jails were intended for rogues and vagabonds, almshouses and poorhouses for the town's needy and workhouses for the idle and disorderly; in fact, the mentally ill wound up in all three, largely willy-nilly (Talbott, 1978). It was Dorothea Dix, arguably the most successful mental health advocate in American history, who convinced the states (after failing to convince the federal government, an irony lost on the framers of federally-financed community mental health centers (CMHC's) a century later) to assume responsibility for the mentally ill, then known as "the insane," or what we would today consider as persons suffering from psychotic illnesses.

Thus, starting in the 1800's, we saw a gradual and steady increase in both the numbers of "asylums" (a good word to recall in its most beneficent definition) and those housed there. That increase continued until 1955, despite the introduction of alternatives to institutional/hospital care beginning in the 1855 (Talbott, 1998) such as:

- The farm of Sainte Anne (Galt, 1855)
- The Illinois Cottage Plan
- The Massachusetts' Boarding out project
- After-care
- Outpatient clinics
- Traveling clinics
- Crisis intervention
- Satellite clinics
- Day hospitals
- Social rehabilitation
- Home care
- Halfway houses
- Vocational rehabilitation

Thus, despite the commonly-held opinion that community care sprung out of policy makers' minds like Venus from the half-shell, by 1955 there were proven, tested examples of all the elements of what we would consider good community care or a community mental health center, granted few and far between, granted unexamined by research and granted unknown in cost.

World War II represented a critical moment for the mentally ill. First, the sheer number of persons reporting for induction in the military who were mentally ill, shocked the medical authorities; indeed, it is held that during one period, more inductees were released on grounds of mental illness than were inducted. Second, physicians in the time-honored military fashion became what the military needed not what they were trained as, thus many unsuspecting, untrained physicians overnight became "psychiatrists." Third, military psychiatry began to learn what Thomas Salmon had learned in World War I, i.e. that persons suffering from combat symptoms could recover and did not need long-term hospitalization. And fourth, conscientious objectors, assigned to state mental hospitals, were shocked by the inhumane crowding and conditions.

Thus, just as we as a nation, exited the War with a changing view of our future, psychiatry saw new directions as well. In short order, a national Joint Commission on Mental Illness was appointed, with leading ex-military and civilian members. Their report, now nearly forgotten, "Action for Mental Health" (1961), called for: "community clinics for outpatient care, psychiatric units in general hospitals for short-term inpatient treatment, 'open communities' for [the] acutely mentally ill but who [could] be rehabilitated, and chronic disease centers for [patients with] long-term illnesses of all kinds."

States took up the call. California and New York as usual, led the charge. In New York for example, legislation called for four of the ten elements that eventually comprised the community mental health center (CMHC): inpatient and outpatient care, consultation and education and rehabilitation. In addition, another group of leaders of the American Psychiatric Association inspected the situation in Europe where they saw and were impressed with: open wards, units in general hospitals and rehabilitation services in the community.

While most citizens and mental health experts mistakenly date the problems of deinstitutionalization to the late 1960's, the downturn in state hospital population actually began half a century ago, in 1955 (Brill & Patton, 1959), and what persons are referring to now is in retrospect the "tilt-point" at which newspapers, cities and citizens became outraged at the sight of the mentally ill flooding the streets, "Bowery's" and the emergency rooms of our nation (Schumach, 1974).

It was at this point, the late 1960's and early 1970's, following a national conference devoted to organizational issues, at which clinical crises, such as deinstitutionalization were introduced, that the American Psychiatric Association acted. It formed a national Blue-Ribbon Committee, held a Conference whose proceedings were published (Talbott, 1978b) and widely disseminated and itself issued a "Call To Action for the Chronic Mentally Ill" (Talbott, 2004b). This "cri du coeur" was not published in isolation; during the same period, the Group for the Advancement of Psychiatry (Committee, 1978) and even the federal government's own watch-dog agency, the General Accounting Agency (Returning, 1977) called for a re-examination of what, by this time, was known as deinstitutionalization, but was widely and correctly seen as depopulation, that is, depopulating institutions without implementing care or funding for patient care in the community.

President Jimmy Carter and/or his staff and family was concerned enough to appoint the second Presidential Commission on Mental Health and Illness in 1977. It devoted considerable attention to the plight of the chronic mentally ill (President's, 1978). However, as is well known, the report, containing dramatic suggestions about reforming the system, died a quiet death between the time when Ronald Reagan's poll ratings began to challenge Carter's and his inauguration as President. Thus from 1978 to now, although Koyanagi and Goldman (1991) insist that small steps have been taken toward the goal, the situation is not really that much better. Indeed, if anything, the private sector and the states so heartedly embraced managed care and privatization in the 1990's that in many states and localities, things got worse, in terms of patient care.

Now, with the release of President Bush's "New Freedom" Commission Report (New Freedom, 2003), we have a new opportunity to change the treatment and care of the chronic mentally ill for the better.

In succeeding sections I will cover the state of the chronic mentally ill in America today, how President Bush's Commission addresses the current situation, and what further needs to be done to fulfill the Report's goals.

What is the state of the chronic mentally ill in America today?

To provide an assessment of how the chronic mentally ill are faring today, I have divided this appraisal of the status quo into systems issues and patient issues.

Systems Issues

Predominant among the problems of the chronic mentally ill today is a "map" showing where they are housed. As we have learned in the last half-century, what was true then, that is, that severely and chronically mentally ill persons were invariably found in large psychiatric hospitals (whether state or federally, that is, VA, run). Soon, however, as Morton Kramer (1975) famously pointed out, the predominant location for this population became "homes," whether board and care, nursing or other "community" homes. The fifty years of scandals in these institutions has not abated and we are still shocked by revelations of the problems when say there is a fire in a home or a homeless person freezes to death, but for the most part we still tacitly support this trans-institutionalization.

The homeless mentally ill continue to constitute a significant proportion of the homeless population in America. Without counting substance abuse, the chronic mentally ill were estimated by Burt in 2001 to constitute 46% of the homeless, just as they did at the height of concern for homelessness in the 1960's and 1970's. Despite all the news accounts and scandalous incidents, they continue to represent the most visible symbol of our failed non-policy of deinstitutionalization. In a much widely quoted figure, UNICEF (1998) estimated that "three quarters of a million people in the United States are homeless. In addition, both their medical and psychiatric problems remain under- or untreated. The Bush Commission (New Freedom, 2003, pp. 30-31) notes in a section entitled "A Shortage of Affordable Housing Exists," that "millions of people with serious mental illnesses lack" "decent, safe, affordable and integrated housing," leading to their cycling "among jails, institutions, shelters and the streets…"

The mentally ill in prisons and other correctional facilities is an equally scandalous situation, although the mentally ill in such institutions at least receive shelter, food and variable medical care, including psychiatric treatment. Lamb and Weinberger (unpublished, 2005) state that "The latest methodologically sound estimates (1995) of the percentages of persons in jails and prisons diagnosed with major depression, schizophrenia and other psychotic disorders, and bipolar disorder range from 15 to 24 percent" (Lamb &Weinberger, 1998). The Bush Commission (New Freedom, 2003, p. 32) reports that 7% of the 1,300,000 persons incarcerated in state and federal prisons have a "current serious mental illness," which they note is 3-4 times the rate in the general population (American Psychiatric Association, 2000). Things are worse regarding children, where "66% of boys and nearly 75% of girls in juvenile detention" (Teplin, Abrahm, McClelland, Duncan, & Mericle, 2002) have "at least one psychiatric disorder."

The mentally ill continue to be housed in various homes that were not intended for and are not able to treat the mentally ill, despite the fact that research time and again has shown that such facilities are unable to care for their psychiatric needs. In such cases, they are often under-, over- and polypharmaceutically-treated. The fashion of sending mentally ill persons to facilities intended to provide medically ill geriatric patients with longer-term care than they are afforded in general hospitals began shortly after 1955. But the states continue to act as if they have to utilize such institutions, in order to move to community care. Recent state budget crises have only aggravated the situation.

In summary, then, regarding where chronic and severely mentally ill persons are living; 50 years after deinstitutionalization began, the evidence has never been stronger that patients continue to suffer from trans-institutionalization.

Other systems issues reported in the New Freedom Commission (New Freedom, 2003, p. 1) include: "stigma," "treatment limitations and financial requirements placed on mental health benefits in private health insurance" and a "fragmented mental health service delivery system," all identified the President Bush's message to the Commission in 2002; as well as an implied lack of coordination and shared decision-making (New Freedom, 2003, p. 4) between families and providers, a lack in understanding that recovery is a goal of the system, disincentives to employment, and access to *health care* (emphasis mine), which were identified in the final report.

Treatment and Care Issues

In addition to these systems problems, what is the treatment and care of the chronic mentally ill like? I will use two sources for my appraisal of the status of these areas, one, my own assessment of what we have learned about treatment and care of the chronic mentally ill since 1955 (Talbott, 2004a); the other, Anthony Lehman et al's many reports from the Schizophrenia Patient Outcomes Research Team (PORT) report (e.g., Lehman et al., 1998). In my assessment, I concluded that we do not implement "what we...know" (Talbott, 2004a, p. 1158) regarding tailoring treatment settings to an individual's needs, recognizing and treating relapse, using hospitalization appropriately, utilizing group and cognitive behavioral treatments, using multiple modalities, maximizing rehabilitation, maximizing community treatment and providing continuity of care. Lehman et al used different words, i.e. "translating research into practice," (Lehman et al., 1998, p. 1) stating that we still do not properly use and monitor antidepressants and antipsychotic medications (in acute and maintenance situations, utilizing clozapine and in using long-acting and targeted intermittent medication) as well as appropriately utilize psychosocial treatments such as: family intervention, supported employment, assertive community treatment, skills training, cognitive-behavioral therapy and token economy interventions."

The Bush Commission takes the findings made by Talbott and Lehman as the status quo, as is obvious by their stating (New Freedom, 2003, p. 5) in Goal #5 that "Excellent mental health care is delivered and research is accelerated," that "New relevant research findings must be systematically conveyed to front-line workers so they can be applied to practice quickly" and that "The Nation must invest in the infrastructure to support emerging technologies and integrate them into the system of care."

In summary, then, treatment and care of the chronic mentally ill still falls far short of the mark, given the incredible findings and innovations in psychopharmacological and psychosocial treatments since 1955. So, given this dismal appraisal of the systems and clinical issues regarding the severely and chronically mentally ill, how did the newest Presidential Commission see and propose to address the situation?

What is the state of the situation at present according to the Commission and what do they propose be done?

Because of the way government reports are written, that is, almost exactly the reverse of their order in contributions to the scientific literature, which proceed from an introduction to the problem, objective, methods, results, discussion and conclusions, we have in this report the conclusions first, then the summary, and finally the statement of the problem(s). In order to help the reader progress from the problems to solutions, I will reframe each of the goals as problems to be addressed and reshape the recommendations as remedies to be sought. In addition, because the task I was assigned was to address the subpopulation of chronic mentally ill, I will largely focus on adults and the elderly and not children, recognizing the importance of screening, referring and treating this population and knowing that other authors will focus on them.

First Issue: Americans don't understand that mental health is essential to overall health.

Why is this so? The Commission states this is the case (New Freedom, 2003, pp. 19-23) because:

1. Too many people "are unaware that mental illnesses can be treated and recovery is possible," that "mental illnesses [are] the leading causes of disability" and thus "many people [50% with severe mental illness] with mental illnesses go untreated."
2. "Stigma impedes people from getting the care they need."
3. Americans are "unaware of suicide's toll" as the "leading cause of violent deaths."
4. Despite the interaction between mental and general health and high degree of co-morbidity, coordination of care between general health and mental health sectors is lacking.
5. Financing is skewed so that insurance does not cover the treatment of mental disorders as well as physical illnesses in the same person. In addition, States don't know how to "cover evidence-based practices, which services may be covered...., which services are allowable under waiver and how to use Medicaid funds seamlessly with....private sources."

6. Services and funding are fragmented between all levels of government and types of medical and social services.
7. Financing is restrictive rather than flexible.

What is their ultimate goal to address the above? Goal 1: [That] "Americans understand that mental health is essential to overall health" (New Freedom, 2003, p. 7). This goal basically says mental health care should be seen equivalent to general health care, stigma will be reduced or eliminated, all populations (e.g. from rural areas, minorities, non-English speakers) will have access and primary care providers will have the *time, training and resources* (emphasis mine) to treat persons with "common" mental illnesses.

How? (New Freedom, 2003, pp. 23-26) 1.1 Through "...*a national campaign* (emphasis mine) to reduce...stigma...." "much like anti-smoking campaigns promote physical health" and 1.2 by "address[ing] mental health with the same urgency as physical health" through "reviewing existing" studies and "initiating new studies" as well as incorporate examination of the "unique needs of mental health financing" in any new efforts at health care reform or transformation.

Comment: The initial recommendation reads as if it is primarily addressed to reduce stigma and barriers to access of the chronic mentally ill, but raises the question of how all these initiatives will be funded. In addition, although they state (New Freedom, 2003, p. 23) that "the most effective way to reduce stigma is through personal contact with someone with a mental illness," instead of recommending a program that would accomplish this, they suggest yet another national public education campaign. Also, although they devote a page and a half to "Swift Action is Needed to Prevent Suicide," no numbered recommendation is made to accomplish this, although in fairness they do cite a model program developed by the Air Force (New Freedom, 2003, p. 25) and say that a national "public-private partnership" should stimulate state projects. Finally, they "punt" the whole issue of restrictive and skewed funding to an as-yet to be announced effort to reform or transform the entire health care system.

Second Issue: Mental health care is not consumer and family driven.

Why is this so? The Commission states this is the case (New Freedom, 2003, pp. 27-34) because:

1. "The complex....system overwhelms...consumers," and instead of being able to use an integrated system, patients and families have to do the integrating themselves.
2. "Program efforts overlap," and the different funding, mission and administration of programs of housing, health care and corrections, to mention but a few, result in a totally disorganized non-system.
3. "Consumers and families do not control their own care."

4. "Consumers need employment and income support[s];" the severely
   mentally ill represent the "largest diagnostic group (35%) on SSI
   rolls...and a quarter (28%) of all SSDI recipients," and "only about 1
   in 3 is employed;" which is not surprising when it turns out that "only
   23% of people with schizophrenia received any kind of vocational
   services."
5. "A shortage of affordable housing exists."
6. "Limited mental health services are available in correctional facilities."
7. "Fragmentation is a serious problem at the state level."
8. "Consumers and families need community-based care."
9. "Consumers face difficulty in finding quality employment," for example,
   "70% of people with serious mental illness with college degrees earned
   less than $10 per hour....and overall....earned...$6...versus $9...for
   the general population."
10. "The use of seclusion and restraint creates risks."

What is their ultimate goal to address the above? Goal 2: [That] "mental health care
[be] consumer and family driven (New Freedom, 2003, pp. 8-9)." The text
supporting this goal says that the diagnosis of a severe mental illness will "set in
motion a well-planned, coordinated array of services and treatments defined in a
single plan of care" with the active participation of consumers and family members.
It will be updated appropriately and place "financial support.... under the
management of consumers and families...." "By allowing *funding to follow consumers,*
incentives will shift (emphasis mine) toward a system of learning, self-monitoring and
accountability" and consumers will use "resources wisely." "The *burden of coordinating care will rest on the system,* not the family or consumers" (emphasis mine).
Redistributing the financing will thus force federal, state and local governmental
agencies into a "partnership." States will be given the responsibility of developing
a grand plan and the "flexibility to combine Federal, State and local resources"
involving "health care, *employment supports, housing and criminal justice*" (emphasis
mine). Creative, innovative programs will result. There is an unstated implication
that all severely mental ill persons *will* (emphasis mine) receive treatment (and with
what the Report says later, that includes psychopharmacology); this is followed by
a stated concern implying over-utilization of seclusion and restraint as a "treatment"
rather than a "safety" issue.

How? (New Freedom, 2003, pp. 35-47) 2.1 By "develop[ing]...individualized
plan[s] of care...," between providers, patients and families that will spell out
options and permit money to follow patients, 2.2 "involv[ing] consumers and
families fully in orienting the mental health system toward recovery" and facilitate[ing]
the utilization of consumers as providers in consumer-run services, 2.3
"Align[ing]...federal programs to improve access and accountability..." as well as
better meet the needs of patients, especially when it comes to employment and
employment services, housing needs and services in correctional institutions and

encourage states to more flexibly utilize Medicaid funding so money does indeed "follow the patient,", 2.4 "creat[ing] Comprehensive State....Plans to coordinate services" that will end fragmentation and facilitate partnerships mentioned before, both aimed at meeting patients' needs optimally, incentivized by federal funding and 2.5 "Protect[ing]...the rights of people....," ending unnecessary institutionalization, employment discrimination and reducing the use of seclusion and restraint."

Comment: With all due respect to the distinguished members of the Commission, none of the first nine "Why" points is new; for at least 30 years, experts and reports, both private and public, have railed about the fragmented system and lack of housing, employment, services in prisons, etc. It is ironic that several of the commissioners and expert scientific consultants are or have been in positions of power in state and federal systems and now, are, in a way, pointing fingers at themselves. How quickly we forget what Pogo said. This goal implies that two giant steps can be easily taken; e.g., merging governmental funds (originally proposed by Talbott and Sharfstein in 1986) and putting them in the hands of consumers and family members; plus it sets up what may be an inherent contradiction between ensuring state of the art, research-proven treatment and consumer preference; take mandatory clozapine treatment or depot medication as examples. And then we come to Point #10, which seems to come out of the clear blue sky, e.g., "The use of seclusion and restraint creates risks." Surely true, but it is a jarring end to their argument about fixing a messed-up non-system.

Third Issue: There are disparities in mental health services.

Why is this so? The Commission states this is the case (New Freedom, 2003, pp. 49-51) because:

1. "Minority populations are [still] underserved....," or inappropriately served, as has been shown by the Surgeon General's Report (United States, 2001), at a time when their population is growing to "40%" by 2025 (Bureau, 2001).
2. "Minorities face barriers...," both due to their misperceptions and beliefs and racism, discrimination and under-insurance.
3. "Cultural issues...affect service providers..." and "much of the existing workforce" lack training in cultural competence.
4. "Rural America [25% of the population] needs improved access...," because it is underserved and its citizens "have...lower...incomes, ...greater social stigma...[and] longer periods without insurance coverage."

What is their ultimate goal to address the above? Goal 3: [That] "Disparities in mental health services [be] eliminated" (New Freedom, 2003, p. 10). This goal presents a Liebnizian scenario in which all Americans *will share equally* (emphasis mine) in the "best available services," regardless of who they are and where they live and those services are "tailored" to ethnicity and need and provided by a culturally competent providers, including emergency room staff and first responders. The only specific suggestion and technology mentioned is videoconferencing to rural areas.

How? (New Freedom, 2003, pp. 49-56) 3.1 Improving "access to quality care that is culturally competent" and that more research and training be provided to translate this research into "culturally competent practices" as well as recommending that State plans monitor access and "set standards for culturally competent care," that "national leadership" needs to improve the bridge between "community health and mental health" and that more "ethnically, culturally, and linguistically competent" providers be created and 3.2 improving "access to quality care in rural and....remote areas" become a high priority for federal interagency cooperation and State plans, with "benchmarks" set and "telehealth" technology more widely utilized.

Comment: No one could disagree with these noble aims, however, I emphasized "will share equally" above because this is the first time in the report that I saw what represents a deft wording to avoid a situation where promises are made that cannot be kept; instead they look towards a situation where all Americans could "share equally" in a much smaller pie.

Fourth Issue: Early screening and referral are not common.

Why is this so? The Commission states this is the case (New Freedom, 2003, pp. 57-60) because:

1. "If untreated, childhood disorders" get worse and "frequently continue into adulthood" where the persons suffering from them use more services and incur higher costs (Knapp, McCrone, Fombonne, Beecham, & Wostear, 2002).
2. Schools, which could help identify afflicted children, are not always equipped and charged to do so.
3. While 7-10 million persons have co-occurring illnesses, they are not "often" identified and treated for more than one illness, (Substance, 2002; Watkins, Burnham, Kung, & Paddock, 2001) providers don't treat dual diagnoses well, and the system is not prepared to cope with the forthcoming doubling of psychiatric illnesses in the geriatric population (Jeste et al., 1999).
4. Psychiatric problems are not well handled in primary care settings, despite the fact that one -half of the care of such disorders takes place there (Regier et al., 1993), the majority of drugs are prescribed in these settings as well as the fact that a great number of patients suffering from mental illnesses who are seen in these settings commit suicide, and finally, the corollary, that general health problems are poorly handled in specialty mental health settings.

What is their ultimate goal to address the above? Goal 4. [That] "Early mental health screening, assessment, and referral to services [become] common practice. (New Freedom, 2003, p. 11)." This goal repeats the *summun bonum* of the 1960's community mental health movement; with all its emphasis on childhood screening in schools and adults in general health settings, etc. and hopes that soon all mental health and general health providers will be adept at such screening and referral.

How? (New Freedom, 2003, pp. 60-66) 4.1 By "promoting "mental health of....children, (which I will not dwell on since my focus in this chapter is chronic mental illness largely among adults, fully recognizing that such screening, assessment, referral and treatment is essential to reducing the numbers of children and adolescents who carry their mental illnesses into adulthood), 4.2 Improving and expanding "school mental health programs," 4.3 Screening for co-occurring...disorders...," and 4.4 Screening "in primary...care, across the lifespan and connect[ing] afflicted individuals] to treatment and supports" as well as encourage "collaborative care models" in the private and public sectors, financed privately and publicly, as well as involving not just the usual federal and state agencies, but the VA in addition.

Comment: Again, no one can dispute this goal, but it falls short of saying how it will be accomplished and with what resources. Our nation's interest in promoting "mental health" as opposed to treating "mental illness" began almost a *century ago* (my emphasis) with one of the driving forces being Clifford Beers' groundbreaking book "A Mind that Found Itself" (1908/1960), whose stress was on health not illness, along with Adolf Meyer's articulation of what became known as prevention (Winters, 1952) and the child guidance (Levy, 1968) movement. The fact that the intent to stress health not illness has been proposed in every report ever written since then, and still appears today, demonstrates how difficult it has been to actually do it. More recently, the goal of *implementing integrated treatment* (my emphasis) was recommended by one of the senior experts to the Commission, Howard Goldman, as well as myself, almost twenty years ago (Ridgely, Goldman, & Talbott, 1986).

Fifth Issue: Excellent care is not delivered and research is not done fast enough.

Why is this so? The Commission states this is the case (New Freedom, 2003, pp. 67-71) because:

1. There is too long a delay between research being done/published and its findings being implemented; "treatments and services.... *languish for years* (emphasis mine), and if implemented are done so unevenly and inconsistently.
2. State-of-the-art treatment, ranging from *medications* (emphasis mine) to *Assertive Community Treatment* (ACT), whether derived from evidence-based practices or "emerging" (a word I think they coined) best practices, such as *jail diversion to multi-family therapy* (emphasis mine)

is not available to all, because of reimbursement, training, too few professionals and the need for more research.

3. Reimbursement policies don't foster translating research to practice, instead they limit paying for some proven treatments and services.

4. Consumers and family members testified that there were too few providers, especially in rural areas, and the current staff, especially BA-level, paraprofessionals and primary care professionals (PCPs) were poorly trained in modern psychiatric, culturally competent, delivery modalities.

5. There has been insufficient research in *minority disparities, long-term effects of medications, trauma and acute care* (emphasis mine).

What is their ultimate goal to address the above? Goal 5: [That] "Excellent mental health care is delivered and research is accelerated" (New Freedom, 2003, pp. 12-13). This goal posits that medications and psychotherapies that are "evidence-based, state-of-the-art...will be standard practice...." The goal involves *adequate training* (emphasis mine) to translate research into practice. It also states that "[t]he nation *will continue to invest* (emphasis mine) in research at all levels." However, they do recommend increased financing of "...new treatments and practices...."

How? (New Freedom, 2003, pp. 71-77) 5.1 They propose that we "Accelerate research to promote recovery and resilience and *ultimately cure and prevent* (emphasis mine) mental illnesses," utilizing a "dialogue among researchers, providers, consumers and family members," 5.2 "Advance evidence-based practices using...projects and create public-private partnership[s] to guide their implementation," as well as "change reimbursement policies to more fully support" evidence-based practices, 5.3 Help providers provide "evidence-based .....services..." and 5.4 "*Develop* (emphasis mine) the knowledge base in four understudied areas: *mental health disparities, long-term effects of medications, trauma and acute care.*"

Comment: I was interested that almost everywhere else, the word "excellent" is used but training need only be "adequate;" and it's pleasant to finally see a federally-sponsored group finally find fault with the 1960's spirited over-reliance on under-trained staff. In addition, increased research is not recommended, the commissioners implicitly merely suggest continuing current levels of funding, e.g. "continue to invest." Note also that while in the rest of the report they call for more clinical applicability of research, here their preference is for clinical over basic research. As for the wish to "develop" research in the four areas of "*minority disparities, long-term effects of medications, trauma and acute care,*" I must presume the commissioners meant to write "increase," since so much research and so many reports already exist in all four areas. As for "*research* [not being] *accomplished fast enough,*" I fear the commissioners have not dealt sufficiently enough with researchers to know that they cannot be forced to work faster and compared to scientists elsewhere in the world, are as quick in publishing worthwhile findings as others elsewhere. While it may be that the Institute of Medicine (2001) found that in general medicine research "*languish*[es] *for years*," in psychiatry, excepting Clozapine's use in the United States, it is untrue regarding other psychopharmacological agents, where profit drives overly rapid dissemination and the fault is not under-dissemination but over-promise. As carefully referenced as most of the report is, I cannot find data to back up these feelings; I'm curious what *medications* have not been rushed to market as soon as FDA approval, (which balances safety with urgency and has exceptions for critical drugs to combat, for example, AIDS and cancer), has been achieved. Regarding psycho-social interventions, the statement holds for some psychosocial interventions such as Fairweather Lodges (Fairweather, Sanders, & Tornatzky, 1974), however, as to others, such as assertive community treatment, this truly revolutionary intervention is a "success story" that I believe the commissioners do not appreciate. In addition, given the current brouhaha about suicides and SSRI antidepressants, would the commissioners really have wanted SSRI's to have been introduced faster, with fewer studies and cautionary notes? Again, in terms of some "emerging" best practices, such as *jail diversion and multi-family therapy*, we do not need more research, they are well and truly proven, we need money and action to implement them. And finally, as for reimbursement policies, several of the commissioners are the very people responsible for not reimbursing some interventions, for example, the 30-year proven intervention of day hospitals/day care.

Sixth Issue: Technology is underutilized.

Why is this so? The Commission states this is the case (New Freedom, 2003, pp. 79-80) because:

1. Health care in general doesn't yet fully utilize technology, and mental health, in particular needs a "telehealth system" and "an integrated health records system."
2. Access to care is problematic, especially in rural areas.
3. Currently available technology can help providers have access to patient information, no matter where both are.
4. Consumers don't have access to reliable information.

What is their ultimate goal to address the above? Goal 6. [That] "Technology [be better] used to [provide better] access [to] care and information" (New Freedom, 2003, pp. 14-15). The key to this is "advanced communication and information technology" available to providers, consumers and family members. This would involve using a "common language," using a common database of "studies" and "breakthroughs," and implementing universally electronic records while preserving privacy.

How? (New Freedom, 2003, pp. 81-85) 6.1 Using "health technology and telehealth to improve access...," and have States eliminate "barriers" such as "restrictive licensure and scope-of-practice restrictions" as well as reimbursing for "e-heath and telehealth services" and 6.2 Have "integrated electronic record[s]....."

to help providers have access to current medical records as well as consumers to have better information to help make decisions about their own care

Comment: Once again, one cannot argue with any of these points, except to point out that the balancing act between easy information exchange among those who should have access to such data and privacy will remain a difficult issue. One statement that is curious is that "access to information will foster continuous, *caring relationships*" (emphasis mine). As someone whose job now is to improve the state of medical humanism among physicians, I'm not at all sure one follows the other at all.

How does the newest Presidential Commission put this all together?

As I mentioned at the start, the report is written backwards, so what I will now summarize actually appears as the "Executive Summary" (New Freedom, 2003, pp. 1-16). The New Freedom Commission's final report has both expected and unexpected emphases that are of particular relevance to treatment and care of the chronic mentally ill: they include a commitment to reduce stigma, eliminate "treatment limitations and financial requirements placed on mental health benefits in private health insurance," fix a "fragmented mental health service delivery system," avoid "patients falling through the cracks," reduce the time and difficulty moving from research to implementation of findings, meet unmet needs such as "unnecessary and costly disability, homelessness,…and incarceration," end "fragmentation and gaps in care" for adults and older adults, prevent suicide, reduce high unemployment, emphasize "recovery" as the most important goal, provide access to quality care tailored to patients' needs and replace "unnecessary institutional care with efficient, effective community services." The Commission notes that "traditional reform measures are not enough" and proposes "fundamentally transforming" mental health care delivery. How?

Before it spells out its goals, the Commission states that the overarching goal of a "transformed system" is the promise of "recovery" (New Freedom, 2003, pp. 4-5) and that universal "easy and continuous access to the most current treatments and best support services" as well as providing consumers and family member "access to timely and accurate information" will facilitate attainment of this overarching goal. In addition, at the time a diagnosis is first made, the commission envisions the formation of a partnership among patient, family members and providers to collectively determine "*who, what and how*" care will be provided, its implementation - to be ensured through an individualized treatment plan, with which patient and family members may agree or disagree. It insists that services and treatments be "*consumer and family centered,*" (emphasis theirs) and that care should not be devoted solely to "managing symptoms" but "*focus on increasing consumers' ability to successfully cope with life's challenges, on facilitating recovery, and on building resilience,…*" (emphasis theirs).

The Commission notes that such a transformation will require (emphasis mine) *changing* "*incentives*…to encourage continuous improvement in agencies that provide care," making research findings available to "front-line providers" quickly so they may apply them sensitively to our diverse population and that treatment and services be reimbursed based on "proven effectiveness and consumer preference – not just on tradition or outmoded regulations...." (New Freedom, 2003, p. 5). It states finally that to achieve this transformation, "the nation must *invest* (emphasis mine) in the infrastructure to support emerging technologies and integrate them into the system of care."

As for the actual implementation, the Commission's Report concludes (New Freedom, 2003, p. 86) that "As has long been the case in America, *local innovations under the mantle of national leadership* (emphasis mine) can lead the way for successful transformation throughout the country."

General critique of the Report

Let me start by saying what I've said several times throughout my "comments" on what the commissioners said, especially as it regards the chronic mentally ill, the population I care most about and about whom I was assigned to discuss; this a noble, well-intentioned, on-target report which contains logical, sensible and necessary steps to fix a broken non-system. Does that mean it will happen and the Goals will be achieved? I'm not sure, but I think we have to examine the issue of reform or transformation more generally first.

How does transformation actually happen in the world? Does it occur from the top down or bottom up? Well, certainly the collapse of the Berlin Wall and election of Viktor Yushchenko, took place because people took to the streets and reversed top-down policy; but most reform comes from above, for example deregulation of the airlines or setting standards for schools.

The commissioners chose a mélange, that is, "*local innovations under the mantle of national leadership.*" As I understand this, this means that the feds will spell out the goals and directions but states and local agencies will actually implement them. But who will pay for the "*invest*[ment] in the infrastructure and who will insist on "*changing incentives*" for public and private reimbursement?

Let's look at past mental health reform or transformation. What drove the move of the chronically mentally ill from asylums to community settings, what stimulated the building of community mental health centers or permitted thousands of chronic mentally ill persons to move to affordable housing?; it was not only national policy but federal funding. Do American institutions change because it is the right thing to do or because there are economic, legal and/or political carrots and sticks? I think the answer is self-evident.

Many organizations and state legislatures insist that proposals and bills carry prices if adopted. This report has none. The implication, idealistic and noble as it is, is that by (someone's) shifting the incentives that currently govern the expenditure of service, research and training dollars, from Medicare, Medicaid, and private insurance as well as moneys spent in schools, correctional facilities, homes, universities, etc., by federal, state and local agencies., money can be moved from existing institutions to patient/family control; from institutions to community care; and from illness treatment to recovery-based interventions.

What have some experts said about the report?

It's too early to have had much discussion of the report and the one published special section in Psychiatric Services (New Freedom, 2003) had a mixture of contributions from the chair of the Commission, who naturally supports the report; the "partners" in the "Campaign for Mental Health Reform," who are committed to help implement the report; and other invitees, who were freer to criticize the report. (Disclosure: I was Editor at the time the section was proposed and papers reviewed and accepted)

What do they add to what I've written above? Michael Hogan, PhD, its chair, notes (2003) that the commissioners were aware of the fate of the recommendations made by the "Carter Commission," the bad news, e.g. that the Mental Health Systems Act was "rolled back" (that is to say in English, "died") and the good news, that Koyanagi and Goldman (1991) felt that *"progress was achieved* (emphasis mine) by staged, incremental, midrange changes in major federal programs such as Medicaid, Medicare and Social Security, rather than "big-bang" reform measures or increased support for specific mental health programs." So these successes "shaped" their "thinking." A page later Hogan states that the group agreed that "the system was *in shambles*" (emphasis mine). One must wonder why the system was/is in such shambles if any progress had been made since 1991. Hogan concludes that implementation will be difficult, but will be aided by: (1) the designation of a SAMSHA director to develop the "implementation approach," (2) "creation of a Campaign for Mental Health Reform," and (3) "the system's strengths – effective treatments, dedicated clinicians, passionate advocates, and the essential ingredient of hope." In the next five pages of the journal's special section (Glover, Birkel, Faenza, & Bernstein, 2003), the founding "partners" representing the National Association of State Mental Health Program Directors (NASMHPD), the National Alliance for the Mentally Ill (NAMI), the National Mental Health Association (NMHA), and the Bazelon Center for Mental Health Law largely laud the report but do have reservations about the possibility for change in the absence of:

- national legislation,
- commitment on the part of non-mental health federal agencies on policy changes,
- uniform state and local "advocacy terrain[s],"
- "opinion research,"
- "communication strategies that target key decision makers in Congress and the Administration,"
- correction of the 10% state "per capita spending reductions,"
- "a single, flexible funding stream,"

- a "real conversation" with the American public on "talk radio," etc.,
- "everyone speaking in a unified voice,"
- "resources to do the job" of "psychiatric rehabilitation or supports for life in the community, such as integrated housing" and "reversing decades of underfunding"
- the willingness of "states and localities" to re-engineer "their own systems."

As I suggested above, the two persons who are outsiders vis a vis the Commission's process and report are a bit more skeptical. The then-President of the American Psychiatric Association, Marcia Goin (2003) notes the necessity to also have:

- "acute care...beds,"
- reimbursement for an adequate period in hospital for stabilization,"
- "additional funding" to support model programs targeting homeless persons, such as the Commission highlighted in California.

And the last commentator, Saul Feldman, (2003) representing "managed behavioral health," suggests we need to also achieve:

- "full parity,"
- funding for the "150,000 units of permanent supportive housing" recommended by the Commission, so necessary to prevent rehospitalization, homelessness, unnecessary institutionalization, etc., (in this portion of his critique, Feldman says what no one has before, i.e. that the Commission was not free "to recommend anything that would cost money.")
- adequate numbers of psychiatrists, (this from a non-psychiatrist, mind you, who runs a managed care company)
- addressing gun control as part of the solution to diminishing suicide,
- standardizing rather than supporting differences among states' efforts.

Surely with time we will see more critique and analysis of the Commission's Report, but the above serves as an introduction to what further needs to be done.

What further steps need to be undertaken to fulfill the Commission's worthy goals?

If one looks back at all my comments about each Goal and in general, as well as those written by the partners in the "Campaign for Mental Health Reform," and the two invited experts (Feldman, 2003; Goin, 2003), there are four critical issues or themes: Good Intentions, Leadership, Funding and Administrative Flexibility and Change.

With all seriousness I propose that there are four axioms that sum up these issues:

1. "The road to hell is paved with good intentions."
2. "No one ever washed a rental car."
3. "You don't get something for nothing," and
4. "You can lead a horse to water but you can't make him drink."
   I will discuss each.

1. Good Intentions. "The road to hell is paved with good intentions."

With some minor exceptions, where the commissioners try to have their cake and eat it too (e.g., provide state of the art treatment for all patients while preserving their right to refuse and direct treatment), or where I think the commissioners are naïve (that American scientists are not working fast enough compared to colleagues elsewhere), wrong (to use the word "develop" rather than 'increase" research in the four areas of "minority disparities, long-term effects of medications, trauma and acute care,"), have dropped a ball ("the most effective way to reduce stigma is through personal contact with someone with a mental illness,"), missed a golden opportunity ("Swift Action is Needed to Prevent Suicide,"), or been too "politically correct ("The use of seclusion and restraint creates risks,") it is hard to disagree with the vision, goals and recommendations of the Report. That is not to say they are wish-washy or banal, although they do repeat many recommendations that have been advocated for at least a century. But let us accept that they are 99% agreed-upon by experts in the field. What now? That is, how is the implementation of these six noble and lofty goals to be achieved?

I was asked to address the manner in which the President's New Freedom Commission proposes that the discrepancies in mental health regarding the "chronically mentally ill patient" were to be remedied from a "policy perspective." Now, my understanding of public policy is that there are two elements of a policy – the articulation of the policy and its implementation. The first part (Good Intentions) is well done. The second remains to be done. How are the nineteen officially numbered recommendations in the Executive Summary (New Freedom, 2003, pp. 7-15) and even more suggestions embedded in the main text to come into being?

2. Leadership (and responsibility). "No one ever washed a rental car."

The commissioners, many of them leaders at either the state or federal level, suggest the solution to implementation will come from: "*local innovations under the mantle of national leadership.*" Once again, Feldman, a former federal leader, put his finger on it: "the significant differences between the states....are a source of confusion and complexity with no apparent benefit." To mix metaphors, letting a "thousand flowers grow" may doom this current effort; separating responsibility and accountability is an administrative nightmare as any textbook on administration will reiterate; they must be linked. That is, the entity that leads and sets policy also has to have the resources and be held accountable for utilization of those resources. Or to return to my axiom, if there's no ownership of the process (the car), it won't be maintained (washed). In the case of CMHC's, for instance, which ironically, Feldman headed up at one time, which gives his comments great credibility, the feds spelled out the guidelines for building, staffing and programs as well as *allocated monies to the CMHC's* (emphasis mine). The feds did not merely articulate one more unfunded mandate.

3. Funding. "You don't get something for nothing."

How are the nineteen officially numbered recommendations in the Executive Summary and even more suggestions embedded in the main text to be funded? As Feldman says in his critique, regarding one recommendation, "No amount of 'collaboration' or 'transformation' or reduced 'fragmentation'…or…'enhanced access' to something that does not exist will produce more low-cost supportive housing." There's a lot to be done, how is it to be funded? That is not clear at this point. Everything the commissioners mentioned needs to be done. Is the money there? Take another example, research. They recommend that we "continue to invest" in it, but do not suggest increased funding. While it is not clearly stated in the report, according to Feldman, the commissioners apparently worked under the clear assumption that they were not "to propose new funding." Well then, maybe funding can be found elsewhere; and there is much mention of monies in other pots: say corrections, social services, education, housing, unnecessary institutionalization, etc. What about that? Which gets me to #4.

4. Administrative Flexibility and Change. "You can lead a horse to water but you can't make him drink."

The commissioners talk a great deal about changing incentives, to have "money follow patients," to shift toward a "system of learning, self-monitoring and accountability," "to encourage employment," "to encourage continued improvement in agencies" and "for public and private reimbursement." Maybe the correctional or educational system will share their monies with mental health if they no longer have to care for the mentally ill, but can mental health manage violent inmates or educate disturbed children? And what is in it for the state and local social service systems, for example, to give huge chunks of their budgets to mental health and lay off staff. I'd like to believe that money is fungible but my sense is that like another maxim: "bureaucracies exist to perpetuate themselves" and it's a rare bureaucracy whose goal is to go out of business or share resources. The commissioners mention time and again "restrictive" and skewed funding, but no solution is proposed.

So what further needs to be done?

A lot. First, leadership and ownership needs to be fixed somewhere. The U.S. Secretary of Defense has the job description, the responsibility and the resources to defend our country and is held accountable; the State Director of Transportation has the job description, the responsibility and the resources to issue drivers' licenses, among other things and is held accountable; the City Commissioner of Sewers has the job description, the responsibility and the resources to run the waste system and is held accountable; why should this huge task be any different; a job description, the responsibility to implement the Report, the resources to do it and being held accountable. The "partnership" can serve as the watchdog, along the guidelines of NIH Advisory Committees.

Second, just like companies and universities and legislatures need business plans and budgets to make decisions, a detailed description of the monetary resources it will take to accomplish this project must be outlined.

Third, a plan that spells out the realities of changing the "incentives" and "disincentives" needs to be written in detail and agreed to by those who will be affected by it. If this requires the President's good offices, so much the better.

Finally, do we need a federal public law or laws to implement some of these goals? Koyanagi and Goldman (1991) seem to indicate that we do. I realize the commissioners were torn between the need to have a banner under which to march (like Kennedy's CMHC Legislation) and the political realities that insist on smaller government, no new taxes and more individual responsibility. But to simply hold aloft a banner, with no where to march and no funds to support the march, is clearly not enough.

Personal addendum

I should end by expressing my gratitude for the hard work and good thinking that went into this report. It may seem that I am overly critical and nit-picking, which may indeed stem primarily from my thirty years of failed advocacy efforts on behalf of the underserved, especially the chronic mentally ill. But I could not agree more with the Commissioner's lofty aims; and I must reveal my conflicts of interest clearly – many of the commissioners and expert consultants and staff are colleagues and friends and are very well intentioned (in the best sense of the word) professionals. I would merely state in my defense that I would be equally skeptical of any reform I had a hand in than one I was outside of. In 1985, when I publicly presented a report of a proposed state mental health reform to then New York Governor Mario Cuomo, which had been written by his own Health Advisory Council, of which I was then the chair, I started with an anecdote about a chronic mentally ill patient who was at this time incarcerated in the "Tombs," New York City's infamous jail. My last words were "Governor, the test of this reform will be whether this patient in the future will receive the treatment and care he deserves, where he should receive it." P.S. He has not.

References

Action for Mental Health: Final Report of the Joint Commission on Mental Illness and Health. (1961). New York, NY: Basic Books.

Alston, P. (1998). *Hardship in the midst of plenty. The Progress of nations.* Unicef Retrieved February 8, 2005 from http://www.unicef.org/pon98/indust1.htm.

American Psychiatric Association's Task Force to Revise the APA Guidelines on Psychiatric Services in Jails and Prisons (Report No. 2). (2000). *Psychiatric services in jails and prisons.* Washington, DC: American Psychiatric Association.

Bachrach, L. L. (1976). *Deinstitutionalization: An analytical review and sociological perspective.* Rockville, MD: National Institute of Mental Health.

Beers, C. (1908/1960): *A mind that found itself.* Garden City, NY: Doubleday.

Brill, H., & Patton, R. (1959). Analysis of population reduction in New York State mental hospitals during the first four years of large-scale therapy with psychotropic drugs. *American Journal of Psychiatry, 116,* 495-500.

Bureau of the Census. (2001). *Profiles of general demographic characteristics 2000: 2000 census of population and housing: United States.* Washington, DC: U.S. Department of Commerce.

Burt, M. R. (2001). *What will it take to end homelessness?* Urban Institute Brief. Washington, DC: Urban Institute.

Committee on Psychiatry and the Community. (1978). *The chronic mental patient in the community.* New York: Group for the Advancement of Psychiatry.

Fairweather, G. W., Sanders, D. H., & Tornatzky, L. G. (1974). *Creating change in mental health organizations.* Elmsford, NY: Pergamon.

Feldman, S. (2003). New freedom commission report: A view from managed behavioral health. *Psychiatric Services, 54,* 1482-1483

Galt, J. M. (1855). The farm of St. Anne. *American Journal of Insanity, 11,* 352-357.

Glover, R. W., Birkel, R., Faenza, M., & Bernstein, R. (2003). New freedom commission report: The campaign for mental health reform: A new advocacy partnership. *Psychiatric Services, 54,* 1475-1479.

Goin, M. K. (2003). New freedom commission report: The commission's report and its implications for psychiatry. *Psychiatric Services, 54,* 1480-1481.

Hogan, M. F. (2003). New freedom commission report: The President's new freedom commission: Recommendations to transform mental health care in America. *Psychiatric Services, 54,* 1467-1474

Institute of Medicine Committee on Quality of Health Care in America. (2001). *Crossing the quality chasm: A new health system for the 21st century.* Washington, DC: National Academies Press.

Jeste, D. V., Alexopoulos, G. S., Bartels, S. J., Cummings, J. L., Gallo, J. J., Gottlieb, et al. (1999). Consensus statement on the upcoming crisis in geriatric mental health: Research agenda for the next 2 decades. *Archives of General Psychiatry, 56,* 848-853.

Knapp, M., McCrone, P., Fombonne, E., Beecham, J., & Wostear, G. (2002). The Maudsley long-term follow-up of child and adolescent depression: Impact of comorbid conduct disorder on service use and costs in adulthood. *British Journal of Psychiatry, 180,* 19-23.

Koyanagi, C., & Goldman, H. H. (1991). The quiet success of the national plan for the chronically mentally ill. *Hospital & Community Psychiatry, 42,* 899-905.

Kramer, M. (1975). *Psychiatric services and the changing institutional scene.* Rockville, MD: National Institute of Mental Health.

Lamb, H. R., & Weinberger, L. E. (1998). Persons with severe mental illness in jails and prisons: A review. *Psychiatric Services, 49,* 483-92

Lamb, H. R., & Weinberger, L. E. (unpublished manuscript, 2005). *The shift of psychiatric inpatient care from hospitals to jails and prisons.*

Lehman A. F., Steinwachs, D. M. & the Co-Investigators of the PORT Project. (1998). At issue: Translating research into practice: The schizophrenia patient outcomes research team (PORT) treatment recommendations. *Schizophrenia Bulletin, 24,* 1-10.

Levy, D. M. (1968). Beginnings of the child guidance movement. *American Journal of Orthopsychiatry, 38,* 799-804.

Musto, D. F. (1977). The Community mental health movement in historical perspective. In W. E. Barton & C. J. Sanborn (Eds.), *An assessment of the community mental health movement* (pp. 1-11). Lexington, MA: Lexington Books.

New Freedom Commission Report. (2003). *Psychiatric Services, 54* (Special section), 1465-1483.

New Freedom Commission on Mental Health. (2003*).* Achieving the promise: Transforming mental health care in America. *Final Report.* Rockville, MD: DHHS Pub. No. SMA-03-3832. Available at www.mentalhealthcommission.gov/reports/final report/fullreport-02.htm

President's Commission on Mental Health. (1978). *Report to the President.* Washington, DC: U.S. Government Printing Office.

Public Law 88-164. (1963). *The mental retardation facilities and community mental centers construction act of 1963.* Washington, DC: U.S. Government Printing Office

Regier, D. A., Narrow, W. E., Rae, D. S., Manderscheid, R. W., Locke, B. Z., & Goodwin, F. K. (1993). The de facto U.S. mental and addictive disorders service system. Epidemiologic catchment area prospective 1-year prevalence rates of disorders and services. *Archives of General Psychiatry, 50,* 85-94.

Returning the Mentally Disabled to the Community: Government Needs to Do More. (1977). Washington. D.C.: General Accounting Office.

Ridgely, M. S., Goldman, H. H., & Talbott, J. A. (1986). *Chronic mentally ill young adults with substance abuse problems: A review of the literature and creation of a research agenda.* Baltimore, MD: University of Maryland School of Medicine, Mental Health Policy Studies.

Schumach, M. (1974, January - April). Series on the problems of deinstitutionalization. *New York Times.*

Substance Abuse and Mental Health Services Administration. (2002). *Report to congress on the prevention and treatment of co-occurring substance abuse disorders and mental disorders*. Bethesda, MD: Substance Abuse and Mental Health Services Administration.

Talbott, J. A. (1978a). *The death of the asylum: A critical study of state hospital management, services and care*. New York: Grune & Stratton.

Talbott, J. A. (Ed.). (1978b). *The chronic mental patient: Problems, solutions and recommendations for a public policy*. Washington, DC: American Psychiatric Association.

Talbott, J. A. (1994). 50 years of psychiatric services: Changes in treatment of the chronic mentally ill. In J. Oldham & M. Riba (Eds.), *Annual Review of Psychiatry 1994* (pp. 93-120). Washington, DC: American Psychiatric Press, Inc.

Talbott, J .A. (1998). Deinstitutionalization, emergency services, and the third revolution in mental health services in the United States. In M. DeClercq, S. Lamarre, & H. Vergouwen (Eds.), *Emergency psychiatry and mental health policy: An international point of view* (pp. 85-105). Canada: Elsevier Science.

Talbott, J. A. (2004a). Lessons learned about the chronic mentally ill since 1955. *Psychiatric Services, 55*, 1152-1159. (Originally published in 1994 in R.J. Ancill, S. Holliday & J. Higenbottam. *Schizophrenia 1994: Exploring the Spectrum of Psychosis*. London: Wiley & Sons.)

Talbott, J. A. (2004b). Position statement: A call to action for the chronic mental patient. *Psychiatric Services, 55*, 1118-1123. (Original work published in 1979, *American Journal of Psychiatry, 136*, 748-752).

Talbott, J. A., & Sharfstein, S. S. (2004). A proposal for future funding of chronic and episodic mental illness. *Psychiatric Services, 55*, 1145-1149. (Original work published in 1986, *Hospital and Community Psychiatry, 37*, 1126-1130).

Teplin, L. A., Abram, K. M., McClelland, G. M., Duncan, M. K., & Mericle, A. A. (2002). Psychiatric disorders in youth in juvenile detention. *Archives of General Psychiatry, 59*, 1133-1143.

United States Public Health Service Office of the Surgeon General. (2001). *Mental health: Culture, race, and ethnicity: A supplement to mental health: A report of the surgeon general*. Rockville, MD: Department of Health and Human Services, U.S. Public Health Service.

Watkins, K. E., Burnam, A., Kung, F. Y., & Paddock, S. (2001). A national survey of care for persons with co-occurring mental and substance use disorders. *Psychiatric Services, 52*, 1062-1068.

Winters, E. E. (1952). *The collected papers of Adolf Meyer*. Baltimore, MD: Johns Hopkins Press.

Chapter 9

The Role of Mental Health Consumers in Leading the Recovery Transformation of the Mental Health System

Daniel B. Fisher and Judi Chamberlin

National Empowerment Center, Inc.

This paper is an adaptation of a paper the authors prepared for the National Summit on self-determination, sponsored by SAMHSA in March, 2004.

Executive Summary

Today's mental health system has failed to facilitate the recovery of people with severe mental illness. Piecemeal approaches focusing on the introduction of specific programs, in the absence of larger shifts in underlying philosophy, have failed to have a lasting impact. Only a fundamental change of the very culture of the system will ensure the recovery called for in the New Freedom Commission on Mental Health Report. Mental health consumer/survivors representing diverse cultural backgrounds have led the recovery movement for many years. Among stakeholder groups, consumer/survivors are the most motivated to bring about a recovery-oriented system because we have the most to gain. This paper provides an outline of how survivor/consumers can play an even larger role in catalyzing the transformation of the mental health system from one based on an institutional culture of control and exclusion to one based on a recovery culture of self-determination and community participation. At the national policy level, this paper recommends that consumers develop and implement a National Recovery Initiative. At the State and local policy levels, State and local Recovery Initiatives are recommended. On the direct service level, the paper provides a road map for developing services, financing, and supports, which are based on recovery.

A recovery-based mental health system would be based on at least the ten fundamental principles of recovery revealed through research at the National Empowerment Center (NEC):

- Trusting oneself and others
- Valuing self-determination
- Believing you will recover; having hope

- Believing in the person
- Connecting at a human level
- Appreciating people are always making meaning
- Having a voice of one's own
- Validating all feelings
- Following dreams
- Relating with dignity and respect

Changing the mental health system to one that is based on these principles of recovery will require a concerted effort of consumers and allies working to bring about changes in beliefs and practices at every level of the system. The building of these alliances will require the practice of recovery principles in every relationship.

Goal: Transformation from the Institutionally-based Mental Health System to a Recovery-Based System through consumer/survivor Leadership

Objective 1: Transform the system to one based on a recovery culture through consumer led development of a National Recovery Initiative (NRI)

Step 1.1: Consumer leaders will set up a National Recovery Initiative Steering Committee, to carry out the recommendations of the New Freedom Commission

Step 1.2: The NRI subcommittee on recovery education will launch a nation-wide pro-recovery, anti-stigma education campaign

Step 1.3: NRI Subcommittee on Policy will develop and synthesize model recovery policies as well as materials for training consumers in board participation

Step 1.4: NRI Subcommittee on Recovery-based Evaluation and Research will develop materials and train consumers in carrying out evaluations of the performance of mental health systems

Step 1.5: NRI Subcommittee recovery-based services and supports will supply the Networking and TA needed to help in the further development of consumer-run state-wide groups to coordinate self-help groups

Objective 2: Consumer-driven transformation to a system of self-determined and recovery- based services and supports

Step 2.1: Shift to person-centered planning

Step 2.2: Shift to financing mechanisms, which support increased consumer control

I. Financing services and supports to allow money to follow the individual

II. Financing consumer-run National Technical Assistance Centers

Step 2.3: Expand the range of choices of services and supports available by creating roles for peers in service delivery and support

I. Expand peer-provided services

A. Peer professionals

B. Peer specialist

C. Peers as staff in consumer-run programs

D. Peers involved in mutual support

II. Expand the use of Personal Assistance Services for people with psychiatric disabilities

Introduction

Though many people with mental illness have been moved from state institutions to community settings, most have not recovered. Although these consumer/survivors are living "in the community," they are not integrated into the community in a meaningful manner. Though state hospital patients have been transported to community settings, and been renamed consumers, their recovery is being impeded by the persistence of institutional thinking by all stakeholders. This institutional thinking persists in the application of an outdated, classical medical model that describes serious mental illnesses as permanent, biological diseases. Institutional thinking considers recovery unlikely, and "good" outcomes are considered to be lifetimes of maintenance on psychiatric drugs, residence in halfway houses or other supervised settings, and repetitive days of mindless "activities" or dead-end, below minimum wage jobs, such as work in sheltered workshops. This system has led to huge costs for maintaining this population, hopelessness for people diagnosed with mental illness, political inertia, and a lack of interest on the part of many professionals for dealing with a population deemed to be incurable. In short, we have taken the people out of institutions but we have not taken institutional thinking out of the people. Institutional thinking persists in all societal thinking about mental illness and severely hampers efforts to facilitate recovery.

Since empowerment, hope, and self-determination are repeatedly cited as the keys to people's recovery (Ahern & Fisher, 2001ab; Anthony & Spaniol, 2002; Chamberlin, 2003; Zinman, 2002), it appears that the underlying institutional medical culture of the present system, with its over emphasis on the narrowly defined version of the medical approach, is actually interfering with recovery. Recently consumer/survivors, administrators, and families have united in the conviction that the mental health system needs a fundamental transformation at the level of its mission and values to one based on recovery. In this paper we present a roadmap for consumer-driven transformation to a recovery-based system that can act as a unifying action plan for citizens and government alike. No longer can people with mental illness wait for government to lead the way to a new system. The leadership for this transformation needs to be taken up by consumer/survivors, families, and other advocates, in partnership with government and mental health authorities.

Many voices have been calling for change, including segments of the professional community, families, political leaders, and, perhaps most importantly, diagnosed people themselves, many of whom have refused to accept the limited roles they were expected to fill. These voices for change have recently received support from the President's New Freedom Commission on Mental Health, whose Report (Mental Health Commission Final Report, 2003, which will hereafter be referred to as the Commission Report) called for a transformation of the mental health system to one based on the principles of recovery, as stated in its vision: "We envision a future when everyone with mental illness will recover"(Commission Report, p. 1). The Report also states that "…care must focus on facilitating recovery and building resilience not just on managing symptoms" (Commission Report, p. 5).

Other government studies have reached similar conclusions. The recently released Veterans' Administration Action Agenda (2003) has called for recovery to be a central principle in the transformation of VA services and supports by recommending that the VA:

• Adopt the Recovery Model in VA Mental Health Programs nationwide
• Develop VA adapted recovery implementation tools as the basis for a national rollout
• Involve consumers who are veterans and families in educating staff/veterans/ family members on recovery

The Surgeon General's Report on Mental Health (Surgeon General, 1999) and the National Council on Disability Report, *From Privileges to Rights* (NCD, 2000) also highlight the importance of having people who have recovered from mental illness play an active role in the policies and services of the system.

Only a fundamental change of the very culture of the system will ensure that the changes made in policy, training, research, and services will lead to genuine recovery. Consumer/survivors must play a leading role in designing and implementing this transformation. Otherwise, we will see people who have recovered playing a secondary role and their work fit into the existing system, rather than their work leading the transformation to a recovery-based system. An example is provided by one mental health center, which pointed proudly to their use of peer counselors. However, rather than using their personal experiences to serve as role models and guides to clients in earlier stages of recovery, these "peer counselors" had been given the job of monitoring medication. In other words, they had to adapt to the existing institutional culture of dependency instead of leading the transformation to a system based on recovery. In addition, the recovery culture needs to be culturally competent as recommended in the Surgeon General's Report on Culture, Race and Ethnicity (Surgeon General, 2001). The existing institutionally based system is narrow in its scope, thereby leaving little room for minority cultures. A recovery-based system would be more accepting and understanding of people from a variety of backgrounds.

The Western New York Care Coordination Program (WNYCC, 2004) provides a further illustration of the importance of culture change to influencing lasting transformation of the system. They stated, "Despite the care taken to develop a template for individual service planning that focused on the interests of individual recipients, a review of the first set of individual service plans developed by care coordinators revealed little change from the 'provider knows best' case management system" (www.carecoordination.org). Their steering committee recognized "culture change as the critical first step to system transformation." (www.carecoordination.org). Therefore, care must be taken to introduce cultural change training, which emphasizes recovery and person-centered planning, into the initial steps of system transformation. Most important, people who have recovered should lead this training.

In a recovery culture, peer support will be seen as a central focus of the services and supports. Peers can transform both the individuals they are helping and those around them. It will be important for survivor/consumers to take the lead because they have the greatest commitment to real change. Although the term "recovery" has come into the lexicon of federal, state, and local reports and plans, there is a concern among survivor/consumers that the meaning of recovery has been subverted. The first example of what we call a limiting version of recovery appeared in the rehabilitation literature of the 90's. According to this limiting version of recovery, people with mental illness can, like people with a spinal cord injury, learn to cope with their illness, but they will never fully recover from mental illness. Since the label mental illness carries the concept that peoples' judgment is permanently impaired, people can never become self-directed adults as long as they remain labeled mentally ill. On the other hand, survivor/consumers and researchers have experienced, researched, and written about complete recovery from mental illness (Ahern & Fisher, 2001ab; Harding, Brooks, Ashikaga, Strauss, & Breier, 1987; Karon & Vanden Bos, 1981). This we will call genuine recovery. The National Empowerment Center has described the path to genuine recovery: the empowerment model of recovery. According to this model, people with mental illness can completely recover by taking control of the major decisions of their life and thereby assuming or resuming major social roles. We emphasize the importance of this distinction because it lies at the heart of the transformation of the system. If the vision of recovery really means limited recovery, the services will still be designed to control consumers' major decisions for the rest of their lives. A system based on a goal of limited recovery is a system with no exit points. It is a system, which is always run from the top down by administrators, doctors, and other clinicians that perpetually make decisions for the consumer. It is, however, important to emphasize that, in the NEC definition of full, genuine recovery, people may continue to experience symptoms or may choose to use medication. The hallmark of genuine recovery is the individual regaining control of his or her own life and filling valued social roles.

The empowerment model of genuine recovery has the following features:

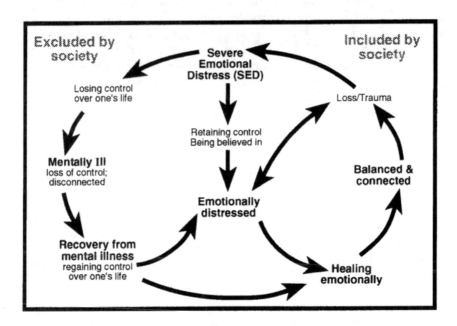

Figure 1. Empowerment Model of Recovery from Mental Illness.
Created by Daniel B. Fisher, M.D., Ph.D. and Laurie Ahern.
Copyright 1999 National Empowerment Center, Inc.

The Empowerment Model is based on the research findings that genuine recovery is possible for most people labeled with mental illness (Ahern & Fisher, 2001ab). Given the right mix of relationships, attitudes, and resources, people with mental illness can fully recover by (re)gaining control of the central decisions of their lives, learning to live with intense emotions, and developing the skills and relationships needed to establish a major social role. According to this model, most people begin life at the right side of the diagram (Figure 1), balanced and whole. However, we all suffer trauma and loss, which lead, to emotional distress and feelings of fragmentation and not being whole. Through coping strategies and social supports most people are able to heal emotional and indeed develop and stronger sense of self. Sometimes, however, a major trauma or loss, such as a failure to adapt to college or the loss of a loved one, can lead to severe emotional distress. At that point (at the top of the diagram) it is crucial that there be sufficient non-institutional supports and coping strategies available to allow the person to heal. During this period it is also vital that people retain their connections with their community and as much control over their life as possible. In the absence of such supports, such as supportive people who believe in her/him, adequate and appropriate housing and finances, and coping strategies, the person's life and controls are taken over by institutional mental health systems and programs and they are labeled severely mentally ill. Once a person is labeled with mental illness they must recover not only from the severe emotional distress, but also from the role and identity of a person with mental illness. The label not only relegates people to a low status and diminished rights, but it also eats away at a person's confidence and initiative to pursue dreams and to lead a full life of one's own choosing. Consumer/survivors have unified around the goal of genuine recovery as outlined in this Empowerment Model.

The report of the Subcommittee on Consumer Issues to the New Freedom Commission (see www.mentalhealthcommission.gov) described genuine recovery very well:

> Mental health research shows that people can and do fully recover, even from the most severe forms of mental illness. Most fundamentally, recovery means having hope for the future, living a self-determined life, maintaining self-esteem, and achieving meaningful roles in society. Most consumers report they want the same things other people want: a sense of belonging, an adequate income, a way to get around, and a decent place to live. They aspire to build an acceptable identity for themselves and in the community at large. These are the essential ingredients of recovery from mental illness.
>
> An emerging literature on the success of the recovery approach comes from the self-help movement, testimony of consumers, the psychiatric rehabilitation community, and research. Public and private sectors of the mental health community are initiating recovery-based programs, services and self-help technologies to overcome the barriers faced by people living with a mental illness in America. Recovery is an organizing principle for mental health services, programs, and supports that is based on consumer values of choice, self-determination, acceptance, and healing.
>
> For recovery to take place, the culture of mental health care must shift to a culture that is based on self-determination, empowering relationships, and full participation of mental health consumers in the work and community life of society. To build a recovery-based system, the mental health community must draw upon the resources of people with mental illness in their communities.
>
> It is widely recognized that changing the mental health system to be more responsive to consumer needs requires the participation of consumers at all levels of policy planning and program development, implementation, and evaluation. Meaningful involvement of consumers in the mental health system can ensure they lead a self-determined life in the

community, rather than remaining dependent on the mental health system for a lifetime.

A recovery-oriented mental health system embraces the following values:

- *Self-Determination*
- *Empowering Relationships*
- *Meaningful Roles in Society*
- *Eliminating Stigma and Discrimination*

We are proposing in this paper a Recovery Initiative Action plan, which would lead to:

Goal: A Consumer/ Survivor Led Transformation from an Institutionally-based System to a Recovery-based System

In order to insure that mental health services are truly empowering and recovery-focused, attention must be paid to the underlying values of each service (e.g., hospitalization, crisis intervention, housing, rehabilitation services, employment services, etc.). Services, which are focused on symptom management or maintenance, for example, must give way to those which stress movement, development, and change (in other words, are recovery-based). Services must provide mechanisms for community integration and promote opportunities to live in ways that non-disabled people live.

It is clear that a massive shift in philosophy, accompanied by changes in funding mechanisms, will be necessary to implement successful self-determination approaches that maximize the ability of people with psychiatric disabilities to gain control of their lives. In the next section, we will describe a proposal for making the necessary shifts to a recovery culture so that the kinds of new programs and funding mechanisms described above can flourish.

Objective 1: Transform the system to one based on a recovery culture through a consumer/survivor led National Recovery Initiative (NRI)

The New Freedom Commission Report recommends that the system "involve consumers and families fully in orienting the system to recovery…local, State, and Federal authorities must encourage consumers and families to participate in planning and evaluating treatment and support services. The direct participation of consumers and families in the development of a range of community-based, recovery-oriented services is a priority (Commission Report, p. 37) "….Every mental health education and training program in the Nation should voluntarily assess the extent to which it…engages consumers and families as educators of consumers, families, and health care providers…about the concepts of recovery (Commission Report, p. 75)."

Over the past two decades, mental health consumers/survivors have started to build such a national presence within the public mental health sector, with growing numbers now participating in research and evaluation (Van Tosh, Ralph & Campbell, 2000) and taking leadership roles in policy and administration of public mental health services (McCabe & Unzicker, 1995). They have led efforts to determine housing preferences (Tanzman, 1993), to define outcome measures (Campbell, 1997; Trochim, Dumont, & Campbell, 1993), and to develop partnerships models with public mental health professionals (Campbell, 1996). Consumers/survivors carved out an expanding role in lecturing, conducting grand rounds, teaching continuing education classes, and offering workshops at national professional conferences. In 1993 consumer-practitioners and psychiatrists engaged in a dialogue in New York regarding coping strategies and recovery from mental illness (Blanch, Fisher, Tucker, Walsh & Chassman, 1993).

To truly transform a system it is necessary to effect changes at all levels. The Commission's Recommendations provide the roles for consumers to catalyze such a transformation because they encompass all levels and activities of the system. Consumers are the best agents to foster the needed changes. In March, 2003, the Report of the Consumers' Issues Subcommittee to the New Freedom Commission proposed the concept of a National Recovery Initiative: "In order to facilitate recovery from mental illness, the Subcommittee urges Federal, state and local governments to together develop a National Recovery Initiative that promotes consumers' self-determination at both the collective and individual levels of recovery" (see www.mentalhealthcommission.gov).

The policy options that follow comprise the key components of the proposed National Recovery Initiative. This idea has captured the imagination of many consumer/survivors across the country because it gives substance to a unifying principle. Recovery inspires consumers to be involved in transforming the system and in their own lives in a manner that the present system has failed to do. A National Recovery Initiative also gives consumer/survivors an opportunity to exercise a degree of control in their lives, which was never before apparent. The vision of recovery has unified consumer/survivors as never before. This is a proposal to form temporary committees, which are centered on shared recovery values and shared implementation, rather than the formation of a permanent national organization.

Step 1.1: Consumer/survivor leaders will set up a National Recovery Initiative Steering Committee, which will carry out the New Freedom Commission's Recommendations

The purpose of this steering committee would be to recommend national goals, policies and actions for carrying out the steps outlined below. The committee would also monitor progress towards these goals through an evaluation component. Since the theme of "nothing about us without us" is a key principle throughout the consumer/survivor community, it will be important to have all the significant segments of that community represented from the outset. Consumer/survivors from diverse cultures have rarely had a voice in mental health policies. Consumer/ survivors from minority cultures have had even less of an impact on the system than consumers in general. Therefore, from the outset, it will be important to assure that representatives from diverse cultures are actively engaged at the table and that attention is given to culturally responsive materials. In addition, it would be important to be inclusive of people from sexual and gender identity/expression minority communities. The criteria for inclusion would include:

- Experience at a state and/national level with development of mental health policies
- An ability to work with a variety of people from a variety of backgrounds
- An understanding and acceptance of the basic recovery premises outlined in the New Freedom Commission Report
- Representation of the various philosophical views, geographic regions, ages, ethnic groups, and sexual and gender identity/expression minority communities

A congress of 40-50 consumer leaders would be the mechanism through which the steering committee is to be established. Although ideally such a congress should take place in person, several teleconferences could be used instead. A primary function of this steering committee would be the development of a National Recovery Initiative Action Agenda. This agenda would consist of a section on the process for bringing such an Initiative into being and a section on guidelines for content guidelines.

The Mental Health Commission's Subcommittee on Consumer issues started the process of developing a NRI Action Agenda in 2002-03. The feedback from consumer leaders received at Alternatives 2002, the 2002 meeting of National Association of Rights, Protection and Advocacy (NARPA), and a meeting of the National Association of Consumer/survivor Mental Health Administrators (NAC/ SMHA) in 2002 was used to generate the paper on consumer issues. The next step is for the steering committee to develop an action agenda to carry out the goals established to date through the New Freedom Commission Consumer Issues Subcommittee.

Since its appearance a year ago, the idea of a National Recovery Initiative has captured the imagination of numerous consumer leaders. This theme has unified factions of the consumer movement and the family movement around a common, positive concern. The proposed contents of the Initiative were outlined in the subcommittee's report, and are divided into two levels of consumer activity. These two levels were collective (systemic) and individual self-determination:

> The Subcommittee recommends increasing collective consumer self-determination by ensuring consumers' significant participation in the development of a National Recovery Initiative. This initiative would

inform policy, evaluation, research, training, and service delivery at local, state and national levels in all systems integral to recovery from mental illness. The Subcommittee urges Federal, state and local governments to employ consumers in leadership roles in the development of a National Recovery Initiative.

The Subcommittee urges the mental health system at the Federal, state and local levels to increase individual consumer self-determination by helping people with mental illness to acquire the self-management skills needed to manage their own lives. To accomplish this, we urge a shift from traditional services to recovery planning services, such as peer support services and services provided by independent living centers (see www.mentalhealthcommission.gov).

The NRI Steering Committee would have an interactive Website on which it would post its membership and its agenda, and on which it would receive feedback. Additional methods of dissemination and dialogue would be provided as well, in recognition that web access is not universal, and is probably more limited for consumers, and even more so for consumers who are members of ethnic and racial minority groups.

The NRI Steering Committee would play a role in implementation of the New Freedom Commission Report at the Federal and State levels. The commission recommends that the fragmentation in funding and services be reduced by the development of a federal mental health policy across department lines. For instance, though SAMHSA is the lead agency in federal mental health policy, it plays a minor role in financing relative to CMS, SSA, HUD, RSA, NIMH, and the VA. The NRI Steering Committee could play a valuable role in assisting these agencies in coordinating the changes in their funding and regulations needed to facilitate the shift to a recovery-based system. If the NRI could have representation on the strategic planning bodies of these agencies, it would allow for representation of a broad cross-section of consumers nationally. In addition, The NRI Steering Committee could give support and coordination of transformation at the state levels.

The NRI Steering Committee would establish subcommittees on recovery education, recovery policy development, recovery-based evaluation and research, and development of recovery-based services and supports. These subcommittees would be selected by the NRI Steering Committee and would lead this systemic transformation to a recovery culture through their education of decision makers and the public about recovery, their participation in setting policies consistent with a recovery culture, in carrying out system evaluation to ensure that changes are carried out which promote the transformation to recovery, and their development of recovery-based peer-run services and supports. These subcommittees would use an NRI Website to interact with constituents.

Step 1.2: The NRI subcommittee on recovery education will launch a nation-wide pro-recovery, anti stigma education campaign

The present mental health system is a top down hierarchy. The culture of the present system is carried by the top decision-makers: administrators, funders, clinical directors, and mental health professionals. These are the people who need to buy into a shift to a recovery culture, and to see that sharing their decision making power will make the system function better and facilitate recovery. These decision-makers need to give inspiration and guidance to their service providers that a transformation to recovery is a desirable outcome. To answer this need, the steering committee would select a subcommittee on recovery education, consisting of representatives of the steering committee and nationally recognized recovery educators. In addition, a national panel of consumer leaders with experience in providing recovery education will be convened to develop a national recovery curriculum. It would be important to ensure that the curriculum is culturally competent to the needs of diverse ethnic, sexual, and gender communities.

Since personal contact with people with first hand experience with recovery is generally the most effective tool for transforming the hearts and minds of people entrusted with mental health policy direction and service delivery, it is proposed that a large scale recovery education project be initiated under the guidance of consumers, in consultation with the top level decision makers. Bassman and Penney established a viable model for such an educational initiative in New York (Bassman, 2000) by pairing consumer recovery educators with local consumers. These teams educated hospital staff on the principles of recovery. The New York Association of Psychosocial Rehabilitation Services (Rosenthal, personal communication) has also used a similar model, which also is used to educate the community. Some states, such as California, have placed a high priority on recovery education and have relied on national and local educators. Current consumer/survivor recovery educators can be utilized as trainers and mentors of emerging leaders, which will build additional capacity, which would be carried out by regional training conferences. These recovery educators could teach recovery competencies to all persons who provide assistance to consumers. This recovery training could also serve to reduce stigma and discrimination among community residents, since a pro-recovery message is usually the best anti-stigma approach. When people speak for themselves it illustrates that they are capable and competent, far more than any message in which others speak for them.

The National Empowerment Center has developed a three part curriculum called the PACE (Personal Assistance in Community Existence)/Recovery Education Program to educate all stakeholders about recovery (Ahern & Fisher, 2001ab; Fisher & Chamberlin, 2004; Fisher, Langan, & Ahern, 2003). This curriculum introduces the research evidence that people recover, enumerates the major principles of recovery, cites recovery literature, and provides training to peer supporters so they can facilitate recovery. An evaluation revealed that PACE training had a positive impact on several of the parameters of recovery such as hope and empowerment (Zahniser, Fisher, & Ahern, in press).

Another responsibility of this subcommittee would be the development, in conjunction with the Consumer TA Centers, of a website and library of self-help materials. In addition, this website could provide information on the four areas which the Commission Report highlighted as needing extra attention: disparities for minorities in mental health, a study of the effects of long-term medication use, an examination of the effects of trauma, and problems of acute care (Commission Report, 2003, pp. 76-77).

Step 1.3: NRI Subcommittee on Policy will develop and synthesize model recovery policies as well as materials for training consumers in board participation

To play a significant role in policy development, consumers/survivors need to understand recovery principles, have ideas of policies for which they could advocate, and have an understanding of evaluation methodologies, so that the effectiveness of the instituted policies could be determined. Many of these materials already exist in different locales. The job of the committee would be to bring together the best materials and agree on a tool-kit for consumer participation in policy development. Consultants can help, but consumers need to play a lead role to ensure that the materials focus on genuine recovery and are presented in formats and languages, which are accessible to a variety of educational levels and are responsive to cultural differences. In addition to people of various racial and ethnic groups, training materials need to consider the needs of people with disabilities other than mental illness. For example this might include material and training accommodations (e.g. Braille, large print, sign language interpretation, cassettes, and CD's).

This committee would also prepare ongoing policy analyses and supply the information to the Steering Committee to assist it in participating in national policy formation.

Step 1.4: NRI Subcommittee on Recovery-based Evaluation and Research will develop materials and train consumers in these areas

This subcommittee will establish a tool-kit for the evaluation of programs to determine the degree to which new programs reflect recovery values and practices. Consumer-run evaluation teams have already shown their ability to evaluate mental health programs in Ohio, Pennsylvania, Georgia, Florida, South Carolina, and Massachusetts (Campbell, 1997). Since consumers are much more candid when speaking to fellow consumers, consumer evaluation teams are capable of eliciting much useful information that is not revealed through other methodologies. Evaluations would supply valuable information to the policy setting committee. In addition, there needs to be much more attention and resources allocated to consumer-driven research in the area of recovery. This need was also highlighted in the Commission report. This activity will require the funding and training of consumer researchers. These researchers should be in a good position to develop baseline data that can be used as the foundation for future collection and evaluation of evidence based data on recovery and recovery-based services.

Step 1.5: NRI Subcommittee on recovery-based services and supports will supply the networking and technical assistance needed to help in the further development of peer-run services

Consumers are uniquely suited to further develop peer-run services. It is very difficult for even the most well-intentioned professionals to start peer-run services without replicating, even if unwittingly, the inequalities and values of the traditional system. The shared experience of being labeled and living on disability benefits, the role modeling afforded by one's own recovery, and the decrease in stigma and discrimination all make consumers much more open to participating in peer-run services than in professionally-run services. The subcommittee would work closely with the National Technical Assistance Centers to survey the statewide consumer organizations, which in turn would assess the extent of peer support groups and determine what they need for further development

The following section will elaborate in more detail the topic of implementing self-determination at the services and supports level.

Objective 2: Consumer-driven transformation to a system of expanded choices of recovery-based services and supports

The existing mental health system is based on an institutional medical model which sees mental illness as a lifelong condition from which it is impossible to fully recover, Therefore, service users have only limited opportunities to fulfill any role other than that of passive recipient of whatever services treating professionals determine they should receive. "Choice," in this context, is limited to, at best, selecting within a pre-determined set of options. Even when service users are allowed such limited choices, they are frequently overruled on the basis of clinical judgment. The implicit message is that service recipients are incapable of assessing or acting on their own best interests, and that disagreement with treating profession-als is evidence of symptomatology rather than of self-assertion and self-determina-tion.

A recovery-based mental health system, on the other hand, would start from an entirely different premise. Each person entering the system would be viewed as undergoing a period of *temporary* distress and disorganization, from which he or she is expected to recover, and given appropriate supports. Each service user would have the full opportunity to select those services and supports, which, in his/her evaluation, would best meet his or her needs at that time.

For a person entering the system in acute crisis, such needs would most likely center on providing safety and security *as defined by the individual*. This would probably involve a small, home-like setting (or the person's own home), with helpers of his or her choice ensuring that basic needs (such as nutritious food and adequate sleep) were met. As the person emerged from an acute state, the range of options and choices would enlarge, based on assisting the individual to resume former roles or move on to new ones. Peer support options should be offered as early as possible on a one on one basis with the goal of moving the person into mutual support. The peer specialist could help the consumer negotiate the systems involved in recovery by providing insider knowledge, hope, and role modeling. Helpers would include the full array of mental health professionals, as well as peer supporters and natural supports (family and friends).

At present there are only a small number of adequately funded consumer-run programs. Even when mental health authorities have funded small projects for peer support, these are seldom well-integrated into the existing mental health system, are usually viewed as adjuncts and "frills," and still leave only very limited avenues for meaningful consumer involvement.

There is currently only a narrow range of clinically based services reimbursable under Medicaid for adults with psychiatric disabilities living in the community. These programs are designed by clinicians and tend to be medically based with little relevance to concepts of independent living, consumer choice, or recovery. Consumers can increase their control by being the author of their own individualized recovery planning which would then form the basis for which supports and services would be covered. Consumers at the individual level need to lead the transformation of their own lives to becoming self-determining adults, by exerting maximal control in the choice and provision of the services and supports they need to integrate into the community. Several states have experimented with new financial models called cash and counseling or self-determination projects. There have been successful demonstrations of such new financing arrangements of money following the person in area of developmental disabilities (Foster, Brown, Phillips, Schore, & Carlson, 2003). Medicaid recipients in Arkansas with developmental disabilities who direct their own supportive services were significantly more satisfied and had a higher quality of life than those receiving services through a home care agency. However, for people labeled with mental illness, only Florida has succeeded in its attempts to provide the opportunity for people to choose their own services and supports, though even that demonstration is on a small scale.

Dr. Thomas Nerney (Nerney, 2004) has described the five principles of self-determination:

- **Freedom**, the opportunity to choose where and with whom one lived as well as how one organized all important aspects of one's life with freely chosen assistance as needed;
- **Authority**, the ability to control some targeted amount of public dollars;
- **Support**, the ability to organize that support in ways that were unique to the individual;
- **Responsibility**, the obligation to use public dollars wisely and to contribute to one's community;

- **Confirmation**, the recognition that individuals with disabilities themselves must be a major part of the redesign of the human service system.

Nerney (2004) noted how these ideas of self-determination are being incorporated into the care of people with a variety of disabilities:

> In the last decade public policy for individuals with physical and cognitive or intellectual disabilities has gradually been coalescing around several important themes. These themes all lead toward greater recognition of community participation, income production or work, control over resources and leading meaningful lives that resemble in all-important respects the aspirations and ambitions that all Americans have for them. This is not to say that these goals have been realized or that the impetus to achieve them does not vary from state to state (Nerney, 2004).

In Michigan in 2003, the Michigan Department of Mental Health issued a directive stating:

> Persons who rely on the public mental health system for necessary supports and services must have access to meaningful options from which to make choices, and be supported to control the course of their lives. Arrangements that support self-determination must be sponsored by the public mental health system, assuring methods for the person to exert control over how, by whom, and to what ends they are served and supported (Nerney, 2004).

Despite this policy goal, Nerney has found that such policies fall short in assisting people with mental illness: "As Michigan attempts to valiantly implement self-determination, people with psychiatric disabilities still fall through the cracks, experience homelessness in great numbers and live in abject poverty in greater numbers than any other population" (Nerney 2004).

The experience in Florida has been more successful, though it only has been provided to 100 consumers. The Florida Self-Directed Care program describes itself as:

> ...an approach to providing publicly funded behavioral health care services wherein the individual has a high degree of self-determination in choosing services and providers necessary for recovery from mental illness. AMHSDC [Adult Mental Health Self Directed Care Program] assists in funding mental health treatment and support services to adults who have serious mental illness allowing the individual to control the public mental health funds allotted for his/her treatment and to directly purchase the services from the vendor of choice. Individuals are offered independent advice and guidance in securing the services they need to begin the recovery process

The AMHSDC program allows individuals with a severe and persistent mental illness to take more personal control of their recovery. It allows them to become less passive and more pro-active in the treatment and recovery process. Those who have the necessary motivation and ability to do so are able to receive the treatment that, in their own judgment, is best for them. Each participant's recovery progress is being tracked carefully in an effort to determine what potential value lies in this approach.

Participants in the AMHSDC program choose from a variety of community-based providers that may or may not already be a part of the current community mental health system. Residential and crisis stabilization services are delivered by existing community mental health providers through the traditional delivery system. Participants are responsible for determining exactly which community-based services they want and by whom these services will be provided. An independent community advisory board comprised of service recipients, their significant others, and advocates, guide the program. Participant recovery is being measured in a number of ways including productive days in the community (productive as defined by each individual), structured self-reports of satisfaction with the program's delivery approach from participants, and structured self-reports about achievement of personal recovery goals and objectives. Standard objective measures are being used to evaluate individual outcomes that will include input from significant others, including recovery coaches. The major difference in measurements between AMHSDC and the traditional system is focused on participant self-reports about personal recovery achievement and satisfaction with the total AMHSDC delivery system (see www.floridasdc.info/Pages/Welcome.html).

Implementing a self-determination approach requires at least three major changes in the system. First, there needs to be a shift away from prescriptive, professionally designed treatment planning to individualized, consumer-authored recovery planning. This has been called person-centered planning in the developmental disabilities field. This person-centered planning maximizes consumer choice (see step 2.1.1). A second element of the change to self-determination is a redesign of financing mechanisms to increase consumer control of their care (see step 2.1.2). The third element is the expansion of the range of available choices (see step 2.1.3).

Step 2.1: Shift to person-centered planning

Existing treatment planning is currently directed by professionals. These plans are based on diagnostic labels and treatment guidelines, which neglect the individualized nature of recovery. The Mental Health Commission recommends "that each adult with serious mental illness…have an individualized plan of care [and] consumer needs and preferences should drive the type and mix of services provided" (Commission Report, p. 35). When people are allowed to fashion their own recovery goals based on their dreams, they are much more motivated to carry them out. In contrast, when their goals are set for them by professionals, they appear unmotivated.

An example of the person-centered approach is provided by the Western New York Care Coordination Program in which "the person's dreams, interests, preferences, strengths, and capacities are explicitly acknowledged and drive activities, services, and supports." The Program further states, "services and supports are individualized and don't rely solely on pre-existing models (www.carecoordination.org)."

Step 2.2: Shift to financing mechanisms which support increased consumer control

I. Financing services and supports to allow money to follow the individual: Current funding mechanisms are inflexible, medically based, and present many challenges to these fundamental shifts in the system toward one that is person-centered and recovery-based. In contrast the Mental Health Commission Report recommends that " the funding for the plan should then follow the consumer, based on their individualized care plan" (p. 35). We will describe two models here; but much more work needs to be done to insure that money follows the person and is used to purchase those services which are desired by the individual and which promote recovery.

In Florida, the Self-Directed Care Program, which covers 100 participants in a four county area, has established individual budgets for program participants, through which they can select and purchase the services they want to fulfill their individual recovery plans. Payment will be made through a fiscal intermediary by means of vouchers. Participants can select from a wide array of traditional and non-traditional services; the criterion is that they must promote the individual's recovery. The program is utilizing a mix of Medicaid and state funds.

In New Hampshire, some Department of Behavioral Health (DBH) funding is planned to be shifted to a "recovery bundle," which includes those services and activities that promote recovery directly through education, vocational training, supported employment, recreation, community involvement, additional treatment, and other activities to be defined. This is in addition to a separate "clinical bundle." Recovery services are non-medical services that do not require supervision by a physician, and are expected to be reimbursable through Medicaid. Participants may use the assistance of a consumer advocate to help develop individual budgets defining the use of available funds, subject to review by the case manager. Through this mechanism, DBH intends to empower consumers to take instrumental action on their own behalf toward their recovery goals. A project oversight group consisting of DBH, participating centers, and consumers will oversee implementation and make reports to all providers and interested parties (Linda Paquette, personal communication, New Hampshire Department of Behavioral Health).

The State of Michigan received a grant in 2003 to begin a consumer cooperative demonstration, which would encourage groups of consumers and their families to pool economic resources to obtain the best set of services for their members. This approach (similar to a food-buying cooperative) is based on market-based incentives and the increase of consumer economic power (Barrie, 2003).

II. Financing consumer-run National Technical Assistance Centers: These TA Centers can play a vital role in the shift to services, which are truly self-determining. Just as the NRI is important in the development of policies which support self-determination, these TA Centers can provide the training and information to providers and consumers to needed to carry out person centered planning, flexible funding such as through individual accounts, and an expansion of consumer-run services.

Step 2.3: Expand the range of choices of services and supports available

I. Expand peer-provided services: The Report of the Consumer Issues Subcommittee to the New Freedom Commission also recommended that peer support services be integrated into the continuum of community care and that public and private funding mechanisms be made sufficiently flexible to allow access to these effective support services. The subcommittee proposed that a carve-out from the Federal Community Mental Health Block Grant funding be established to support the integration of community-based peer support services within the continuum of community care, stating "We encourage the inclusion of billable peer services under the Medicaid Rehabilitation Option [as has been carried out in Georgia]" (see www.mentalhealthcommission.gov).

In order to expand the range of choices of services in the NRI Action Plan, an increase in the involvement of consumers in the four major peer roles is recommended:

> *A. Peer professionals.* A peer professional is someone who has professional training (e.g., psychiatrist, psychologist, nurse, or social worker) who has also recovered from a personal experience of mental illness, and who is open about his/her experiences. A peer professional combines both academic and experiential knowledge, and brings both aspects to his or her work. By improving the supports for consumers entering professional schools and by recognizing recovery from mental illness as a positive asset, the field can be greatly enriched. The enthusiasm and knowledge of people who have recovered is a valuable and underutilized asset. An example is provided by a 26 year old man who has recovered from schizophrenia, and who recently wrote to the NEC, "Since I have made a miraculous recovery, I want to go into the field, get my graduate degree in social work, and share my recovery process with as many schizophrenics as I can and help them recover too."
>
> *B. Peer specialists.* A peer specialist is someone who has recovered or is in recovery (see above distinction between limited and genuine recovery) and who has received specialized training to provide peer support services. In a number of states, such as Georgia, programs have been developed in

which peer specialists receive training and certification, and their services are reimbursable through Medicaid .

The Georgia Consumer Network proposed an idea for peer-led services, and the state mental health authority formulated a plan for peer specialist services that would be supervised by professionals and would meet all the parameters of a Medicaid-financed service. In discussions with the Medicaid authority it was determined that the state should shift its delivery practices from the Medicaid Clinic Option to the Rehabilitation Option in order to better facilitate the promotion of rehabilitation principles. Negotiations through the state plan process with the federal Medicaid agency yielded results, and in July of 1999, service delivery began. New Peer Support Services as well as other more recovery focused day services were made available. Georgia has the distinction of being the first state to gain approval from the Centers for Medicare and Medicaid Services (CMS) to offer "Peer Supports" as a billable service in the state plan for Medicaid Mental Health Services. On Feb. 1, 2004, South Carolina became the second state to approve of Peer Support Services as Medicaid billable services.

C. Peers as staff in consumer-run programs. Most states now have at least a few consumer-run programs. Some states, such as Michigan and New Hampshire, have funded large numbers of them. Most consumer-run-programs are drop-in centers, where people can come to spend time meeting with others and participating in activities. Other examples of consumer-run programs include a smaller number of housing programs, job-finding programs, warmlines and a few crisis centers. In all cases, people who participate in the programs have a major role in running them and making decisions about them. People who work in these programs are usually paid, with funding sources including state and local governments, private foundations, and individual donations. Two recent reviews of the literature (Davidson et al., 1999; Solomon & Draine, 2001) established that there is preliminary evidence to support the effectiveness of peer-run support services to help people with mental illness. Consumers in the consumer-run support centers had better social functioning than the ones in community mental health centers (Yanos, Primavera, & Knight, 2001). Dr. Jean Campbell has recently concluded a multiyear study of consumer-operated services (COS). The preliminary results show an increase in well-being by the consumers attending the COS as compared to the control group (Campbell, personal communication).

The Ruby Rogers Advocacy and Drop-In Center in Somerville, Massachusetts, provides an example of a peer-run program. The Center was started in 1984 under the auspices of MPLF, Inc., a freestanding consumer-run advocacy program, which applied for funding from the Massachusetts Department of Mental Health. The Center's budget included funds for a part-time (eventually full-time) director, who was specified to be a person who had recovered from mental illness, as well as a number of part-time staff positions that enabled members to take on leadership roles while still being able to collect benefits. The Center provided informal peer counseling, and a wide range of member-led activities that engaged the interests of members and went far beyond the typical "busy work" of traditional day treatment.

Funding and bureaucratic limitations created constant obstacles. Because the Center did not fit into any existing Department of Mental Health program descriptions, there were a number of funding crises. Eventually the Center was put under the auspices of a professionally run program, limiting its autonomy. Nonetheless, the Ruby Rogers Center, along with literally hundreds of consumer-run drop-in centers on the country, provide models of how consumer/survivors take on leadership roles in helping their peers toward recovery.

D. Peers involved in mutual support. This is the most informal kind of peer support, which can evolve into ordinary friendship. In addition to peer support that is provided on a one-to-one basis, there are also informal networks of support, involving larger numbers of people. For example, many people participate in support and discussion groups over the Internet, as well as face-to-face groups. Every year, hundreds of people get together for the annual Alternatives Conference, which provides not only information and knowledge about peer support and other important learning experiences, but also gives people the opportunity to network informally.

II. Expand the use of Personal Assistance Services for people with psychiatric disabilities: In addition to services provided by peers, there are other models, which increase consumer choice. A model that should be carefully examined is that of Consumer-Directed Personal Assistance Services (PAS). PAS is widely available for people with physical and (to a certain extent) developmental disabilities. In 1999, the National Blue Ribbon Panel on Personal Assistance Services stated:

> ...people with disabilities should have meaningful and informed choices regarding types of long-term services and supports they receive. This choice should include choice of setting (home vs. institution) in which long-term services are received. After this choice has been made, consumers should have control over the extent to which they will manage and direct those services. This emphasis on consumer choice and control is congruent with core American values that put a priority on personal independence and responsibility.

The Commission recommended that PAS be available for a number of different population groups, including both those with physical disabilities and those diagnosed with mental illness. Nonetheless, the availability of PAS for people with psychiatric disabilities continues to be extremely limited.

In Oregon, the state mental health authority runs the C-PASS program for people with psychiatric disabilities, which funds personal care services (PCS) through the Oregon Home and Community Based Waiver. Eligible individuals (who must be Medicaid recipients who live in independent settings and require assistance with basic life tasks) are eligible for up to twenty hours a month of PCS services. These services are consumer-directed and are received by approximately three hundred individuals statewide. The consumer has the power to hire, train, and fire the personal assistant, and payment is by means of a voucher, which is signed by the service recipient and paid by the state using Medicaid waiver funds. A study is currently underway in Oregon to study the ways in which consumers use these services, and to greatly increase the number of people utilizing these services (currently only about 4.3% of eligible individuals statewide).

PAS is only one methodology for making mental health services responsive to individual needs. It is being described in such detail here because it is a method which already has a long and successful track record for serving people with disabilities in a self-determined manner, and for which Medicaid funding is already available (although significantly underutilized for people with psychiatric disabilities).

Conclusion

In conclusion, changing the mental health system from its dependency-oriented institutional thinking to one that is based on the principles of recovery will require a concerted effort of consumers and allies working to bring about changes in beliefs and practices at every level of the system. Without fundamental changes in the overall culture of the system, none of the most clever funding schemes or peer-run services will significantly alter the traditional, institutional medical model approach. The President's New Freedom Commission Report is a start in the right direction. However, to make the vision of that report a reality there will need to be a core of national and state level consumer leaders who embrace it and are supplied with the resources to carry it forward. Alliances must be developed with all stakeholders who believe in the recovery approach, to enable the implementation of transforming activities, which will make possible the Commission's vision of a system in which every person can recover.

References

Ahern, L., & Fisher, D. (2001a). *PACE a recovery curriculum*. Lawrence, MA: National Empowerment Center.

Ahern, L., & Fisher, D. (2001b). Recovery at your own PACE. *Journal of Psychosocial Nursing, 39*, 22-32.

Anthony, W., & Spaniol, L. (2002). *Psychiatric rehabilitation* (3rd ed.). Boston, MA: Boston University Center for Psychiatric Rehabilitation.

Barrie, P. (2003). *Talk given on flexible financing at SAMSHA/CMS sponsored conference on Self-Determination*. College Park, MD.

Bassman, R. (2000). Consumers/survivors/ex-patients as change facilitators. In F. J. Reese (Ed.), *The role of organized psychology in treatment of the seriously mentally ill* (pp. 93-102). San Francisco, CA: Jossey-Bass.

Blanch, A., Fisher, D., Tucker, W., Walsh, D., & Chassman, J. (1993). Consumer-practitioners and psychiatrists share insights about recovery and coping. *Disability Studies Quarterly, 13*(2), 17-20.

Campbell, J. (1996). Towards collaborative mental health outcomes systems. *New Directions for Mental Health Services, 71,* 69-68.

Campbell, J. (1997). How consumers/survivors are evaluating the quality of psychiatric care. *Evaluation Review, 21*(3), 357-363.

Chamberlin, J. (2003). *On our own.* Lawrence, MA: National Empowerment Center.

Davidson, L., Chinman, M., Kloos, B., Weingarten, R., Stayner, D., & Tebes, J. K. (1999). Peer support among individuals with severe mental illness: A review of the evidence. *Clinical Psychology-Science & Practice, 6,* 165-187.

Department of Veterans Affairs. (2003). *Achieving the promise: Transforming mental health care in the VA.* Washington DC.

Fisher, D., & Chamberlin, J. (2004). *PACE/Recovery peer training recovery curriculum.* Lawrence, MA: National Empowerment Center.

Fisher, D., Langan, T., & Ahern, L. (2003). *PACE/Recovery reader.* Lawrence, MA: National Empowerment Center.

Foster, L., Brown, R., Phillips, B., Schore, J., & Carlson, B. (2003). Improving the quality of medicaid personal assistance through consumer direction. *Health Affairs* Web Exclusive, March 26, 2003. Bethesda, MD.

Harding, C. M., Brooks, G. W., Ashikaga, T., Strauss, J. S., & Breier, A. (1987). The Vermont longitudinal study of persons with severe mental illness, I. Methodology, study sample, and overall status 32 years later. *American Journal of Psychiatry, 144*(6), 718-726.

Karon, B. P., & VanDen Boos, G. R. (1981). *Psychotherapy of Schizophrenia.* New York, NY: Aronson.

McCabe, S., & Unzicker, R. (1995). Changing roles of consumer/survivors in mature mental health systems. *New Directions for Mental Health Services, 66,* 61-73.

Nerney, T. (2004). The Promise of Freedom for Persons with Psychiatric Disabilities. In J. Jonikas & J. Cook (Eds.), *UIC NRTC'S national self-determination and psychiatric disability invitational conference papers* (pp. 129). Chicago, Il.

New Freedom Commission on Mental Health. (2003). *Achieving the promise: Transforming mental health care in America. Final report.* Rockville, MD: DHHS Pub. No. SMA-03-3832.

Solomon P., & Draine, J. (2001). The state of knowledge of the effectiveness of consumer provided services. *Psychiatric Rehabilitation Journal, 25*(1), 20-7.

Tanzman, B. (1993). An overview of mental health consumers' preferences for housing and support services. *Hospital and Community Psychiatry, 44*(5), 450-455.

Trochim, W., Dumont, J., & Campbell, J. (1993). A report for the state mental health agency profiling system: Mapping mental health outcomes from the perspective of consumers/survivors. *Technical report series.* Alexandria, VA: NASMHPD Research Institute, Inc.

US PHS Office of the Surgeon General. (1999). *Mental health: A report of the surgeon general.* Rockville, MD: DHHS, PHS.

US PHS Office of the Surgeon General. (2001). *Culture, race and ethnicity a supplement to: Mental health: A report of the surgeon general.* Rockville, MD: DHHS, PHS.

Van Tosh, L., Ralph, R., & Campbell, J. (2000). The rise of consumerism. *Psychiatric Rehabilitation Skills, 4*(3), 383-409.

Western New York Care Coordination Program. (2004). *Care coordination.* Retrieved February 10, 2005 from http://www.carecoordination.org/.

Yanos, P. T., Primavera, L., & Knight, E. (2001). Consumer-run service participation, recovery of social functioning, and the mediating role of psychological factors. *Psychiatric Services, 52,* 493-500.

Zinman, S. (2002). *Testimony before the President's New Freedom Commission on Mental Health.* Washington, DC.

Chapter 10

An Exemplar of One State's Implementation of the New Freedom Commission Report: Nevada

Sheila Leslie
Assemblywoman for District #27, Reno, Nevada
Carlos Brandenburg
Nevada State Division for Mental Health and Developmental Services

The creation of the New Freedom Commission on Mental Health in April of 2002, had a significant, demonstrable impact in Nevada. The appointment of state Senator Randolph Townsend, R-Reno, to the New Freedom Commission as the only state legislator in its membership, created a special linkage back to Nevada, inspiring the passage of Senate Bill 301 in the 2003 Legislative session (Chapter 445, *Statues of Nevada 2003*). SB 301 established the Nevada Mental Health Plan Implementation Commission, (NMHPIC) charged with creating and delivering an action plan to the Interim Finance Committee, the Legislative Committee on Health Care, and the Governor by January 1, 2005.

The structure of NMHPIC was a consensus decision, featuring a membership of six key legislators – balanced by political party and geography, all of whom had a deep interest in the topic of mental health services – and key state administrators from four divisions of the largest department of state government, the Department of Human Resources (DHR). These divisions are Mental Health and Developmental Disabilities, Health (Bureau of Alcohol and Drug Abuse), Child and Family Services, and Division of Health Care Financing and Policy (Medicaid). The strategic decisions around selection of the NMHPIC membership were carefully considered in an effort to maximize the opportunities for successful implementation of its recommendations. The Senate Majority Leader and the Speaker of the Assembly were responsible for appointing three members from their respective chambers to serve.

At the first meeting in September 2003, the NMHPIC elected Senator Townsend to serve as Chair, based on his national experience serving on the New Freedom Commission and his long history of leadership on mental health issues in Nevada. Senator Townsend has worked closely with statewide Mental Health Coalitions in Nevada for many years to improve the quantity and quality of available services, resulting in the construction of a new inpatient facility in Sparks, appropriately christened as the Dini-Townsend Hospital.

Assemblywoman Sheila Leslie, D-Reno, was elected to serve as the Commission's Vice-Chair. Assemblywoman Leslie also has a long history of working with mental health advocacy groups to promote mental health services and has a professional background in non-profit human services. She also serves as the Assembly Chair of the Joint Budget Subcommittee on Human Resources, which oversees the budget for the Division of Mental Health and Developmental Services.

The four remaining legislators represent communities in the Las Vegas area. The two Senators, Bob Coffin, D-Las Vegas and Ray Rawson, R-Las Vegas, have decades of legislative experience and both serve on the Senate Finance Committee, with Senator Rawson serving as the Senate Chair of the Joint Budget Subcommittee on Human Resources. The two Assemblymen are freshman legislators, both serving on the Assembly's Health and Human Services Committee. Dr. Joseph Hardy, R-Boulder City, is a family physician and William Horne, D-Las Vegas, is a lawyer.

Four state administrators were selected to serve, representing the state agencies most closely linked to the provision of mental health services in Nevada. Dr. Carlos Brandenburg, is the long-time Administrator of the Division of Mental Health and Developmental Services and has a deep understanding of the needs and resources of the state in this area. Charles Duarte, the Administrator of the Division of Health Care Financing and Policy is responsible for Medicaid spending in Nevada. Jone Bosworth, the Administrator of the Division of Child and Family Services oversees children's mental health issues for Nevada while Maria Canfield, the Chief of the Bureau of Alcohol and Drug Abuse, located in the state Health Division, is the primary source of funding for substance abuse services.

These Administrators served as *ex officio* members of the Commission, voting on all policy matters but abstaining from any votes on fiscal recommendations.

Supporting the Commission's work were research, legal, and fiscal staff from the Legislative Counsel Bureau. During the 2003-2004 interim between legislative sessions, the Commission held seven meetings and received many hours of testimony from national and state mental health experts, consumers, and advocacy groups.

The Commission chose to organize its meetings around the six goals outlined in the New Freedom Commission's final report, *Achieving the Promise: Transforming Mental Health Care in America*. Each meeting featured a number of national experts on specific topic areas as well as local practitioners who could translate the national work into projected impact in Nevada. The public was invited to actively participate in the Commission's work by presenting their views on the current status of programs, services, and needs in Nevada in the specific topic areas, ideas regarding the most optimal methods of improving mental health in Nevada, and public testimony.

All participants and members of the public were invited to submit written suggestions for action by the Commission in addition to the recommendations provided during the meetings focused on the six national goals. At a work session in January of 2004, the Commission adopted its top recommendations as outlined below. A subsequent meeting held in June 2004 focused on the deferred recommendations that would have a fiscal impact on the state budget.

Summary of Recommendations

The Nevada Mental Health Plan Implementation Commission

Senate Bill 301

(Chapter 445, *Statutes of Nevada 2003*)

The following recommendations were approved by the Nevada Mental Health Plan Implementation Commission and its Subcommittee to Continue the Work of the Commission, established by the Commission at its work session on January 26, 2004. All bill draft requests were adopted by the full Commission. All other recommendations for actions were adopted by the full Commission, unless noted as an action by the Subcommittee.

Recommendations for Legislation

The members of the Nevada Mental Health Plan Implementation Commission adopted the following recommendations for legislative measures:

Goal 2: Mental health care is consumer- and family-driven.

1. Request the drafting of legislation to establish a subcommittee of the Interim Finance Committee (IFC) to address housing in Nevada that is funded in whole or in part by public funds, including, but not limited to, housing for those persons who are mentally ill, elderly, disabled, low-income, or who otherwise need housing assistance, with special focus on persons reentering the community, including those from correctional institutions. Further, the creation of such a housing subcommittee of IFC would (1) establish a coordinated approach to all housing dollars entering Nevada; and (2) ensure there is a connection between housing and services. (BDR 277)

2. Request the drafting of legislation that would require consumers to be active participants in the development of their mental health treatment and care plans. (BDR 280)

Goal 3: Disparities in mental health services are eliminated.

3. Request the drafting of legislation requiring a consumer, past or present, of mental health services in the state system be included as a member of Nevada's Commission on Mental Health and Developmental Services. (BDR 279)

Recommendations for Commission Action

The following recommendations for action were adopted by the full Commission or its legislative subcommittee.

Goal 1: Americans understand that mental health is essential to overall health.

1. Establish a subcommittee of the Nevada Mental Health Plan Implementation Commission to meet with designees appointed by the Governor, including representatives from the broadcast industry, radio, television, and newspaper publications to develop a plan for public service announcements in English and Spanish. Direct school districts to report on implementation of programs that focus on de-stigmatizing mentally ill persons.

2. Urge, in its report, the Governor to include in the Executive Budget funding for comprehensive, statewide suicide prevention and intervention programs that include survivors of suicide. Support and maintain a statewide suicide prevention plan that will include evaluation, prevention, and post-intervention services; education and training for gatekeepers, professionals, the media, and the public; youth suicide prevention in schools; and careful attention to the relationship between suicide and co-occurring disorders.

Goal 2: Mental health care is consumer- and family-driven.

3. Recommend, in its report, that the Governor provide for the development of a Comprehensive State Mental Health Plan. The plan will be designed to overcome the problems of fragmentation in the mental health delivery system and will provide important opportunities to leverage resources across multiple agencies that administer both state and federal funds. The Commission envisions a single entity coordinating the plan. The planning process should support a dialogue among all stakeholders and reach beyond the traditional state mental health agency to address the full range of treatment and support service programs that consumers and families need. The final result should be an extensive and coordinated state system of services that work to foster consumer independence and support consumers' ability to live, work, learn, and participate fully in their communities and provide for specific items such as standardized formularies to address co-occurring disorders.

4. Express, in its report, support for the concept of the Behavioral Health Plan System Redesign of the Division of Health Care Financing and Policy (DHCFP), Department of Human Resources (DHR), and urge the Executive Branch and DHR to go forward with the funding and implementation of the proposed redesign plan. The Behavioral Health

Plan recommendations include, but are not limited to, standardizing the infrastructure of the system, developing specialty clinics, eliminating state-devised reimbursable codes for Nevada Medicaid, delivering targeted case management services through state agencies, and defining mechanisms for utilization management. The recommendation includes incremental costs that may come through DHCFP and the Division of Mental Health and Developmental Services (DMHDS).

5. Recommend, in its report, that Nevada should take steps to promote, encourage, and facilitate greater access to safe and affordable community-based housing and support services by using an array of resources within the United States Departments of Housing and Urban Development (HUD), and Health and Human Services (HHS), and the Veterans Administration (VA) as leverage. To accomplish this, the Commission approved the following actions:

- Send a letter to Nevada's Congressional delegation urging the members to support restoration of Residential Substance Abuse Treatment funds in the federal budget.
- Include this recommendation in the Commission's report along with a statement regarding the need for housing funds specifically for mentally ill persons.
- Request the DMHDS, DHR to update the inventory of available housing that was completed two years ago.

6. Urge, in its report, the Executive Branch to research and provide to the Interim Finance Committee recommendations for a person or firm to provide contract services for the purpose of securing grants that lead to funding mental health, housing and other health-related services.

Goal 3: Disparities in mental health services are eliminated.

7. Urge, in its report, DMHDS to develop a rural recruitment and retention program that acknowledges difficulties in hiring and retaining qualified professionals in rural Nevada. Include rural recruitment and retention in the state's cultural competency plan.

8. Urge, in its report, all state agencies and local governments to develop a cultural competency plan for the state and urge DHR to provide effective assistance for minorities, particularly those who face cultural barriers and lack English proficiency, to receive in-patient and out-patient mental health services.

Goal 4: Early mental health screening, assessment, and referral to services are common practices.

9. Express, in its report, support for the concept of increasing medical staff at the state's mental hospital to accommodate mentally ill patients with physical health issues, and allow DMHDS the flexibility to address the fiscal concerns in the agency's budget through contract services.

10. Express, in its report, support for the crisis triage center concept throughout the state, including the development and implementation of formalized training for staff that interacts with offenders with mental health disorders, including correctional officers and staff of the Division of Parole and Probation, Nevada's Department of Public Safety.

11. Express, in its report, support for funding of psychiatry fellows from the University of Nevada School of Medicine (UNSOM) and Adolescent Psychiatry Fellowship Training Program for the purpose of reducing the shortage of child and adolescent psychiatrists.

12. Express, in its report, support for the concept of maintenance of UNSOM's psychiatry residency training program in northern Nevada and support for the establishment of a new psychiatry residency training program in southern Nevada.

13. Express, in its report, support for the establishment of residency training, fellows, and paid internships that include alcohol and drug training to increase qualified mental health staff. To accomplish this, the Commission approved the following recommendations:

- Broaden the pool of qualified geriatric clinicians through the licensing of professional counselors in Nevada;
- Expand the scope of practice for licensed alcohol and drug counselors to assess for and oversee the treatment of Axis II mental health disorders;
- Require certification of professional staff working with older adults, such as completion of a Providers Certificate of Specialization in Aging offered by the Geriatric Education Center at UNSOM; and
- Enhance the state's ability to provide integrated substance abuse and mental health services to persons with co-occurring disorders.

14. Express, in its report, support for the enhancement of senior mental health services.

Goal 5: Excellent mental health care is delivered and research is accelerated.

15. Urge, in its report, the University and Community College System of Nevada (UCCSN) to assist governmental agencies with behavioral health data collection issues.
16. Urge, in its report, DMHDS to establish mechanisms to monitor the effectiveness of mental health services efforts.
17. Urge, in its report, DHR to establish funding mechanisms or incentives to implement an evidence-based practices agenda.
18. Urge, in its report, DHR to seek funding to purchase materials and train clinicians in evidence-based psychological practices

Goal 6: Technology is used to access mental health care and information.

19. Urge, in its report, DMHDS to implement electronic medical records for all DMHDS clients and urge DMHDS and the Division of Child and Family Services (DCFS) to establish a computerized medical information system to increase coordination, communication, and continuity between and within state and private agencies.
20. Urge, in its report, DMHDS to develop tele-mental health capacity for rural Nevada for all disciplines, including psychiatry, psychology, social work, juvenile justice, marriage and family therapy, dually licensed (substance abuse and mental health) providers, service coordination, and nursing. Additionally, include in the final report a statement regarding the need to establish telehealth guidelines to protect the public health.
21. Urge, in its report, DCFS to establish telehealth-based psychiatric services at each of the three state-operated youth (correctional) training facilities: the Northern Nevada Youth Training Center in Elko, the Caliente Youth Center in Caliente, and the Summit View Youth Correctional Center in Las Vegas.

In 2005, the Nevada Mental Health Plan Implementation Commission will seek to implement the proposed legislation and recommendations outlined in its final report. It is likely that a joint mental health subcommittee will be appointed by the Assembly and Senate to thoroughly review the report and recommend legislative action as needed. It is anticipated that many of the enhanced budget items will be included in the Governor's 2005-2007 budget, to be reviewed by the Legislature's budget committees for implementation in the next biennium.

It is important also to note that local governments and advocacy groups have actively monitored and participated in the Commission's work over the past year, and are proceeding on their own to implement appropriate action through program planning, budget advocacy, and community awareness.

In Northern Nevada, a Co-Occurring Disorder Work Group is planning a Community Triage Center to be incorporated into a new homeless shelter. The group also facilitated training of local law enforcement officers in the Community Intervention Team model. This training will be offered on a regional basis in Northern Nevada on a bi-monthly basis in 2005.

In Southern Nevada, a Mental Health Coalition composed of 39 public and private groups has issued an "action agenda" to guide funding of mental health services during the 2005 session of the Nevada Legislature. The action plan was developed in response to a "mental health emergency" declared by the Clark County Manager in July 2004 when fully one-third of all emergency room beds were filled with mentally ill patients.

It is clear the work inspired by the national New Freedom Commission and Nevada's State Commission has just begun. By gaining the commitment from policy-makers to address these complex and serious issues, focusing public awareness on the issue, and galvanizing the advocacy community and consumers, the Commissions will have fulfilled an historical role in erasing the stigma of mental illness and transforming mental health care in America.

The Afterword

A Short List of Dreams and Schemes to Fix Healthcare

Nicholas A. Cummings
University of Nevada, Reno and
The Cummings Foundation for Behavioral Health, Inc.

The United States seems to be entering an era of self-reliance, reflecting a rapidly declining confidence by younger Americans in both government and corporations to provide for either their healthcare or retirement needs. A spendthrift Congress has dissipated the so-called social security "lockbox," leaving a spate of unfunded IOUs. Do the arithmetic; social security is bankrupt because of demographics. When first created seventy years ago there were 40 workers paying into the system for every retiree. In 2005 it is somewhere between three and four, and soon to be only two paying for everyone drawing out. Part of the problem is that people are living up to ten years longer today than they did when social security was enacted. By 2018 or 2020, social security will be paying out more than it receives, and the theoretical (i.e., IOU) reserve, even if replenished by the Democrats' plan to lift the $90,000 annual payroll tax ceiling, it will be gone by 2040. Not only would this constitute a very large tax increase, a $90,000 income may in a few years be average, having been eroded by inflation. In its present state social security will not be there for the under thirties generation.

American corporations have plundered workers' pension plans for their own needs, leaving similarly unfunded IOUs. No wonder late 2004 opinion polls reveal that over 50% of Americans favor personal ownership of healthcare and retirement, in the form of medical savings accounts and personalization of social security. This percentage grows as the age cohort declines, with an astounding 77% of the respondents in their twenties preferring self-reliance to government or corporate responsibility. Paradoxically, those over 55 who will not be effected by personal savings accounts tend to oppose the idea, while those under 55 who will be effected tend to favor them (Tumulty & Roston, 2005). But even for those under 55, to participate in personalized accounts or remain in the current system would be a matter of choice, and younger Americans like the freedom to choose for themselves.

A number of proposals, some already enacted and others likely to become law, seek to respond to both the crisis and the growing shift in voter sentiment. The White House certainly intends to push for an ownership society in both healthcare and social security reform, believing that personal savings accounts hold the promise of enabling the working class for the first time to acquire wealth. This was successfully demonstrated in the Galveston, Texas experience. Opting out of social security through a loophole, these civil service employees now have legendary nest-eggs of several hundred thousand dollars on retirement. Similarly, Chile privatized its retirement system in the 1980s, doubling and tripling the amount of money available on retirement over that of the old government pension (Kadlec, 2004). Stated succinctly, this view holds that capitalism works best when everyone has capital. These changes will certainly permeate mental healthcare, impacting on practice and redefining the doctor-patient relationship. The influence of these schemes is predictable, as is the likelihood of their implementation, and the mental health practitioner would do well to heed the harbinger of change.

Health Savings Accounts

Health Savings Account (HSA) legislation was enacted late in 2003 and implementation gained momentum late in 2004. It allows companies and employees to set aside, tax free, money in accounts that remain individually owned by employees, to meet medical expenses. The money in the accounts grows tax-free, and companies or individuals can buy high deductible healthcare insurance policies significantly cheaper than traditional policies (Forbes, 2004). These can be coupled with the HSA, and the amount that can be set aside tax-free is equal to the deductible on the insurance, up to a limit (Coolidge, 2004). The individual can take money out of the HSA to cover doctor, dentist, orthodontist, pharmacy, optical, laboratory and hospital bills, and money not spent accumulates and grows tax-free. In the event of employment change, the HSA follows the employee. The minimum deductible allowed is $1,000 for singles and $2,000 for families, and the maximum is $5,000 and $10,000 respectively. However, the HSA tax-free contribution ceiling is $2,600 for singles, $5,150 for families, and with $500 added for those over 55. The administration is committed to expanding these amounts as indicated by the President's State of the Union speech of 2005.

The rapid acceleration of HSAs will, over time, presage a number of changes. (1) The plan is attractive to healthy individuals who are sick of paying premiums kept high by the 20% who utilize 80% of the healthcare. An often expressed sentiment is typical: "Why should I pay for the diseases of smokers?" There is no question that having high deductibles will save a bundle on insurance, and the deductible payments come out of tax-free money. (2) Now in charge of one's own healthcare, the prospective patient will avoid unnecessary healthcare, be selective in the choice of provider, and demand more service and quality for the dollar. This empowerment of the individual means both free choice and personal responsibility. (3) The doctor-patient relationship suffered with the advent of third-party reimbursement, and severely damaged by managed care, is largely restored. For the behavioral care provider, "psychotherapeutic drift" (the attitude that in the absence of progress, as long as someone else is paying, why not keep coming in the hope something therapeutic will happen) will disappear. It will no longer be managed care, but the patients, spending their own money, who will determine what treatment is applicable, what it should cost, and what constitutes progress. (4) Healthy life styles are inherently encouraged in this plan, with amelioration of today's prevailing attitude that "I can do anything to my body because the doctor will fix it and my insurer will pay for it." (5) Some authorities believe the empowered patient might well save healthcare (Forbes, 2004; Friedman, 2004).

The debate over future schemes to fix healthcare will be contentious and fraught with political motivations on both sides of the Congressional aisle, but these will be overshadowed by the contentiousness and political in-fighting over fixing social security. When social security will go broke is a matter of whose creative math you use, but there is no such ambiguity about the cost of healthcare which is spinning out of control. It has now reached the double-digit inflation rate that in the 1980s ushered in managed care. For about 15 to 20 years managed care tethered rising healthcare costs, but the managed care companies made the mistake of seeing the purchaser (government, corporations, employers) as their customer rather than regarding the patient as the ultimate consumer. As a result, they overly focused on cost cutting, and became "managed cost" instead of managed care. As patients revolted over the severe cuts in service and access, as well as the intense micromanagement of their healthcare, the implosion of managed care was inevitable. Managed care lost its teeth, became essentially a payment mechanism, and costs again began to escalate. For example, General Motors, America's largest corporation, is preparing for a $1 billion dollar rise in healthcare costs, reducing earnings substantially, and adding $1400 to the cost of each vehicle produced (Hawkins, 2005). So make no mistake, healthcare costs will be brought under control. The only question is how extensive and how draconian the changes will be?

Fixing Medicare and Medicaid

It is beyond the scope of this volume to address social security, but Medicare and Medicaid, Titles XVIII and XIX of the Social Security Act, fall squarely within the purview of healthcare. Curiously, these programs are in much greater trouble than is social security, as their costs are already out of control, yet no one in Washington seems to be debating their fate. We are now spending $572 billion a year on these two entitlements, approaching half of the total $1.4 trillion annual healthcare expenditure of the United States (Kotlikoff, 2004). With the costs of Medicaid already out of control, and with 77 million baby boomers moving inexorably into Medicare, the healthcare portion of social security is destined to crash much before social security itself does so. One economist, Laurence Kotlikoff of Boston University, proposes a unique system of individual specific vouchers, based on each persons health status, provided by the government and used to buy health insurance. The way it would work, a perfectly healthy 85-year-old might get $8,000, whereas an 85-year-old with pancreatic cancer might get $75,000. If the latter patient needed more, the difference would be made up by the insurance company. If less was needed, the insurance company would pocket the difference. Because those in the worst medical shape would have the largest vouchers, instead of shunning them, the insurance companies would be as happy to sign them up as they would their healthy contemporaries. The government would, of course, have to keep extensive and up-to-date confidential electronic records on each participant. According to this economist, the key cost element is that the government could set total expenditures at an affordable level and then allocate the amount to participants so that those with the greatest medical need get the largest vouchers. Competition among insurers would ensure that participants got the best care per voucher or dollar spent (Kotlikoff, 2004).

Whether an idea that would totally eliminate the current fee-for-service system in Medicare is even a possibility, such examples indicate that the debate over solving the healthcare crisis will not only be contentious, but also innovative.

Medical Errors

Medical errors are now the third or fourth leading cause of health deaths in the United States, depending on whose statistics you are reading. But these medical errors are usually not thought of as part of tort reform. Consider that the cure for medical errors is transparency, permitting a system to evaluate its procedures and thus correct the errors, is impossible in a litigious society in which doctors and hospitals regard any disclosure as open game for trial lawyers. Even such matters as infection rates in various hospitals is a tightly guarded secret, in defiance of state laws designed to force such disclosure (Rundle, 2005). Transparency, coupled with electronic records, would eliminate most medical errors, but this is unlikely in an atmosphere of run-away liability judgments.

The $27 billion a year that is added to the health system annually from lawsuits is only about a third of the estimated $75 billion cost of defensive medicine, defined as unnecessary healthcare expended to eliminate even the remotest possibility of professional liability. Tort reform is a major thrust of the White House, and possibilities range from capping non-economic judgment awards to concentrating class action suits in federal courts, thus eliminating the current practice of seeking out remote rural counties where so-called "plaintiffs juries" are eager to give the store away. Another idea is the creation of a system of medically knowledgeable "health courts." Some manner of tort reform, such as that extant in California that ended its healthcare crisis and doctor drain of two decades ago, is inevitable. Trial lawyers are raising an unprecedented war chest, and are seeking to expand their support among mostly Democrats in the Congress. This battle, too, will be contentious, mostly along partisan lines, but finally a full debate will take place.

An HMO That Got It Right

Although Health Maintenance Organizations (HMOs) continue to provide the healthcare of tens of millions of Americans, they have been sharply criticized for their emphasis on costs over care. A notable exception has been Kaiser Permanente in Northern California, the nation's first HMO founded in 1946 long before the appellation HMO was coined, and an organization owned by several thousand physicians whose approach has consistently been that effective, efficient care is cost-effective care. Rather than concentrating on cost-cutting, the emphasis has been for nearly half a century that of keeping the patient healthy. Recently the Permanente Medical Group (PMG) was featured in a NBC Special Report, "An HMO That Got It Right," (Thompson, 2004), revealing that an expensive but effective emphasis on prevention has resulted in a 30% lower heart disease rate in its several million subscribers as compared to national averages. Reducing heart disease by one-third more than made up the costs of the aggressive program of prevention that promoted life style changes.

PMG accomplished this and similar feats by its system of capitation where rather than fee-for-service, the physician group is reimbursed through a capitation that pays a flat monthly premium per subscriber. These funds can be expended for prevention and wellness, whereas a fee-for-service model only reimburses for sickness. In the 1970s the federal government encouraged the capitation model through a series of grants and other incentives, and physicians responded by forming large capitated group practices. Soon it became apparent that these physicians continued to practice as if they were on a fee-for-service basis, without taking advantage of the flexibility for innovation accorded by a capitated system. Consequently, most failed to operate profitably within a capitation that was designed to streamline services, promote effective prevention, and provide care at lower cost than the inflexible fee-for-service system. To this day Kaiser Permanente stands as a unique model that can solve much of healthcare's problems if only providers could bridge their knowledge gap in healthcare economics as the PMG physicians have done. That Kaiser care is appreciated care is demonstrated by the experience with an enlightened population of faculty and employees at Stanford University. Year after year 76% of this population chooses the Kaiser plan over alternative fee-for-service plans (Enthoven, 2004).

A Hospital That Got It Right

The last time you were in a hospital, either for yourself or to visit someone, did you notice how many healthcare personnel are obese or otherwise look unhealthy, while still others are huddled at outside entrances during their breaks smoking cigarettes? Did the system seem to resemble organized chaos? Were you sometimes treated with less than courtesy? From the way they dressed, was it difficult to differentiate the doctors, nurses, and clerical staff from each other and from the janitors? Did you secretly wonder what happened to professionalism? Given that there are more or less many exceptions, this seems to picture our healthcare facilities today. If you want to see a different picture, however, visit the Mayo Clinic and Hospital in Scottsdale, Arizona. Specializing in secondary and tertiary care, meaning the patients often require specialized and advanced care, nonetheless the facilities are more than impressive, equipment is state of the art, records are electronic, the décor is beautiful, doctors and nurses look and dress as doctors and nurses, and efficiency, politeness and courtesy are pervasive. No wonder patients, looking for a level of care they cannot get at home, flock there from all over the United States and Canada. Recently this writer traversed the system in awe, culminating in a routine colonoscopy done by a gastroenterologist dressed in a suit and tie, whose expertise was so facile that I was comfortable in having refused a sedative, thus enabling me to watch my own examination on a monitor. This is a model of healthcare delivery and a resurgence of professionalism that cries to be emulated.

An MBHO That Got It Right

Recently a former president of the American Psychological Association referred to managed behavioral health organizations (MBHOs) as a "joke," highlighting that backlash legislation and public pressure have relegated them to the level of being nothing more than an annoyance to the practice of psychotherapy (Fox, 2004). Neglecting the patient as it pursued cost cutting, they have become essentially payment mechanisms that seek to pacify the purchasing employers with low cost, a buffer to malpractice exposure, and little noise (i.e., as few complaints as possible). MBHOs stormed on the scene with intensity in the early 1980s, made draconian changes in mental healthcare, and seemed to fizzle in strength by the turn of the 21st Century. Relying on bean counter techniques (pre-certification, session limits, denial of care, provider profiling) instead of effective behavioral interventions, it was a failed model from the beginning. Only one MBHO stands as a notable exception.

American Biodyne, as described by Bloom (1992), from its founding was clinically driven, using effective, focused and targeted psychotherapy, as well as greatly expanded behavioral services of which many were not covered under other plans. It had its research and demonstration base in twenty years at Kaiser Permanente, and eventual refinement in the Hawaii Project. Managers were clinicians trained in business, so that when a difficult decision had to be made, it fell on the clinical rather than the business side. All clinicians were trained in an exhausting two-week, ten-hours a day model that its hundreds of psychology, social work and psychiatry participants affectionately dubbed the Biodyne Bootcamp. In perpetuity, 15% of all clinicians' time was spent in clinical case conferencing and quality assurance. By extensive use of behavioral interventions, the need for psychotropic medications was reduced by as much as 80% (Cummings & Wiggins, 2001). Astoundingly, under its clinical founders and in the decade in which American Biodyne grew to 14.5 million enrollees in 39 states, there was not a single malpractice suit or patient complaint that had to be adjudicated. It demonstrated that effective and greatly expanded behavioral interventions reduced mental health costs and saved medical dollars as well. When this unique plan then passed to its successors, business managers who had no idea of how to continue the original clinically driven model, it became just another MBHO. Nonetheless, the model has been described extensively in the literature and stands as a once effective delivery system in mental healthcare that one day can be replicated or adapted to the future.

Mental Health Screening

Mental health professionals have long advocated early detection and screening of mental and emotional conditions, arguing that early treatment accelerates recovery and prevents these conditions from becoming chronic. The President's New Freedom Commission on Mental Health concluded that psychiatric conditions are far more prevalent, especially among children and adolescents, than previously thought, and accordingly has recommended national screening to detect these (Hogan, 2003). Once this announcement was made, a storm of controversy erupted, often from among the very groups that have for decades advocated early detection. Privacy issues have been raised, with fears that there would be a "big brother" data bank of the mentally ill. Others have criticized that this is merely trolling for patients in an era in which the practice of psychotherapy is in decline. Perhaps the most valid concern is that such national screening will result in millions more Americans, and especially children and adolescents, merely being remanded to taking psychotropic medication instead of having their psychological problems addressed with behavioral interventions and counseling (Cummings, 2004).

Behavioral Health as Primary Care

There is considerable discussion in healthcare about moving behavioral health into primary care, particularly the model that has behavioral care providers (BCPs, primarily psychologists and social workers), co-located in the primary care setting. This model has been described extensively (see for example, Cummings, Cummings & Johnson, 1997; Cummings, O'Donohue, Hayes, & Follette, 2001; O'Donohue, Byrd, Cummings & Henderson, 2005). A number of factors are fueling this thrust, principally that 60% of all patients seeing PCPs are somaticizing stress into physical symptoms, or a physical illness is being exacerbated by emotional factors. Referrals for psychotherapy are most often resisted by patients, and only 10% of those referred ever go into psychological treatment. On the other hand, when the PCP has merely to walk the patient down the hall to a BCP's office, over 90% engage in treatment. In such settings, the cost of behavioral care is more than offset by savings in medical/surgical care, and furthermore, the PCPs' time can be leveraged to perform higher paying procedures. Finally, in the co-located model as much as 80% of mental healthcare can be treated in the primary care setting where the cost is less than when referred out to specialty psychiatry/psychology.

To date several health systems serving millions of Americans have adopted the co-located integrated behavioral/primary care model, but these are mostly staff models in which co-location can be readily implemented. These settings include the worldwide medical facilities of the U.S. Air Force, Kaiser Permanente in California, several Veterans Administration hospitals, and some community health centers. Hampering progress toward behavioral/primary care integration is the current carve-out arrangements where mental health services are delivered by a different company than the one that delivers medical/surgical care.

In a timely article, Barlow (2004) notes that "recently healthcare policy makers have established that evidence supporting the efficacy of these [behavioral] interventions is more than sufficient for their inclusion in health care systems around the world" (page 869). He proposes that psychologists label these procedures *psychological treatments* so as to differentiate them from the more generic psychotherapy.

Dramatic changes in mental healthcare delivery, especially one that would end the mind-body dualism of centuries and disrupt entrenched, prestigious departments of psychiatry and medicine toward a combined primary/behavioral care service, are bound to encounter strong resistances. But as cost effective data emerge from the systems that have already integrated, the treatment will characteristically gravitate toward the dollars. What will it mean economically for the declining practices of behavioral care providers? Consider a 900% increase not just in referrals, but in those entering treatment. Instead of sagging practices there suddenly could be a shortage of behavioral care providers.

References

Barlow, D. H. (2004). Psychological treatments. *American Psychologist, 59*(9), 869-878.

Bloom, B. L. (1992). *Planned short-term psychotherapy: A clinical handbook.* Boston, MA: Allyn and Bacon.

Coolidge, C. (2004, December 13). Saving for your health. *Forbes,* 240-244.

Cummings, N. A. (2004). Mental health commissions: Achievements, setbacks and hopes. *National Psychologist, 13*(6), 12.

Cummings, N. A., Cummings, J. L., & Johnson, J. N. (Eds.). (1997). *Behavioral health in primary care: A guide for clinical integration.* Madison, CT: Psychosocial Press.

Cummings, N. A., O'Donohue, W. T., Hayes, S. C., & Follette, V. (Eds.). (2001). *Integrated behavioral healthcare: Positioning mental health practice with medical/surgical practice.* San Diego, CA: Academic Press.

Cummings, N. A., & Wiggins, J. G. (2001). A collaborative primary care/behavioral health model for use of psychotropic medication with children and adolescents. Report of a national retrospective study. *Issues in Interdisciplinary Care, 3*(2), 121-128.

Forbes, S. (2004, September 20). Insuring healthcare coverage. *Forbes,* 33.

Fox, R. (2004). It's about money: Protecting and enhancing our incomes. *Independent Practitioner, 24*(4), 158-159.

Friedman, M. (2004). Keynote address to the World Health Care Congress. January 28. Washington, DC.

Enthoven, A. (2004, January 28). *Personal communication.* Washington, DC.

Hawkins, L. (2005, January 14). GM expects big drop in 2005 profit. *Wall Street Journal,* A3.

Hogan, M. F. (2003). New Freedom Commission Report: The President's New Freedom Commission - Recommendations to transform mental health care in America. *Psychiatric Services, 54,* 1467-1474.

Kadlec, D. (2004, November 22). Taking the plunge. *Time,* 65-67.

Kotlikoff, L. J. (2004, December 13). Fixing Medicare. *Forbes,* 50.

O'Donohue, W. T., Byrd, M. R., Cummings, N. A., & Henderson, D. A., (Eds.). (2005). *Behavioral integrative care: Treatments that work in the primary care setting.* New York, NY: Routledge (Taylor and Francis Group).

Rundle, R. L. (2005, February 1). Some push to make hospitals disclose rates of infection. *Wall Street Journal,* A1-6.

Thompson, A. (2004, December 20). *NBC Nightly News/An HMO that got it right* [Television Broadcast]. New York

Tumulty, K., & Roston, E. (2005, January 24). Social Security: Is there really a crisis? *Time,* 22-29.

The Last Word

New Thoughts on Social Security

Herbert Dörken

Scientific Director, Cummings Foundation for
Behavioral Health, Reno, Nevada

To become workable, Social Security requires a major and complete revision to deliver its benefits, be age appropriate, be fiscally solvent and offer some rational choice. The model developed by FDR was quite like that advanced in Germany by Kaiser Wilhelm decades before. Pay a tax on your wages to be invested for you and at age 65 you will be entitled to benefits. Of the majority of workers then, mostly men, more than half died before they reached 65, so therefore, they collected nothing. If that plan had been advanced by a private financial corporation with such an outcome they would likely have been sued for fraud. Any competent life insurance company can tell you the average life expectancy by sex and years of future life expectation from any given age. Instead social security plans were based on a hope and a promise not on the facts of life expectancy. What can be done now? Plenty, if you follow the demographics of worker life expectancy the current system is also regressive and discriminatory since the poor and African Americans tend to die younger.

1. Terminate any congressional access to Social Security trust funds other than payment for benefits due. There is no way to have any fiscal resources if Congress will not cease plundering them. The public should know this.
2. Begin a 15 year payback from general revenue, 1/15 a year until the so called "borrowed" funds have been fully restored. If Congress will not agree to replace "borrowed" funds on schedule without any tax increase for it, then Social Security should be phased out with the funds available and replaced with a fully privatized system.
3. Limit the payment of any benefits to U.S. citizens or permanent U.S. residents and to no other and payable only in the U.S.
4. Limit the payment of supplemental security income (SSI) to U.S. citizens or permanent U.S. residents in the U.S. and drawn from social welfare funds not SS trust funds and payable only to those who have paid social security payroll taxes for at least 20 quarters (5 years). Moreover, the

disability benefit is to have a thorough medical review every 2 years to determine what continuation is warranted.

5. Reset the age to be entitled to full benefits to age 70. Enable "early" partial benefit from age 65, but at an actuarially determined 25% to 30% reduction and "very early" benefits from age 60, but at a 50% to 60% reduction of the full benefit. For those who elect early and very early retirement for each year beyond 60 or 65 there would be a 5% or 6% increase in benefit. At age 67, the benefit reduction would be only 15% or 18% of the full benefit. The employee needs more flexibility in the age of retirement.

6. Full benefits at age 65 now require 40 quarters of coverage (10 years of payable taxes). The full benefit requirement should be doubled, that is 80 quarters or 20 years of Social Security payroll taxes.

7. Social Security benefits paid from the trust fund should no longer be subject to any income tax.

8. The current Social Security payroll tax is 12.4% on the first $90,000 of taxable income. The rate should not be changed (6.2% employee, 6.2% employer or self-employed) but the taxable income limit should be slightly raised to $100,000. This increase will only add some solvency if Congress is stopped from raiding the "trust fund".

9. For those 45 years of age or older they would continue on Social Security benefits as adjusted above but could have a one time choice of privatization in which up to the last ten years of employee payroll taxes would be transferred from the trust fund to their new private account.

10. For those under 45 years of age, they would have no choice of continuing in the present system as modified above but must adopt a private plan. In it an amount equal to 12.4% of Social Security taxable income would be registered in the name of the employee electing to privatize but would be payable only when the employee has accumulated 80 quarters of coverage (20 years). An employee who began at age 30 could therefore "retire" at age 50 or any year thereafter and could, if so elected, continue to pay into the privatized personal account up to the age of 70.

11. Except for those 45 years of age or older, those electing to privatize would forego any benefit from the trust fund, except for the transfer in number 9 above.

12. The capital in a privatized retirement account would grow tax free while invested and be subject to income tax as withdrawn like an IRA account. However, they would be registered in the name of the employee (including employer's payroll taxes) and not subject to the community property state laws.

13. For an employee with a $40,000 payroll taxable income for 20 years, the private retirement capital would equal 12.4% of $40,000 for 20

years, or $99,200 plus any gain from compounding plus an estimated gain of 5% a year, say $200,000. And this would be in addition to any IRA or 401k or other retirement savings account. For those who began work at age 20 and worked to age 70, at an average of $30,000 a year that would generate $186,000 of income provided capital potentially doubled by investment gain.

14. If the employee dies before collecting any or all benefits, the residual balance is payable in full to his or her beneficiary or estate. The privatized account is owned by the employee. For those employees who continue living at any time after accumulating 20 years of contribution, the employee can elect to withdraw a minimum based on year of life expectancy and may continue to work and payroll contribute if he or she so chooses.

15. The privatized accounts are invested only in a Federal Thrift Savings plan (wherein millions of federal workers currently get their choice of well-diversified funds that are regulated for safety and soundness). This would have a secondary public benefit of increasing the investment of our economy.